BEAUTIFUL
FACES

BEAUTIFUL FACES

The Architects of Enhanced Attractiveness and Improved Human Breathing

Dr. Richard Downs   Dr. Joseph Zelk

Copyright © 2024 by Dr. Richard Downs, Dr. Joseph Zelk

All rights reserved. No part of this book may be used or reproduced by any means, graphic, electronic, or mechanical, including photocopying, recording, taping, or by any information storage retrieval system without the written permission of the author except in the case of brief quotations embodied in critical articles and reviews.

ISBN (paperback): 979-8-9917588-0-2
ISBN (ebook): 979-8-9917588-1-9

Book design and production by www.AuthorSuccess.com
Cover art by www.stock.adobe.com

Dedication for the Haiti International Dental Institute Vision

To Caleb and Debbie Lucien, whose steadfast faith in Christ and leadership have illuminated a path of hope and opportunity for the people of Haiti.

To the dreamers and doers of Hosean International Ministries, who tirelessly invest in education, economic growth, and life-changing opportunities, shaping a future where every child has access to learning and every individual is empowered to thrive.

This vision for the Haiti International Dental Institute stands as a testament to the transformative power of faith, compassion, and collaboration. It is dedicated to restoring smiles—not just through dental health but by nurturing dignity, confidence, and the promise of a brighter tomorrow.

Through advanced training in dental implantology and community outreach, we aim to bring sustainable solutions to a nation filled with potential, resilient hearts, and unshakable hope.

May this endeavor honor the extraordinary people of Haiti and the enduring commitment of those who believe in their limitless possibilities.

With profound gratitude and purpose,
Richard Downs and Joseph Zelk

Contents

INTRODUCTION
Unlocking Airway Wellness and Facial Radiance   1

1	Tortured Faces	12
2	What's Wrong with Our Faces?	32
3	Contributing Causes – The First Assault	44
4	The Concept of Facial Beauty	111
5	What are Sleep-Related Breathing Disorders? The Second Assault	131
6	The Problem of Dental Profession Awareness	157
7	The Dawning Awareness of the Dental Profession	169
8	The Transition from Traditional to New Approaches	199
9	The Transition in Orthodontic Care	235
10	Emerging Science and Healthcare	242
11	Children and Sleep Suffocation	256
12	Nasal Breathing	280
13	Child Growth & Facial Beauty – Dr. Felix Liao	298

14	Case Studies by Kamran Fattah DMD, Airway a Vivos® Practitioner	319
15	Combination Vivos® & Clear Aligner Care Kevin Goles, DDS, D-ASBA	334
16	The Air Institute: Geoffrey Skinner, DDS, D-ABDSM, D-ASBA	348
17	Conclusions	365

INTRODUCTION

Unlocking Airway Wellness and Facial Radiance

Welcome to a journey of discovery and transformation, where the intricate interplay between airway wellness and facial radiance takes center stage. This book explores the fascinating realms of breathing, facial harmony, and overall well-being, exploring the profound connections that shape our appearance and health.

The commonly heard advice to strive for the best version of yourself has never manifested in such a transformative manner, affecting your physical and mental well-being. Nothing is more crucial in achieving this goal than grasping a genuine foundation to construct the house of self-improvement.

In pursuing facial elegance and optimal health, we often overlook the crucial role played by our airways, especially during sleep. *Beautiful Faces: The Architects of Enhanced Attractiveness and Improved Human Breathing*, seeks to unravel the intricacies within, connecting the dots between the breath we take, the sleep we need, and the radiant beauty we exude. This book is a guide that bridges science, aesthetics, and holistic well-being.

A Reality Check:

The information we provide in this book is for educational and informational use only. The information is not intended to be used by the readers for any diagnostic purpose and is not a substitute for professional medical advice. You should always seek the advice of your physician, dentist, or other healthcare providers with any questions regarding the diagnosis, cure, treatment, mitigation, or prevention of any disease or other medical condition or impairment or the status of your health.

It is also important to note that increases in openings for airways shown on photos, X-rays, or CT scans do not mean that obstructive sleep apnea (OSA) has been improved, treated, or cured. There still is no definitive science to show that mouth expansion improves sleep apnea. However, an excellent new FDA-cleared mouth-widening treatment strongly suggests that expansion does help with obstructive sleep apnea. We will discuss that in more detail later. Also, our contributing authors are documenting cases with excellent metrics on how jaw enlargement affects sleep apnea. Additional combination therapies are presented, too.

Facial appearances can be improved with and without enhanced airways and sleep disturbances. Anecdotal evidence can be helpful but not proof that the sleeping disease is improved or cured. In like manner, sometimes facial appearances can be made worse while airway metrics might be enhanced, and sleep disturbances helped.

We believe, though, that the cases you will see presented in this book represent an improved approach to airway health and beauty. Sleep specialists are also now prescribing these instead of just CPAP therapies because they see consistent results that help those with sleep apnea. Sleep specialists, including Dr. Zelk, are, for example, prescribing NightLase®, myofunctional therapy, oral airway expansion, including orthodontic and clear aligner care that creates space for the tongue, oral sleep appliances, ExciteOSA® electronic tongue toning devices, iNAP® negative pressure devices, oral dental sleep appliances, EPAP therapy (expiratory positive airway pressure), positional sleep therapy, surgical airway opening procedures, nasal and airway opening surgeries, weight loss and much more. We will explain these treatments later in the book.

Finally, readers should know that even though this book is primarily written by a dentist and a Doctor of Nursing Practice Board Certified in

Behavioral Sleep Medicine, no dentist, chiropractor, or other allied health professional can diagnose sleep apnea. That is reserved for sleep specialists, MD, DO, NP, and PA health practitioners in the medical profession who diagnose and then prescribe treatment for the conditions. Dentists are rapidly assisting in screening and caring for these patients with our medical colleagues.

One more thing to be aware of is that those readers who are not healthcare professionals are likely to know more about sleep disorders and sleep health than your primary care physician or dentist after completing this book. That is fine with us. We will be delighted if it pushes my colleagues and all healthcare professionals to better address this epidemic.

The Authors

The two principal authors of this book, Dr. Richard Downs, DDS, and Dr. Joseph Zelk, DNP, are unique in their experiences. Joe will tell his story a bit later. I am knowledgeable in general dentistry. I retired from practice, but my years of experience and passion for uncovering the intricacies of dental and airway health have led me to share this knowledge with you. During my professional journey, I have observed instances where my dental care fell short, and previously inexplicable failures have been answered as to cause. Now, I comprehend the transformative influence that understanding and nurturing the airway can exert on facial aesthetics, dental health, and overall health. Based on this new understanding, I have pioneered forming two companies for oral and nasal airway health products. I have pursued and attained a Diplomate credential in the American Sleep and Breathing Academy to further that understanding. I am still learning.

My interest in becoming a dentist began around the age of six. My interest in dental sleep medicine began with my increasingly loud snoring that was interfering with my wife's sleep and health. I had no idea of the significance of the health consequences of my sleep disorder for both of us until I began to take courses on the subject of dental sleep medicine about seventeen years ago. Like most people, I thought snoring was just a primarily annoying male distraction. When I attended these courses, my eyes were opened to a world that hugely impacted dentistry and myself. I had a sleep test, and it turned out I had moderate-grade obstructive sleep apnea, which I treated with a dental sleep appliance. It worked wonderfully to get the nighttime sleep breathing issues under control.

My first oral appliance was called a TAP®. I have had several different types since that time, including the Elastic Mandibular Advancement device and Somnomed® dorsal wing style device, and I will soon have an Invisasleep®, developed by Joseph Zelk. We will explain these treatments later in the book.

Joe is unique as a champion of the dental profession in sleep medicine. I think he knows more about dental sleep medicine than anyone else. He is not a dentist, yet he has personally administered over 15,000 oral sleep appliances to treat obstructive sleep apnea. This is unique, and we are fortunate to have a sleep specialist working as a partner in the dental profession.

My Childhood

I spent my childhood in a tiny Iowa town, and my earliest memories are of sharing a house with my aunt and uncle. The house was split into two halves, with my brother Jim, myself, and my parents on one side and my uncle's family on the other. We shared a bathroom. During winter, the house was heated by a basement furnace fueled with wood, using a convection-driven circulation system. Concepts like black mold, dust, or allergies were unknown to us; the house had no air filters on registers. This house was on my grandfather's farm. We had well water.

During that time, we drank unpasteurized milk from the cows, consumed the new-to-market oleo, and occasionally took Geritol® as a supplement. Meat and potatoes were staple foods, and my dad's janitorial job at the local school provided us with leftover canned food. To this day, I still prefer the taste of canned peas and green beans over frozen or fresh ones. There was a notable absence of a genuine understanding of proper nutrition. The advent of pre-sliced, fluffy white bread, claiming to build bodies in many ways, resulted in a generation of children who preferred this magical white cloud of bread. Consequently, many children developed an aversion to whole grain bread and even sought to remove the crust from the less substantial and preferred fluffy center of the slice.

Back then, not only was information on nutrition lacking, with little awareness about the impacts of new types of fats, increased sugar in foods, and toxins, but there were also astonishing practices by today's standards. It was an era when cigarettes were promoted as beneficial for health, the sugar industry had a significant influence on science publications and public nutrition practices, and DDT insecticide was considered harmless to humans. Glyphosate and other herbicides and insecticides had minimal precautions for use and handling.

In these times, children, including myself, used to run behind tractors as they moved through town, releasing white clouds of DDT vapors to combat mosquitoes. We found joy in darting in and out of these white gaseous billows of DDT as if playing in ground-level cumulus clouds. It's stunningly challenging to fathom such activities being tolerated compared to today's awareness.

One of the first books I read in college was *Silent Spring* by Rachel Carson. I was alarmed only then about my early experience with this DDT.

One day, early in my life, we moved to our new house one block away from the house we had shared with my aunt and uncle. It lacked a furnace, indoor plumbing, gas, or electric stove. The basement had a dirt floor, and my mother manually pumped water from a pump on the back porch for laundry. I was told the water came from an underground spring. The water was never tested for any bacteria or toxins. Bathing happened in a metal tub reminiscent of a small cattle watering container, with an outhouse serving as the bathroom. Mornings involved us boys gathering corn cobs from the garage for fuel in our cook stove, and I vividly remember the red glowing warmth they provided as my mother cooked a meal.

With now four boys in the family, all four of us slept in one upstairs bed, warmed only by the heat of each other's bodies and warm air rising from a hole in the floor looking down into the downstairs dining room. The dining room had an oil burner stove, the sole source of warmth for the entire house.

Sharing a bed seemed warmer, although the challenge was my brother Gerry, who frequently wet the bed and walked in his sleep. I often tried to wake him during these episodes, realizing now that these likely would have been signs of a sleep disorder. Unfortunately, in 1958, testing and treatment for sleep disorders were unheard of.

We only went to the dentist if someone had a toothache or pain. No preventive dental care was ever offered. Crowded teeth were prevalent, and almost no one had orthodontic care. I remember getting toothpaste for the first time in a metal tube. It was Crest®.

I do remember, as a child, being taken to my local ENT physician at about age twelve for what turned out to be a polyp in my right nostril, which was later removed at around forty-five years of age. I also remember someone, maybe a doctor, saying that I had a "high arch," referring to the roof of my mouth. I thought at the time that was a good thing because I had high arches in my feet, which was better than flat feet. Little did I know that was abnormal. I was also self-conscious of my crowded teeth and receding chin. I did not like my profile, nor do I like it today.

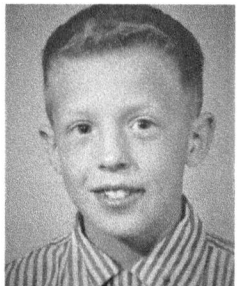

Figure 1

The above photo of myself was taken at about age ten. You can already see the teeth crowding and the narrow face. At this age, an intervention to broaden the dental arches has huge benefits. No one at the time was doing that. It was assumed this was genetics and nothing could be done but make room by removing permanent teeth.

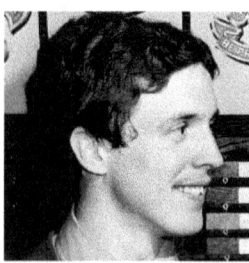 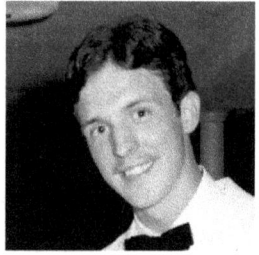 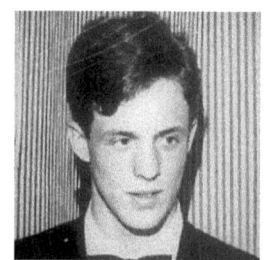

Figure 2　　　　　　　Figure 3　　　　　　　Figure 4

Left is a near profile photo showing my crowded teeth. The middle photo is my 1969 wedding photo of overcrowded teeth. Both images are at age twenty. The right is high school, age eighteen. In all these photos, you see crowding, a narrow face, and a steep jaw angle downward, yet the lips only become dished (a look of receded upper and lower jaws) once braces are administered later in dental school.

Later in life, I had the crooked teeth straightened in dental school, with four premolar teeth removed to help create space for that alignment. Premolars are the teeth just behind the "eye teeth," as they are commonly referred to. I also wore headgear to pull my upper front teeth back into the spaces created by the extracted teeth (Figure 5): this reduced the space for my tongue. That was the standard of care at the time. Little did I know that it likely also made my compromised airways even worse. It also made my profile worse, not better. The smaller mouth contributed to my receded chin looking more receded and my cheeks less supported.

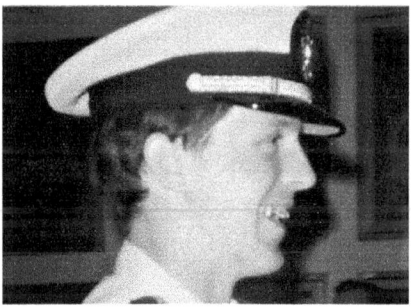

Figure 5

In this photo, I am an ensign in the Navy, still in dental school, and wearing orthodontic bands and wires. As mentioned in the text, I have had four teeth removed in this photo, and the front teeth are being retracted (pulled back) to close the spaces behind the eye teeth with the assistance of headgear. You can already see a flattening of the face and lips and a worsening profile. The front teeth are not back yet because the eye teeth are being retracted first. The already small chin is allowed to recede backward, too. The tongue has less space to function within. This is a photo of me getting off the jet back from Newport, Rhode Island, to see my newborn son for the first time.

Some dispute that smaller faces, crowded teeth, and smaller mouths contribute to ill health and disease. They will also claim that few good scientific studies support creating larger jaws to help with health issues. This stand is becoming a less sustainable argument as the studies become more numerous and the new FDA recognition of Vivos® jaw-widening appliances has been cleared. Improving the structural airway has now been established with this clearance. This FDA clearance means that this type of care can be used to treat obstructive sleep apnea, a medical condition treated by dentists with enormous health implications.[1]

In this book, we will maintain that jaw widening and nasal opening for health and beauty are the new standards of care that need to be adopted. Some still say no definitive science has proven that misaligned teeth cause medical problems. We find those statements irresponsible. That argument that we do not have to widen airways is not as potent as it once was because now, if the best care is improving both airway and beauty, that is what you should do. You should do both.

All these signs in my mouth became more clearly linked together as I realized this was a complex of related disorders of modern stunted jaw and nasal growth that led to my sleep apnea. Now, I know and want to help others not only recognize but be able to do something about it. At age seventy-five, I have to do more work than some to get my sleep apnea under control, and the therapies that work well on younger people do not work on me. It is almost as if I and many others are dealing with a chokehold of our existence.

What you can expect from this book

You will meet actual patients in the book who have struggled to find someone to help them, and when they finally did find that person, they delightfully discovered better-looking faces.

You will learn why modern faces are getting smaller and less attractive and how this also devastates our health through nighttime suffocation.

---

[1] Julie Gannon, "Vivos Therapeutics Receives First Ever FDA 510(K) Clearance for Oral Device Treatment of Severe Obstructive Sleep Apnea," Globe Newswire, November 29, 2023, accessed February 21, 2024, https://vivos.com/vivos-therapeutics-receives-first-ever-fda-510k-clearance-for-oral-device-treatment-of-severe-obstructive-sleep-apnea/.

Embark on an enthralling journey of discovery, where beauty meets health, and the secrets of the breath are unmasked. *Beautiful Faces* promises an enlightening expedition into aesthetics, airway health, and the evolving landscape of human care.

The Chokehold Chronicles: Faces Unmasked in the Toxic Abyss

Dr. Joseph Zelk, DNP, FNP, CBSM, DBSM, is a sleep specialist with a double board certification in behavioral sleep medicine from the American Academy of Sleep Medicine (AASM) and the Board of Behavioral Sleep Medicine. Dr. Zelk has a Doctor of Nursing Practice, is a board-certified family nurse practitioner, and has completed a residency covering sleep medicine and dental sleep medicine training.

Dr. Zelk discovered early in his career that only a small group of patients with OSA can tolerate CPAP due to its air pressure. Humans "suck" in air to breathe, and CPAP "blows" pressure out, which is very disruptive to sleep in the majority of people. This understanding led him very early in his career to seek out CPAP treatment alternatives. Dentists pioneered this treatment. The dental appliances (synonyms include oral appliance/device, dental appliance/device, sleep appliance/device, mandibular advancement device/splint, and more) provided by dentists trained in OSA management are much more likely to be worn by patients regularly, which led Dr. Zelk to initiate a campaign to train more dentists nationally in recognizing snoring and sleep apnea so they could become partners in treating this epidemic of sleep apnea. He has been a champion of dentists being involved in sleep medicine and a pioneer in that field. He has been doing that for more than twenty years.

He helped with the FDA introduction and clearance of the eXciteOSA® tongue-stimulating device. Dr. Zelk also has patented dental oral sleep appliances to treat sleep apnea. He was also instrumental in bringing awareness of the iNAP® negative air sleep apnea device. Dr. Zelk and I are passionate about getting this information out and improving the world with proper facial structures and wellness.

Dr. Zelk tells about his journey with sleep-disordered breathing, upper airway resistance syndrome, obstructive sleep apnea (UARS/OSA) and his ill health as a child. It is a tale of multiple airway illnesses and antibiotic exposure from a formative age. He speaks about his impeded growth and facial development, which are both similar in ways to mine but also unique to him that his genetic and environmental circumstances dictate.

This book is organized to take you on a step-by-step exploration, beginning with fundamental concepts in "Breathing Basics" and leading you through the science of growth and development, facial harmony, airway disorders, breathing science, and beyond. Each chapter does not necessarily build upon the last. Still, there is a general flow from problem to history to solution, creating a cohesive narrative that empowers you to embrace the symbiotic relationship between your airway and facial improvements in form and function.

You will see a lot of citations. These citations include peer-reviewed science references and more common articles from popular magazines and websites. Not all anecdotal observations are unimportant or invalid, but peer-reviewed science papers should also not always be taken as settled science. The only actual proof areas of knowledge are in mathematics. The other fields of knowledge of science in health and biology are to be considered the best knowledge at present. They almost always change. We included the citations because it is proper to credit the sources and allow the readers to look further into subjects that pique their interest.

By the end of this journey, you will gain insights that extend far beyond conventional beauty standards. You will discover practical strategies, backed by scientific research and practicing clinicians, to enhance your dental, airway, and overall health and elevate your facial elegance.

While this book is written for the general public, professionals, and healthcare workers interested in the field and seeking more resources and knowledge, it offers actionable steps for lasting transformation for them and their patients. It may also be beneficial for professionals to recommend to their patients.

Imagine a World—What to Expect

Imagine a world where every breath you take, whether awake or asleep, contributes to your vitality and the sculpting of your facial features. As you embark on the pages that follow, prepare to unlock the secrets that connect the rhythm of your breath to the radiance of your face. This journey is more than a quest for beauty; it explores the profound harmony between developmental and conventional airway wellness, sleep, and facial elegance.

Get ready to breathe life into your appearance.

Welcome to *Beautiful Faces: The Architects of Enhanced Attractiveness and Improved Human Breathing.*

CHAPTER 1

Tortured Faces

A Silent Crisis

In a world constantly spinning with ever-accelerating change, distractions, and the relentless march of innovation, an epidemic festers in the modern morass—its presence so subtle, its impact profound. These assailants have orchestrated a two-phase offensive, launching relentless attacks against our well-being and health twenty-four hours a day.

The first front of this assault is a barrage that weakens our defenses, leaving us vulnerable to the second devastating attack. The second attack is insidious only because it is so common that few realize it is not normal. This second front is a nocturnal offensive and strikes under the cover of darkness, exploiting our vulnerability when vigilance is absent. These night attacks unleash systemic and often violent acts, penetrating the very core of our lives both physically and mentally. They happen during sleep, and since we are asleep when they occur, they are not recognized. If any of them were to happen while awake, ambulances would be summoned, and if these assaults were done by other people, they would be arrested and put behind bars.

Yet this second assault has created unwilling physiological saboteurs within our bodies with complex systems, structures, and interactions. These submissive confederations of body system collaborators have relentlessly worn down our health to finally perform a sabotaging role that helps the epidemic's monolithic power destroy us.

This coordinated battle plan hinges on the continuous weakening power of the overlying offensive, the modern lifestyle—a strategic orchestration of deforming forces that renders us susceptible to the night's hypoxic onslaught. It's not a pandemic of a single pathogen, nor does it grab headlines with catastrophic flair. Instead, it's a gradual and insidious multifront siege on our airways and facial structures, creating ripples of consequences that stretch far beyond our appearance. It is like the frog in the kettle that does not realize the water is gradually warming up to the point of danger.

As we explore the depths of this concealed erosion of our health in this book, it will become evident that we're not merely facing a health challenge; we're confronting a meticulously coordinated attack on our vitality, resilience, and even the structure of our society and the health of our civilization.

While some of the forces of this siege are capricious, most are unintended by-products of the speed and expedience of modern living. We have ignored it and let it happen for the most part. It is a challenge we can confront and control.

Join us as we unveil the layers of this silent battle and chart a course toward reclaiming how we look and the essence of our well-being. Welcome to the frontline of unmasking and confronting what we believe is the single most unrecognized and under-treated epidemic of modern times. A journey that can be addressed and reclaimed by the average person. A journey that reclaims our innate repressed genetic potential for not only facial beauty but transcends appearance and beckons us to reclaim the essence of a thriving life. It is a quest to recover the beauty of our physical and spiritual selves.

The Problem: A Silent Crisis Unveiled

You might ask, what is this about how we look? Faces are shrinking, not just physically but in vitality and resilience. For the most part, we are not noticing the rapid change in modern faces. We are even becoming so accustomed to these changes that our modern notions of beauty and structure are changing, making the awareness much more difficult to unveil.

Modern attacks on our bodies, from less sleep, altered foods, and dietary habits to compromised breathing patterns, are reshaping the very foundation of our facial structures. These changes are being incorporated into our development, growth, and genetics. The consequences are far-reaching, affecting our appearance and overall health.

We will not go into too much detail about sleep, nasal and mouth anatomy, brain anatomy, and sleep deprivation. However, there will be some technical science that some may find tedious. Writing for the fourth-grade level educated audience, recommended by some, does not show enough respect and confidence for readers. We have tried to explain the science wherever possible in understandable terms. However, some of this technical information is best gained or enhanced by reading other well-written texts and books like *Why We Sleep* by Matthew Walker, PhD, a professor of neuroscience and psychology at the University of California, Berkeley. You will find many reasons why we need not just sleep but "restorative" sleep in this book, and other authors who build on this need. As Walker says, healthy sleep is your most potent health measure.

In a 2024 *Nature Neuroscience* paper, Keith Hengen and his interdisciplinary team introduced a theory that melds principles from both physics and biology to highlight the profound importance of sleep. Your brain is like a computer, explains Hengen. Sleep recalibrates the brain to a computational state called criticality. It is something like a computer. Throughout waking hours, memory and experiences gradually modify their code, deviating from an ideal state. The primary objective of sleep is to return the brain to an optimal computational condition.[2]

The scientists posit that sleep functions as a vital reset button for the brain, enabling it to attain a "criticality" that enhances cognitive functions and optimizes information processing. They witnessed "neural avalanches," representing cascades of activity that illustrate the flow of information in the brain. At criticality, avalanches of various sizes occurred, akin to a diverse vocabulary in a book.

However, as waking hours advanced, the cascades leaned toward smaller sizes, signifying a deviation from criticality. Scientists could predict the moments when rats were about to fall asleep or awaken by studying the distribution pattern of these avalanches in the brain.

Hagen suggests that during wakefulness, our brain circuits gradually move away from a state of criticality, where they are optimally balanced and

---

[2] J. D. Shavit, "Groundbreaking Study Uncovers Why Humans Need Sleep," *The Brighter Side of News*, January 11, 2024, https://www.citationmachine.net/chicago/cite-a-website/search?q=The%20Brighter%20Side%20of%20News.%20January%2011%2C%202024.

responsive. Sleep then acts as a reset mechanism, returning these circuits to a state of balance. This balance is crucial for efficient cognitive function and overall brain health.

This criticality is deeply affected by loss of sleep. Dr. Walker says that about one in ten people experience insomnia. He also makes a distinction in his book between sleep deprivation and true insomnia. If sleep deprivation is considered, then the numbers must include almost anyone. I have read articles that say 30 percent of the population suffers from insomnia. His point that our modern lifestyle indicates that most are not getting enough sleep is devastatingly true. That could be defined as including self-imposed insomnia. When I say self-imposed," I'm referring to a situation where individuals consciously choose to limit their sleep duration due to personal decisions or lifestyle habits that reduce the amount of time they spend in bed consistently.

Dr. Walker mentions the need to create an optimal environment for sleep. He includes having no light in the sleeping area, having a cool room, turning off electronic devices at least two hours before bed, getting eight hours of sleep for adults, later public school start times for children, staying away from alcohol, caffeine, and insomnia drugs, getting exercise, avoiding sugar, going to bed and arising at the same time every day, and clearing your mind of concerns of the day. This last point brings to mind another missing feature of modern society: the spiritual benefits of sleep.[3]

Even though this book is not primarily about insomnia, sleep deprivation, and sleep hygiene, it is essential that we do a short segment on this because the structures of the face have a bidirectional relationship with a lack of restorative sleep in all its forms.

In discussing sleep, we will acknowledge both its physical and spiritual aspects.[4] As Blaise Pascal aptly put it, something like this: Within every person's heart exists a void shaped like God—a void that cannot be filled by anything created.[5] We must recognize that neglecting the spiritual side of sleep can have profound psychological, physical, and existential consequences for our health. When we concentrate on only the physical components of

---

3 Maya Goldman, "Health Care Needs More Spirituality, Experts Say," *Axios Vitals*, last modified February 1, 2024, https://www.axios.com/2024/02/01/health-care-spirituality-public-health.

4 Ibid.

5 Blaise Pascal, *Pacal's Pensees*, (New York: Dutton, 1958).

sleep and overlook this aspect, we may inadvertently contribute an incomplete solution to self-imposed insomnia. This insomnia may stem from a more profound yearning for meaning and purpose in life, a yearning that may manifest itself in frenetic striving for material values, depression, and anxiety to quell that yearning, resulting in less restorative sleep.

Considering the mechanical framework for health is incomplete, I will include this spiritual insight from Brian Hall, M.Div., about how a mechanistic approach to human health imparts no meaning to one's life. Hall's insights complement Dr. Walker's findings. He is a spiritual life coach with Brianhallcoaching.com. I want to introduce his insights on spiritual sleep health. I have paraphrased his words with his permission.

The Sacred Gift of Sleep: Rest, Renewal, and Encountering the Divine—Brian Hall

In the hustle and bustle of modern life, sleep often feels like a luxury we can't afford. Yet, within its quiet embrace lies a profound treasure—a spiritual symphony orchestrated by God, offering renewal, vulnerability, and a path to divine encounter.

Rather than viewing sleep as lost time, let's see it as a divine gift from a loving Creator who understands our needs. As the Bible says, "It is useless for you to work so hard . . . for God grants sleep to those he loves" (Psalm 127:2). Each night, we're encouraged to release our worries and entrust our well-being—body, mind, and soul—to a compassionate Father.

Falling asleep is an act of faith, acknowledging our limitations, and trusting in God's care. As we rest, we echo the psalmist's words, "In peace, I will lie down and sleep, for you alone, O Lord, will keep me safe" (Psalm 4:8). This surrender is a powerful affirmation of our trust in God's protection. Prayer before sleep helps clear the mind of anxiety and stress, and allows a psychological shift to prepare for sleep with fewer concerns. It prepares you for God's messages, too. Even praying this psalm can help calm the mind for sleep.

Sleep can be a metaphor for spiritual complacency. Romans 13:11 urges us to awaken from spiritual slumber and embrace God's purpose for our lives. Let's open our hearts to God's transformative work, ready to receive His guidance. A clearer mind gained from restorative sleep allows us to see our purpose more clearly and gives us more energy, emotional intelligence, and motivation to pursue it. Knowing your purpose is a fulfilling emotion, improving sleep-calming effects.

Throughout the Bible, dreams serve as channels for God's communication. While not every dream holds deep meaning, approaching sleep with openness allows space for divine messages. Consider keeping a dream journal to capture these moments and seek God's wisdom.

As night falls, sleep becomes a sanctuary of trust in God's promises. Like the Sabbath rest, it reminds us of God's faithfulness. Let's release our burdens and anxieties, resting in the assurance that God's mercies are new every morning. Rhythms are built into our lives. Sabbath rest and circadian rhythms are just two that are essential for health.

Sleep humbles us, reminding us of our dependence on God. In our vulnerability, we echo the Lord's words, "Apart from me, you can do nothing" (John 15:5). This humility grounds us in God's strength.

Prioritizing rest is an act of faith, honoring God's design for work and rest. Let's care for our bodies as temples of the Holy Spirit, recognizing the importance of physical and spiritual rest.

Sleep is a vital spiritual and physical discipline, enhancing our capacity to hear God's voice and resist temptation. Let's cultivate healthy sleep habits as part of our spiritual journey.

Sleep reminds us of the eternal rest promised to believers. Just as falling asleep leads to waking up refreshed, death ushers us to everlasting life in Christ.

- Set the tone for sleep with prayer, meditation, or scripture reading.
- Create a restful environment with dim lights and soothing sounds.
- Cultivate gratitude to dispel anxiety and foster peace.
- Keep a dream journal to capture divine messages.

Sleep is more than a biological function; it's a sacred journey into the heart of God's love. May your nights be filled with rest and renewal, awakening each day refreshed and ready to walk in His purpose.[6]

---

6 Brian Hall, M.Div. This article was written for this book and does not appear on his website. https://www.brianhallcoaching.com.

Lack of sleep

Support for what Dr. Walker says about lack of sleep also comes from the book's co-author, Joseph Zelk. Dr. Zelk says epidemiologists have illustrated a significant decrease in the average nightly sleep duration among Americans over the past few generations. For instance, in 1950, the average nightly sleep duration was eight and a half hours, which declined to seven and a half hours by 1970 and further decreased to six and one-quarter hours by 2000, continuing to diminish over subsequent years.[7] Dr. Walker laments that the lack of sleep devastates our health, and Hagen adds that this deficit impacts our critical thinking ability, agreeing with Walker.

Insomnia in Contrast with Sleep Apnea

The definitions of insomnia and sleep apnea are also somewhat clumped together in some of the studies of sleep disorders. Sleep apnea can cause insomnia. The reader needs to know that insomnia and sleep apnea are different. For example, in the *Medical Journal of Australia*, published 25 June 2023, the lead author studied 552 people with sleep studies and found 90 participants, 17 percent of whom had insomnia. Additionally, 5.4 percent of the participants, totaling thirty individuals, were diagnosed with "clinically significant" obstructive sleep apnea. Finally, only two participants, which account for 0.4 percent of the total, were found to have restless leg syndrome. All these are different sleep disorders that may or may not coexist.

They concluded that individuals with these sleep disorders contribute to a 40 percent loss in workplace productivity. The problem is that they conclude that insomnia did this. What I mean is they conclude that insomnia, as an all-encompassing category, contributes to less workplace productivity without mentioning that the other disorders are included.[8] This conclusion confuses sleep apnea with insomnia. They also only included moderate or severe sleep apnea in the data when the largest segment of those suffering from sleep apnea are in the mild range. They also only studied young people.

---

7 Danielle Pacheco, "Pain and Sleep." Sleep Foundation, May 23, 2023, accessed Feb 9, 2024. https://www.sleepfoundation.org/physical-health/pain-and-sleep.

8 A. C. Reynolds, et al. "Insomnia and workplace productivity loss among young working adults: a prospective observational study of clinical sleep disorders in a community cohort," *Medical Journal of Australia* 219, no. 3 (2023): 107-112. doi: 10.5694/mja2.52014.

If we are speaking about chronic insomnia disorder that is pernicious and uncontrollable and affects some unlucky individuals, then the number of those affected drops a great deal. This type of insomnia is called "primary" insomnia. Primary insomnia is a sleep disorder recognized by difficulties initiating or maintaining sleep without an identifiable cause. In contrast to secondary insomnia, which can be attributed to factors such as medication, sleep apnea, work schedules, poor sleep habits, or underlying health conditions, primary insomnia occurs independently, without any apparent external triggers. People with primary insomnia usually get around six hours of sleep per night, which is less than the usual eight hours people need. Insomnia can increase the chances of experiencing major depression, anxiety, substance abuse, thoughts of suicide, high blood pressure, and diabetes.[9]

As a side note: Even though this book is not about insomnia, I will mention a promising treatment for primary insomnia I found while writing this book, and it is cited here in an article by lead author Yating Wu in the journal *Brain Science*, in which one group of test subjects with primary insomnia received a treatment called 20 Hz t-VNS (transcutaneous vagal nerve stimulation) for twenty minutes twice per day in the auricular concha area (the hollow bowl-shaped part of the outer ear located just outside the ear canal), while the other group received a sham treatment. There was a greater than 50 percent reduction in the Pittsburgh Sleep Index Scale (PSQI) after treatment. This means there was a good result in reducing primary insomnia with a safe device.[10]

Dr Walker believes we must address this lack of sleep early in life. I agree. I also think he is right that the numbers who suffer, whether they are due to people choosing not to give themselves enough sleep time or those with chronic uncontrollable insomnia, are epidemic. I highly recommend you read his book *Why We Sleep*.

More support for what Walker says regarding insomnia comes from Talker Research. They say in sleep, the average American achieves an ideal night's rest a mere 132 times annually. A routine of 120 nights of average

---

9 S. Schutte-Rodin, et al. "Clinical Guideline for the Evaluation and Management of Chronic Insomnia in Adults." *Journal of Clinical Sleep Medicine*, 4/5, (2008), 487-504.

10 Y. Wu, et al., "Transcutaneous Vagus Nerve Stimulation Could Improve the Effective Rate on the Quality of Sleep in the Treatment of Primary Insomnia: A Randomized Control Trial," *Brain Sciences*, 12/10 (2022), 1296. doi: 10.3390/brainsci12101296.

restful sleep is also attained, but the remaining 113 nights unfold as restless tosses and turns or staying wide-eyed many hours or until dawn. The villains in this drama are often stress and anxiety, keeping the mind awake before they can sleep to sabotage the prospects of deep restorative sleep. As the night wears on, stress acts as stubborn self-talk, keeping individuals awake for an additional three hours past their intended bedtime. This nighttime wakefulness casts its influence into the dawn, affecting the ability to greet the new day with alertness. A survey from the sleep-deprived discloses that nearly two-thirds of those questioned agree with the statement that a night of poor sleep can potentially ruin the following day.[11]

This research from Talker Research says nothing about any of these sleepers having obstructive sleep apnea. It places every person in a category of getting a good night's sleep or not getting that good sleep, depending on stress and anxiety. This is a simplified list of two causes of lack of sleep. However, it does point out that about one-third of Americans are not getting "restorative" sleep.

Dr. Zelk, a sleep specialist, explains insomnia this way. The initial step in addressing insomnia involves its accurate diagnosis. Clinicians can typically make a straightforward assessment with appropriate training and sufficient time. Four key indicators guide this process: First, patients who are experiencing difficulty initiating sleep or staying asleep. Second, some form of illness, whether physical or mental, should be associated with sleep disturbances. If an individual experiences sleep challenges but remains in good overall health without feelings of fatigue or lethargy, intervention may not be necessary. Third, the duration of sleep difficulties is crucial, as the American Academy of Sleep Medicine defines chronic insomnia as recurring trouble sleeping at least three nights per week for a minimum of three months.

Finally, patients must have adequate opportunities and conducive circumstances for sleep to accurately diagnose insomnia.

We define insomnia so the reader knows what we are and are not addressing in this book. We are primarily concerned with sleep apnea and physical

---

11 Talker Research, "How Many Times Per Year Do Americans Get a Perfect Night's Sleep?" January 9, 2024, MSN, retrieved from https://talker.news/2024/01/09/how-many-times-per-year-do-americans-get-a-perfect-nights-sleep/.

facial features, not insomnia. One common cause of insomnia is untreated and undiagnosed UARS/OSA.[12] We will address both but emphasize the distinctions in Chapter 5. Indeed, if you are chronically tired from insomnia, your face will not be radiant; however, treating insomnia most often includes a sleep coach and what is called cognitive behavioral therapy. Insomnia patients are more likely to be prescribed sleep medication.

Those with sleep apnea are generally not prescribed sleep medication unless they have problems with restless leg syndrome and need something to control that. The therapies and issues for insomnia do not necessarily involve the approaches we explore in this book unless the undiagnosed sleep apnea (sleep suffocating) is causing insomnia, which is more common than most understand. This is a reason Dr. Zelk and I believe any person with insomnia should first get a sleep study to rule out obstructive sleep apnea before they have any sleep coaching, cognitive behavioral therapy, or medications for insomnia prescribed because we need to ask why they have insomnia. Medication for insomnia can be dangerous for those with sleep apnea. Until we exhaust those questions of why, medication may be considered a stopgap while further investigation occurs.

Restorative Sleep

You might get eight, nine, or even ten hours of sleep. However, if it is fragmented, suffocating, and consists primarily of light stages of sleep rather than deep sleep and regularly occurring sleep, it is not restorative sleep. We want "restorative sleep." This is an important distinction.

We are going to address the problem of lack of restorative sleep caused by obstructive sleep apnea and our shrinking faces, which, in my opinion, are the most devastating sleep disorders of our modern era. And because this is about sleep, I believe this is the most critical health issue ever. Sleep is the most important foundation of health we have. Nothing else comes close. However, sleep disorders are not treated as the most important health foundation in the current medical treatment planning by the average primary care providers and even medical specialists.

---

12 Katherine Zheng, "What Is Upper Airway Resistance Syndrome (UARS)?" Last modified February 1, 2024, reviewed by Dr. Michael Breus, https://www.sleepfoundation.org/sleep-apnea/upper-airway-resistance-syndrome.

The American Academy of Family Physicians notes that up to 10 percent of U.S. adults meet the criteria for chronic insomnia disorder. In comparison, obstructive sleep apnea impacts as many as 38 percent of adults in the United States, particularly men, postmenopausal women, and those with a higher body mass index.[13] Although chronic insomnia and OSA aren't directly correlated, insomnia-induced sleep deprivation may reduce oxygen saturation (not enough oxygen in the blood), predisposing individuals to more OSA events.[14] If insomnia leads to lighter sleep, individuals may be more prone to waking up when experiencing episodes of interrupted breathing, such as those occurring in obstructive sleep apnea.[15] Yet even these statistics do not emphasize enough the sleep issues children are facing.

We will explore the structural changes to our faces and the hypoxia they cause. Hypoxia refers to a condition where there's insufficient oxygen in the bloodstream, typically occurring during suffocation. Some individuals have oxygen desaturation to levels of 80 percent or less! Yet, because they are asleep, they do not notice it. This is crash cart emergency suffocation levels! People typically cannot hold their breath while awake to go below 90 percent. Supplemental oxygen is usually needed if your oxygen levels go below 89 percent. People routinely experience less than 89 percent during events in sleep apnea. Ninety-five percent or more is the level considered normal.

While hypoxia might occur in some instances of insomnia, it's not common as it is in obstructive sleep apnea. Dr. Walker discusses the serious repercussions of sleep deprivation, even if it's just one hour less per night, outlining its impact on our body and overall health. Discussion of losing this crucial hour of sleep also highlights the significant effects of daylight savings time.

The ramifications are profound. He agrees that sleep is the foundation of health. Walker speaks about the upset in the sleep stages, such as REM and non-REM sleep (sleep architecture) and its relation to disease, our ability to concentrate, and our learning ability and mental health. His descriptions of the brain and how it works are profound and beautiful. We will touch on these subjects occasionally as we develop our points.

---

13 J. Drowos, "Obstructive Sleep Apnea and Chronic Insomnia Disorder: Updated Guidelines from the VA/DoD," *American Family Physician* 103, no. 7 (2021): 442-443. PMID: 33788525.

14 Ibid.

15 Ibid.

Even though obstructive sleep apnea can cause insomnia, it is not the leading cause of insomnia. OSA often creates the same pathologies noted in Dr. Walker's book. Sleep architecture is upset, sleep fragmentation is produced, sleep time is lowered, and the stimulation of the fight and flight response, the raising of blood pressure, the impact on mental health, learning, aggressive behavior, cancer, and many other diseases are the same.

Sleep is the supreme health foundation. We believe the structures of the airway are the main obstacles to healthy sleep. We want to address the causes of modern airway collapse rather than just place a mask on the face and blow air into the mouth and nose. Sure, we will address traditional care, and we certainly believe these methods have saved and improved millions of lives. However, most of you will be introduced to new airway and sleep health approaches you have never seen or heard of before.

We emphasize the structural changes being negatively impacted by our modern lifestyle. The ideas presented in the book *Jaws* by Paul Ehrlich and Sandra Kahn deeply explore this theme.[16] We highly endorse this book and its insights. While we will touch upon some developmental causes discussed in *Jaws*, our main objective is to provide actionable solutions as the next step forward.

Dr. Walker briefly touches upon the concept of beauty in his book. We expand on this important human quality by emphasizing our individual and unique genetic potential for improving our aesthetically pleasing facial structure, which is closely intertwined with the health-versus-disease aspects of sleep deprivation.

Additionally, we emphasize the emerging role of dentists and allied health-care professionals in the airway and sleep health treatment team. These new team members possess unique capabilities that other professions do not. We explore the evolution of this new role of these professionals, the benefits it brings, and the pathway they have paved to address the modern predicament of sleep-related issues. While our focus is not directly on treating insomnia, our therapies and knowledge can aid individuals grappling with improper growth and development, as well as head and neck structural disorders that lead to suffocation during sleep.

---

16 Kahn, Sandra, and Paul R. Ehrlich. *Jaws: The Story of a Hidden Epidemic.* Stanford University Press, 2018.

The Vicious Cycle: Unraveling the Medical Domino Effect

As faces melt and the modern assault on them continues, a vicious cycle is set in motion. The airways, designed by nature to be free and open, become constricted. This constriction leads to a myriad of medical problems, from sleep disorders and chronic fatigue to cardiovascular issues. Burdened by the aftermath, the healthcare system teeters on the brink of unsustainable costs.

According to CBS News, in 2016, the annual cost of undiagnosed sleep apnea was $149.6 billion in the United States. The article further stated, according to Dr. Ronald Chervin, president of AASM, if every individual in the United States with sleep apnea were identified and treated, it could lead to yearly economic savings exceeding $100 billion. He emphasized that the top-notch, patient-focused care delivered by certified sleep medicine specialists has the potential to substantially alleviate both the health and financial impacts of sleep apnea.[17] They also stated that the productivity of these patients increased by 40 percent in the workplace with treatment. We don't have enough sleep physicians to address this epidemic.

Automobile accidents and disasters like the Exxon Valdez and Three Mile Island nuclear accidents are not figured in these losses. A person who has just one night of four hours of sleep has a blood alcohol concentration (BAC) equivalent to sleepiness of 0.095 percent! This is over the legal limit of alcohol impairment, and yet the penalties for this impaired driving do not exist as they do for alcohol. These people will experience microsleeps that they have no awareness of, and that result in more deadly accidents than those caused by alcohol. Alcohol-impaired people are often late in reaction time, while microsleep-impaired individuals often do not react or slow down at all.

The estimates in this CBS article were calculated based on the 30 million Americans affected by sleep apnea. Today's forecast is that more than 70 to 80 million Americans will be affected, and care costs will dramatically increase. These costs can be tackled.

---

17 Ashley Welch, "This Sleep Disorder Costs the U.S. Billions of Dollars a Year," CBS News, CBS Interactive, 8 Aug. 2016, www.cbsnews.com/news/undiagnosed-sleep-apnea-costs-billions-of-dollars-per-year/.

The Human Toll: Misery, Mental Health, and Misdiagnosis

The toll extends beyond the physical. This is not to diminish the physical, including those most affected by the facial disfiguring impacts of the assault. Picture the agony of sick children with open mouths, ear infections, irritability, struggling to breathe, placed on endless regimens of antibiotics, their tiny faces bearing the weight of a medical crisis often misunderstood. Mental health epidemics surge as breathing difficulties intertwine with anxiety and depression. Worse yet, misdiagnosed situations perpetuate the cycle, rendering our healthcare system ill-equipped to address the root causes. I also wonder if the modern phenomenon of rampant impatience, road rage, political impasse, drug use, narcissism, and violence is not related to increases in sleep disorders. It would be worthy of study, in my opinion.

A Painful Reality: Our Healthcare System at a Crossroads

We stand at a crossroads, facing a painful reality that demands urgent attention. The traditional approach to healthcare, fixated on symptoms rather than causes, has brought us to this precipice. It's a narrative of misery and escalating costs. This crisis calls for a profound shift in how we perceive and address the interplay between airway wellness, whole-body health, and facial radiance. It also calls for a profound shift in addressing the healthcare system.

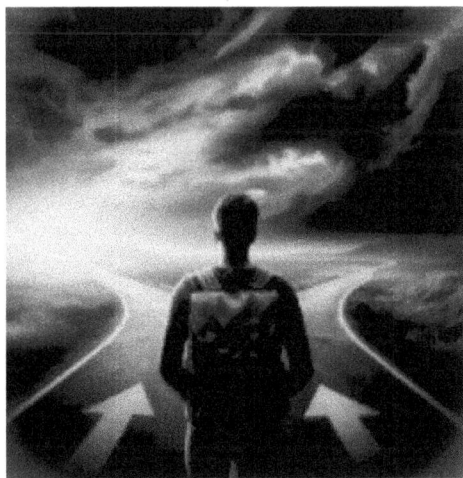

Figure 6: DALL E 3® using Bing® Copilot®

We also must address the disconnect between the professions of dentistry and medicine. This disconnect has impeded the recognition and adoption of dental contributions to the health of the whole body, not just oral health. It has resulted in the slow adoption of very effective therapies in airway health and sleep apnea to the underrecognized role it plays in oral health and many of our most devastating diseases, such as heart disease, cancer, dementia, diabetes, and stroke.

Nicole Spector and Gary Glassman have said that the distinction between dental and medical fields has long been acknowledged, but there's a growing trend toward convergence. Dentists strive to bridge the gap between dentistry and medicine, recognizing their role as oral medicine practitioners.[18] Termed the "historic rebuff" within dental circles, the rift between medicine and dentistry originated in 1840. At that time, physicians at the University of Maryland College of Medicine declined a suggestion from peers to integrate dental education into the medical program. Consequently, the College of Dentistry emerged as a separate entity. The refusal of dentistry to participate in Medicare during the 1960s further deepened this divide, leading to the present disparity in reimbursement systems for medical and dental services.[19]

Dr. Kevin Boyd, a pediatric dentist with a master's degree in Human Nutrition, says we collaborate within a familiar realm alongside otolaryngologists, speech-language therapists, dental hygienists, chiropractors, and osteopaths.[20]

Dentistry has traditionally maintained a certain degree of separation from medicine, explains Dr. Michael Tischler, a specialist in reconstructive dentistry and the implant editor for *Dentistry Today*. He highlights the historical separation in 1840 between dental and medical fields, suggesting that this division seems arbitrary given the direct relationship between oral health and overall health.

---

18 Nicole Spector, "Pain and Sleep: The Reason Your Dental Work Isn't Covered by Medical Insurance," NBC News. October 24, 2017, https://www.nbcnews.com/better/health/reason-your-dental-work-isn-t-covered-medical-insurance-ncna813666.

19 Chad M. Rasmussen, et al., "Education Solutions to the Medical-Dental Divide," *AMA Journal of Ethics*, vol. 24, no. 1, 2022, pp. E27-E32. doi: 10.1001/amajethics.2022.27.

20 Kevin L. Boyd, DDS, M.Sc., "Board-certified Pediatric Dentist in Chicago. Holds an M.Sc. degree in Human Nutrition and Dietetics. Teaches in the Pediatric Dentistry residency training program at Lurie Children's Hospital and serves as a dental consultant to the Lurie Sleep Medicine service." American Dental Association - Speakers.

Dr. Gary Glassman, an endodontist practicing in Toronto, Canada, and the U.S., echoes this sentiment, emphasizing that the oral cavity is a gateway to the body. He points out that various oral health issues can serve as indicators of underlying conditions, such as kidney disease, heart disease, diabetes, HPV, and cancer, underscoring the crucial role that dentists play as the first line of defense in identifying these potential health concerns. This awareness of oral health's impact on general health may begin as early as the first trimester of gestation.

There's also mounting data that the healthcare industry could benefit from covering dental as part of medical. Consider those 800,000 ER visits per year for dental-related problems. Wouldn't more people get preventative dental care if their medical insurance covered it?

Even the World Health Organization overlooked Noma, a severe oral disfiguring disease involving facial gangrene with a staggering 90 percent mortality rate. It wasn't categorized as a neglected tropical disease (NTD) until 2023, despite meeting all the criteria for such a designation for many years.[21] This omission occurred simply because the disease starts as a gum disease.

At present, dentists are classified as DME or durable medical equipment providers. This was done because a piece of hardware, namely an oral sleep appliance, was the only way dentists were treating obstructive sleep apnea patients in the past.

This DME designation can still be helpful for therapies such as iNAP® negative airway therapy, EPAP therapy, and eXciteOSA® tongue muscle electronic myotherapy (these will be explained later), but it does not encompass the newer medical therapies being developed within dentistry. In my view, this DME designation was and is unfortunate. The fact that dentists are now treating with other therapies, such as lasers, orthodontic care, and other airway opening therapies, will not lend itself to a DME categorization.

Dentistry should be seen as another medical specialty care profession. This artificial distinction between medical and dental care does not just affect sleep disorders care but also the care of the teeth and periodontal tissues (gums) when a person needs treatment of these tissues caused by medical conditions like cancer treatment with radiation and chemotherapy,

---

21 John Button, "The WHO Recognizes Noma after Years of Medical-dental Disconnect." *STAT*, December 16, 2023, https://www.statnews.com/2023/12/16/noma-who-neglected-tropical-disease-dental-health/.

Sjogren's syndrome, which dries the mouth, creating increased dental decay and gum disease, autoimmune diseases, car accidents, and other accidents, scleroderma, and many more connecting and causative medical diseases. It is becoming more recognized that dental diseases affect the patient's overall health.

Organizations such as the American Board of Sleep Medicine (ABSM) offer valuable information regarding the certification and training of sleep specialists, providing insights into their expertise and qualifications. Similarly, the American Academy of Sleep Medicine frequently releases reports and data pertinent to sleep medicine and professionals in the field, contributing to understanding and advancing sleep-related healthcare. Additionally, government health agencies like the U.S. Department of Health and Human Services play a crucial role in tracking healthcare workforce trends, including those related to sleep specialists, offering comprehensive data for informed decision-making and policy development. And finally, the American Board of Dental Sleep Medicine and the American Sleep and Breathing Academy work diligently to bring a coordinated professional approach to sleep-breathing disorders.

The Call to Action: Crafting a Narrative of Solution

As we unravel this narrative of pain, let's not treat it as a tale of despair but a call to action. In the following pages, we embark on a journey of understanding, exploration, and transformation. *Beautiful Faces* isn't just a book; it's a road map to reclaiming the vitality and radiance that modern life has sought to erode. In the face of crisis, we find an opportunity for healing and transformation.

The Challenge of Recognition in Our Healthcare System

Recognizing sleep apnea can pose challenges due to its inconspicuous and often misunderstood symptoms. Symptoms such as snoring, daytime fatigue (excessive daytime sleepiness or EDS), feelings of depression, high blood pressure, morning headaches, body pain, loss of libido, and concentration difficulties are frequently observed. For example, despite being prevalent, snoring is often overlooked as an ordinary and normal annoyance rather than a potential indicator of a more significant underlying issue. Snoring in and of itself can cause diseases such as demyelination and axon nerve damage in the soft palate,[22] elongating the uvula, and plaque accumulation in the carotid arteries.[23] Demyelinating diseases[24] encompass various conditions that harm the protective fatty coat (myelin sheath) surrounding nerve fibers. This damage results in slowed or halted nerve impulses, leading to neurological issues.

Elevating the soft palate is attributed to the levator veli palatini muscle. This muscle receives innervation from the pharyngeal plexus of the vagus nerve, or cranial nerve X. Demyelination of the nerve fibers that innervate the levator veli palatini muscle can lead to the nerve not functioning, which can result in difficulty in elevating the soft palate and opening the airway [25] In other words, the soft palate becomes floppy and dysfunctional, leading to even more snoring and louder snoring. That's what happened to me. (By the way, this can be repaired.)

Snoring was the first sign that I might have sleep apnea. My wife complained about it, and it did get worse the older I got. In my case, you could easily hear my snoring through a closed door and in other rooms of the house.

Snoring is closely linked with obstructive sleep apnea in over 80 percent of cases.[26] Some experts say it is closer to 100 percent. These signs caused by snoring and sleep apnea might be erroneously attributed to other causes, emphasizing the crucial need for careful diagnosis through clinical evaluations and sleep studies.

---

22 Farhan Shah, Thorbjörn Holmlund, Eva Levring Jäghagen, Diana Berggren, Karl Franklin, Sture Forsgren, Per Stål et al., "Axon and Schwann Cell Degeneration in Nerves of Upper Airway Relates to Pharyngeal Dysfunction in Snorers and Patients With Sleep Apnea." *Chest* 154, no. 5 (2018): 1091-1098, accessed March 1, 2024. https://doi.org/10.1016/j.chest.2018.06.017.

23 John Button, "Snoring Can Affect The Carotid Artery," *Medical News Today*, December 27, 2013, https://www.medicalnewstoday.com/articles/best-mattresses-for-snoring#when-to-see-a-doctor.

24 Sarah Lewis, PharmD and Seunngu Han, M.D., "What Are Demyelinating Diseases?" *Healthgrades*, August 30, 2022, https://www.healthgrades.com/right-care/brain-and-nerves/demyelinating-disease.

25 Roberto Grujicic, M.D. and Jana Vaskovic M.D., "Levator Veli Palatini Muscle." Kenhub, November 3, 2023. https://www.kenhub.com/en/library/anatomy/levator-veli-palatini-muscle.

26 Mudiaga Sowho, et al. "Snoring: A Source of Noise Pollution and Sleep Apnea Predictor." *Sleep*, 43, 6 (2020), zsz305. doi: 10.1093/sleep/zsz305.

Rachel's Story

Although many causes are implicated in our airway constrictions, we are not focused solely on those contributing factors involving misdiagnosis or mistreatment of the medical and dental professions. We will, however, not leave those subjects out of the overall narrative. My experiences with my airway issues and Dr. Zelk's experiences with his airway issues existed at birth and persisted throughout our growth and development. Yet, Dr. Zelk and I experienced different degrees of unrecognized sleep disease caused by improperly formed faces and jaws. I also experienced what I consider misapplied traditional treatment for my crowded jaws and teeth, which made my condition worse. This story about Rachel, linked below, is a particularly heart-wrenching account of our unrecognized modern epidemic. It is presented because this story is all too common today, and we believe it can be changed for the better.

You can read an unfortunate story about early childhood orthodontic care in England. The entire article from her online posting can be reached in our resource folder by accessing this QR code to the folder and then going to the URL or QR code for Rachel's story.

Figure 7: This is the QR code link to the Beautiful Faces Website and Resource folder. Here is the hyperlink as well. https://drive.google.com/drive/folders/1dnkRBpAwMcqLtMQTaM4Ms8lUsz1_NbBb?usp=drive_link

How do you reclaim five years of growth stunted during such a critical period? You can read Rachel's story at the following website. Note: while writing this book, this site became a pay-to-access website at https://karin-badt.medium.com/the-science-of-orthodontics-511e94795aa.

Noel Stimson, Dr. Ben Miraglia, and Dr. Skip Truitt made this comment on https://karinbadt.medium.com/; I will paraphrase their comment. They said there's a longstanding concern within the orthodontic field regarding "Premolar Extraction/Retraction" (PER) and its potential impact on facial structure. This debate has persisted for over eighty years, originating from Dr. Charles Tweed's advocacy of the controversial PER technique at a 1940 orthodontics conference. A review of this subject by Karin Badt is located on YouTube.[27]

To emphasize this point, a recent 2023 conclusion on premolar extraction is presented in the study entitled "Evidence Supports No Relationship between Obstructive Sleep Apnea and Premolar Extraction: An Electronic Health Records Review."[28] This study is often cited as justification that premolar extraction is not harmful. The article is not about airway enlargement or decreases in airway volume; it is not intended to be a statement about improving or harming facial beauty. We will discuss this again in the book.

To be clear, readers need to understand that increases or decreases in airway volume do not directly mean sleep apnea can be improved or worsened each time they are impacted. We believe airway volume is important, though. You will understand the distinctions better as we move forward.

---

27 Karin Badt, "Extracting Premolar Teeth for Orthodontic Treatment: What are the Risks? (Article Review)" Whole Body Breathing, accessed July 24, 2024, https://www.youtube.com/watch?v=0tUH-NElvcqQ.

28 Ann J. Larsen, et al. "Evidence Supports No Relationship between Obstructive Sleep Apnea and Premolar Extraction: An Electronic Health Records Review." *Journal of Clinical Sleep Medicine*, 11, 12 (2015), 1443-1448.

CHAPTER 2

What's Wrong with Our Faces?

What is unique about our human airways is best explained by Dr. Marc Abramson, DDS, member of the Air Institute of Portland, Oregon. We will discuss this before we discuss what is wrong.

Dr. Marc Abramson graduated from the University of Maryland School of Dentistry in 1975 and did a general practice residency at the Palo Alto VA Hospital from 1975 to 1976. He is an adjunct professor and founder of the Mindfulness Clinic at Stanford University and has spent a lifetime examining, treating, and teaching TMJ disorders, headaches, and sleep apnea. He is board-certified in orofacial pain and sleep medicine, treating and teaching a holistic approach to human health, especially as it relates to dental, jaw joint health, and oral health.

His approaches to health and function have gained recognition in institutions such as Harvard, Columbia, and Stanford. He is the developer of the OASYS oral sleep apnea device that has been FDA-cleared for sleep airway care.

His insights help us understand what is happening to our faces and airways. I will paraphrase his thoughts on human evolution and the unique way our airways and jaw function in the animal kingdom. I have added some brackets to explain some terms for those who may not know what they mean.

Here is a short history of Dr. Abramson's journey into the world of sleep medicine and jaw joint disorders.

Reflecting on my childhood, I recall struggling with breathing difficulties, which led to frequent and painful visits where radium rods were inserted into my nostrils to expose me to radiation, all in an attempt to alleviate sinus issues. These experiences not only underscored the medical practices of the early 1950s but also emphasized the need for safer and more effective treatments.

Another significant event occurred at the age of fourteen when I was struck by a car while walking on the sidewalk, resulting in a fractured femur that required an extensive ten-week hospitalization period in traction. This prolonged ordeal provided first-hand insight into pain management and the importance of the mind-body connection in healthcare.

At age fourteen, I was hit by a car while walking on the sidewalk one Sunday afternoon and was hospitalized with a fractured femur. I was in traction for ten weeks, and during this time, I had to manage the pain of this injury and its repercussions. I recognized then, as I do now, that using my insights and ability to tune in to the sensation rather than fight it allowed me to control it.

I grew to realize the importance of the mind-body connection in healthcare. This made me appreciate using one's inner skills to manage pain in general health.

In dental school, I felt disappointed that I was not being taught any of the skills in this area of interest that I knew were valuable and was only taught the answer to pain was to prescribe medication. In my residency, I looked for alternative health courses and practices not taught in my advanced educational programs. This pursuit began my exploration into integrative medicine and how to use my dental skills to help in healthcare by understanding the intricacies of orofacial growth and development and how it affects many areas of a person's total health.

A pivotal moment in my journey came when I encountered *The Dental Physician* by Dr. Al Fonders. This insightful book illuminated the systemic implications of dental conditions and inspired me to explore innovative treatment modalities. One of the observations he emphasized in his book was a patient who was treated by supporting and freeing up his mandible, which corrected scoliosis of the spine. The book showed skeletal X-rays of his spine before and after the treatment, which showed significant improvement in his alignment.

One notable case I had involved a young boy suffering from significant TMJ dysfunction. Using a lower flat plane splint as part of his treatment, I witnessed an unexpected correction in his spine alignment and documented this transformative outcome with photographs, and informed the boy's physician. Instead of looking at the patient and evaluating what I reported, the physician reported me to the medical board for practicing medicine without a license. I had a visit from examiners and the medical board, threatening to arrest me for practicing medicine without a license. I informed them that I was not practicing medicine but had simply treated the mandible and observed its impact on the rest of the body.

This incident underscored the challenges within the medical model and highlighted the need for a more holistic approach that recognizes the interconnectedness of the body's systems. As a dentist, I often advocate for a broader understanding of the oral system's critical role in overall health.

Dr. Abramson on the uniqueness of the human airway:

The human oral facial system stands out among other mammalian species due to our upright posture and ability to articulate speech. Let's delve into the evolutionary changes that have made us so unique. As humans evolved to walk upright and communicate through speech, remarkable changes unfolded, harmonizing to create our complex and beautiful system. Two key components of this evolution are the transition to upright posture and the changes in the oropharynx (the throat) brought together through the intricate process of evolution.

We must examine four-legged mammals like dogs or cats to understand this transformation. In these animals, the airway, throat, and spine align horizontally through the body, with the jaw situated at the anterior (forward) end of the cranium (head) and the spine extending to the posterior end. As we move up the evolutionary ladder to chimpanzees, we see a partial transition to upright posture as they descend from trees to walk on the ground. While their spinal cord remains aligned for walking, they adapted to operate at a 45-degree angle instead of horizontally.

Comparing this to human posture, we observe significant differences. Our feet feature a forward-pointing big toe and arch support to accommodate upright posture, while our pelvis has developed buttocks to stabilize and support the upper body. Additionally, our spine requires a lordotic (sway in) curvature in the lower and cervical regions to maintain upright posture.

In the cranium, critical changes are needed to facilitate upright posture. The foramen magnum (the hole in the bottom of your skull through which your spinal cord emerges) shifts forward for an upright posture to sit at the base of the skull, aligning vertically with the spinal cord. This vertical alignment extends down the neck, with the airway and esophagus also adopting a vertical position just in front of the spinal cord.

However, this transition presents challenges, particularly concerning the temporomandibular joint (TMJ or jaw joint). In previous mammals, the TMJ operated in a simple hinge movement, but in an upright posture, this movement would compromise breathing. To adapt, the human jaw joint evolved to allow anterior translation, enabling the jaw to move forward without obstructing the airway. Our jaw joint head and the disc on that jaw joint head actually have the ability to move out of the jaw socket and move forward. If one side moves but not the other, you get a clicking or popping noise, and some people develop pain and dysfunction. They must be coordinated together when they move.

Another significant adaptation involves the mandible. In chimpanzees and other four-legged animals, the mandible features a Simian shelf, providing thickness to support the jawbone. The Simian Shelf is an extra thick bone on the tongue side of the anterior lower jaw to provide strength. However, in humans, this strengthening of the bone had to evolve differently to accommodate upright posture, resulting in the development of the human chin. We are the only animals with a chin.

Simultaneously, advancements in the airway occurred to accommodate speech. Up to this point, all mammals had an epiglottic lockup, where the epiglottis is connected to the soft palate, blocking the back of the throat. Human babies are born with this lockup, allowing them to nurse and swallow while breathing through their nose. However, around three months of age, the human larynx descends into the throat, creating an opening behind the tongue known as the oropharynx.

This evolution in the anatomy of the human cranium, with the spinal cord exiting vertically at the base, the TMJ allowing anterior translation, the descent of the larynx, and the floating hyoid bone, creates ideal conditions for upright posture and speech. The hyoid bone is the only bone not attached to other bones. It floats and holds muscle bundles in place. However, these changes also make the jaw joint more susceptible to temporomandibular disorders (jaw joint and muscles) and increase the risk of airway compromise, leading to conditions like obstructive sleep apnea.

The tongue is unique, too, and is called a muscular hydrostat or a bundle of muscles that work with little or no bone assistance. If a hydrostat shrinks and depresses in one area, it must bulge in another. We can do something about oversized tongues by treating the fat cells in the tongue, which is called pyroptosis. We will cover this later.

Unfortunately, many aspects of cranial, facial, and dental growth management have been misunderstood within dentistry, resulting in harm to some patients. Dentistry initially adopted convenient but incorrect positions for the jaw. They tried treating it like a simple hinge, like that of other animals, leading to nerve compression, inflammation, and pain conditions. Similarly, many in orthodontics wrongly believed that dental arches could only be contracted, leading to unnecessary tooth extractions and facial growth restrictions.

Regrettably, this discourse sheds light on numerous inadequacies in managing craniofacial dental growth and the treatment philosophy surrounding temporomandibular joint dysfunction (TMD). As dentistry has evolved techniques for tooth alignment and replacement, it has sometimes taken approaches that run counter to healthy growth, development, and function.

One such misstep occurred in the treatment of edentulous (people with no teeth) patients, where the repeatable and simple approach of pushing the jaw back against the rear wall of the jaw joint space was mistakenly assumed to be the physiological positioning for all restorative treatments, like crown and bridge. This erroneous positioning exerted pressure on nerves near the ear, sometimes resulting in inflammation, various pathologies, and pain conditions such as TMJ pain, headaches, and neck pain while compromising the airway.

The advent of orthodontics sometimes compounded these issues, with the belief that dental arches could only contract, not expand. This led to the extraction of bicuspids and retractive headgear, which can hinder facial growth and development, exacerbate breathing and sinus problems, and further jaw joint compression.

Upon completing my residency and sensing my calling to address jaw joint problems and facial pain globally, I observed what I believe are the shortcomings in current practices. I developed a treatment philosophy focused on freeing the mandible, relieving jaw joint pressure, and promoting facial and throat growth. Despite encountering resistance from some individuals within the profession I cherished, my approach yielded significant success.

My exploration into sleep medicine revealed another overlooked aspect: the impact of jaw and throat irregularities on sleep and airway function. Incorporating principles of craniofacial health, I identified a gap in addressing nasal breathing problems and resistance when using oral appliances for sleep apnea. This led to the development of the OASYS (Oral Nasal Airway System), a groundbreaking oral appliance recognized by the FDA's ENT (ear, nose, and throat) division for its ability to simultaneously address nasal dilation and mandibular repositioning and effectively treat the entire upper airway at once. This oral sleep appliance is unique in its ability to open the nasal valve airway and move the tongue out of the throat.

Understanding the intricacies of craniofacial development and adopting holistic approaches to treatment are crucial steps in improving patient care and addressing the complexities of the human orofacial system.

Thank you, Dr Abramson, for this insight into the unique human orofacial complex.

Some variations of human face structures are related to abnormal modern trends:

Most people don't know that our jaws have become narrower and shorter. Modern faces are more dolichocephalic (narrower and longer) than they used to be. This change, even in ethnic groups where it's more normal, has occurred measurably since the technology age began about 150 years ago. Actual evolutionary changes take thousands of years or more to create measurable changes. Just think of the kids you knew in high school who needed braces, as compared to now. Here are three definitions that may help you understand future discussions. It is also important to note that any head shape or face type a person has does not exempt them from sleep airway blockages.

1. **Dolichocephalic** refers to a specific face type characterized by a long and narrow head shape. The forehead is prominently developed in individuals with dolichocephalic features, extending vertically. The narrow jawline creates a distinctive elongated appearance, and the chin has a more pointed shape. The eyes typically have an almond-shaped contour, contributing to the overall slender look of the face. The nose tends to be long and narrow, complementing the general elongation of facial features. Additionally, the lips are often thin and have a straight configuration, enhancing the characteristics of a dolichocephalic face type.

    The dolichocephalic head shape is primarily associated with the length and narrowness of the skull rather than specific details of jaw position or head posture. While the description of a dolichocephalic face highlights features such as a prominent forehead, narrow jawline, and pointed chin, it doesn't necessarily imply a receded lower jaw or a forward head posture.

    Individual variations in jaw position, head posture, and other facial features can occur independently of the basic head shape. Therefore, someone with a dolichocephalic head shape may or may not exhibit characteristics like a receded lower jaw or forward head posture. Yet, I often see them linked to dolichocephalic head shapes, as I have. This narrow facial profile results in V-shaped dental arches not allowing enough space for the teeth to stay straight and aligned. This is a significant reason for the crowding of teeth. This is why some researchers believe over 90 percent of children in the U.S. would need orthodontics to correct crowded and crooked teeth.

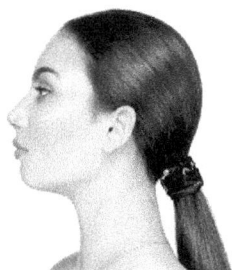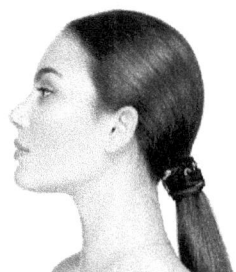

Figure 8: This is a profile of a woman with a receded jaw and chin on the left and a normal jaw and chin on the right. Note also that there is a bulge under the jaw near the neck on the left. The curve from the jaw to the neck should be closer to a right angle than a gradual curve. Shutterstock licensed photo

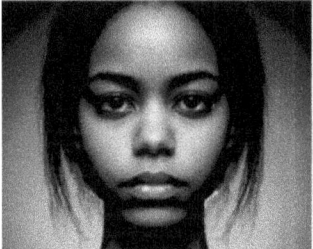

Figure 9: Woman with a narrow face and receding chin. Dall E 3® Bing® and Copilot®

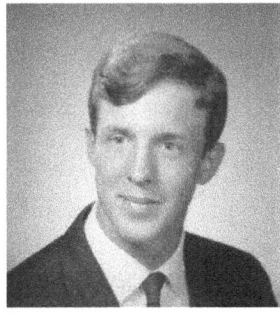

Figure 10: This is Richard's high school senior photo. I am a classic dolichocephalic face form. I am not just dolichocephalic but also an abnormally accentuated dolichocephalic with a narrow and long-faced and recessed chin. I nearly always kept my lips closed for any photo at that age due to crowded teeth.

2. **Mesocephalic:** This depicts a face with a medium head shape. The face has a more average forehead, jawline, and chin proportion. The eyes are round, and the nose is straight. The lips are full and slightly curved.
3. **Brachycephalic:** This depicts a face with a short and wide head shape. The face has a broad forehead, a wide jawline, and a rounded chin. The eyes are round, and the nose is short and wide. The lips are full and slightly curved. Even in this facial type, where the dental arches look broad and rounded, and the teeth are not crowded, if the dental arches have narrowed slightly, the back teeth have inclined toward the tongue, and the tongue is more oversized, airway issues can occur.

All the face types described—dolichocephalic, mesocephalic, and brachycephalic—are normal variations in human facial morphology. These terms refer to different head shapes and proportions, and individuals can naturally exhibit any of these characteristics without it being indicative of abnormality.

These face types are part of the natural diversity seen in human populations, influenced by genetic factors and the interplay of various environmental factors during development. It's important to note that variations in facial features do not necessarily indicate health issues, and people can have different face types while remaining within the range of normal human variation and health. People also exhibit beauty with any facial type.

The trouble is that this can become problematic if the change to a more dolichocephalic face structure is more about environmental influences than normal genetic guidance. A trend to a more dolichocephalic face structure today also affects changes in the entire body.

It is typical to see this type of face now, and it is also changing some of our perceptions of beauty. According to Dr. Steven Park, there seems to be a preference for face type to softer and narrower faces over previous preferences that tended toward rounder faces with stronger jaw shapes.[29] These changes are often, but not always, problems accompanied by this list of abnormalities that were not associated with dolichocephalic faces in the past:

---

29 Steven Park, "Doctor Steven Park," last modified June 15, 2022, accessed April 8, 2024. https://doctorstevenpark.com/.

1. forward head posture
2. sloping forward shoulders
3. hunched upper back (Kyphosis)
4. open-mouth breathing and open open-mouth
5. abnormal swallowing with chin muscle contraction
6. dry mouth
7. tooth decay
8. crooked & crowded teeth with or without overbite, underbite, and overjet
9. periodontal disease (gum disease)
10. tongue ties (a condition that restricts the tongue's range of motion)
11. speech impediments
12. elongated and floppy uvula
13. scalloped tongue
14. tori (excess bone in the roof of the mouth or the tongue side of the lower jaw)
15. teeth grinding
16. broken teeth, crowns, dentures, and fillings
17. failed dental implants
18. TMJ disorder includes jaw joint pain, headache pain, neck pain, and clicking
19. sunken cheekbones
20. narrow noses with deviated septum, upturned nose
21. excessively curved in lower backs (Lordosis)
22. receded chin
23. uneven eyes
24. dark circles under the eyes. (adenoidal facies)

Chiropractors call the spinal profile kyphosis on the upper back and lordosis for the lower back. See the figure below.

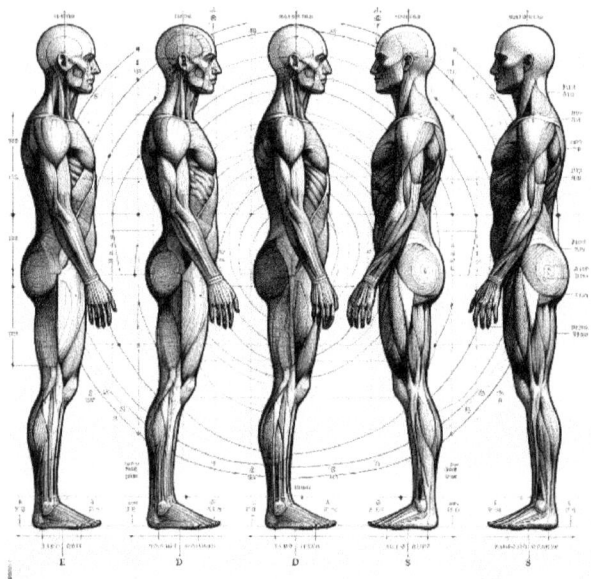

Figure 11: Ideal Posture (Dall E 3® Bing® and Copilot®)
The text and muscle images in this AI-generated graphic have no meaning.

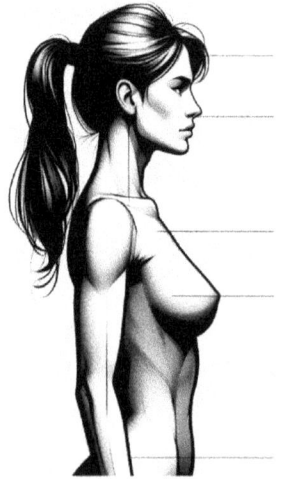

Figure 12: Dall E 3® Bing® and Copilot®
To Show Near Ideal Posture

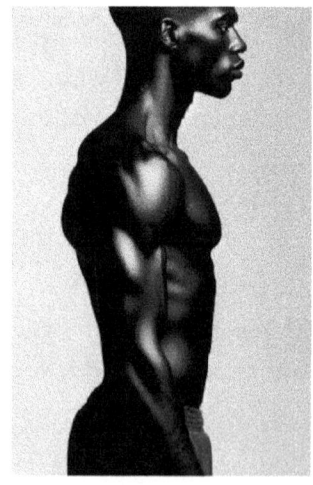

Figure 13: AI image Near Ideal Posture
Dall E 3® Bing® and Copilot®

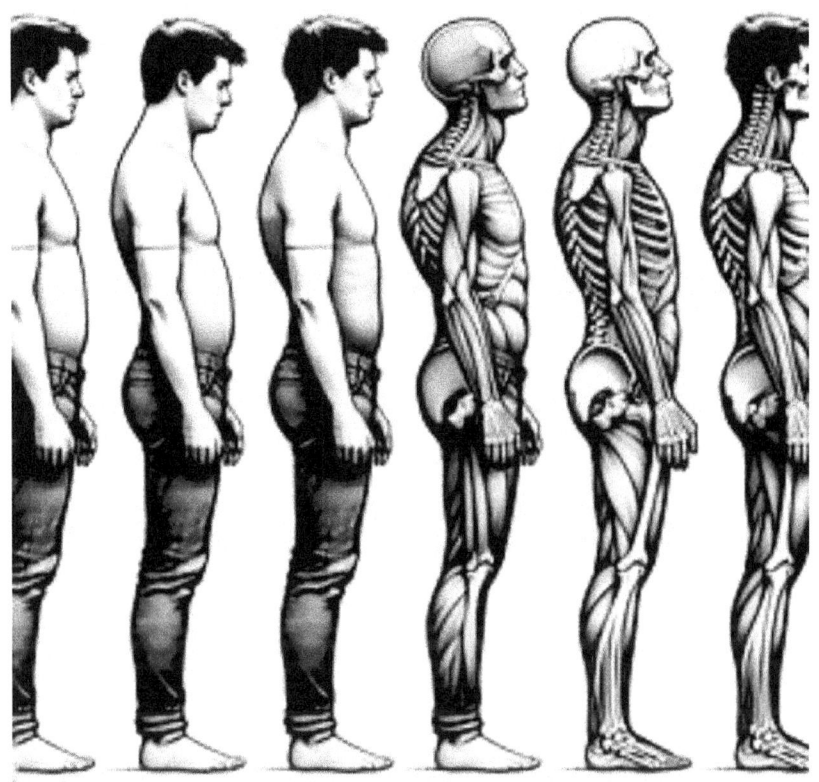

Figure 14: Forward head posture with excess Kyphosis and Lordosis
Dall E 3® Bing® and Copilot®
The details of Bones and Muscles are inaccurate in AI graphics

CHAPTER 3

Contributing Causes – The First Assault

The causes behind facial changes remain open, with many factors contributing to facial and airway deficiencies. While isolating a single or primary cause proves challenging amidst the many potential culprits, we aim to outline some commonly cited influences. Many of these influences interact with others to modify what they might do if isolated in their actions.

We've categorized these influences into fourteen general categories, recognizing that each could warrant extensive exploration. However, our objective is not about exhaustive detail, as numerous resources already exist on this topic, which we will reference throughout this book. Instead, our focus is to provide insight and tools to manage these developmental challenges for yourself and your loved ones rather than be utterly dependent on healthcare providers who generally treat you after the damage has occurred.

This book will primarily discuss solutions aligned with current healthcare practices to address these issues in affected individuals. We'll also explore how individuals can proactively shape their futures and how government initiatives can foster improved public health systems.

1. WESTON A. PRICE AND CONTEMPORARY DIETS

We begin this section by going back more than 100 years to a book and study by Weston A. Price, DDS. We still have not learned from his warnings.

Western or modern diets have been implicated in destroying our faces and were probably most famously documented in Dr. Weston Price's book, *Nutrition and Physical Degeneration,* published in 2009.[30] The book contains arresting photographs of handsome, healthy indigenous people worldwide. It documents the changes in facial structure and disease before and after modern Western diets were introduced to these populations. A similar subject documentary was recently introduced to Netflix by Dan Buettner, called *The Blue Zones.*[31] Here are some images of facial deformities caused by modern diets. Dr. Price documented these over several years before publishing. They were from his book about modern diets being introduced to Indigenous or ancestral living people with damage to their faces in astonishingly short time spans, not 10,000 years, as some assert.

Even though the images are not professionally captured, and Dr. Price uses language that is not politically correct for today, the points that modern diets have impacted facial structure, dental health, and whole-body health are powerful. It is worth reading because it is much more thorough than we can show in this book section.

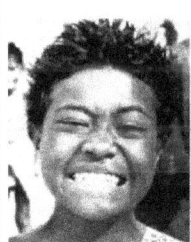
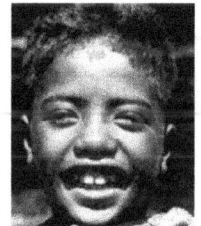

Good dental health begins with the diet of the parents. The Samoan boy on the left was born to parents who ate nutrient-rich native foods. The Samoan boy on the right was born to parents who had abandoned their traditional diet. He has crowded dental arches, and will be more susceptible to dental decay.

A Comparison of the Diets

(Compiled from *Nutrition and Physical Degeneration* by Weston A. Price, DDS)

Photos Copyright ©
Price-Pottenger
Nutrition Foundation®,
All Rights Reserved,
www.ppnf.org

Figure 15: This image and text were printed with permission from Price Pottenger Nutrition Foundation.

---

30 Weston A. Price, *Nutrition and Physical Degeneration: A Comparison of Primitive and Modern Diets and Their Effects (*Lemon Grove, CA: Price Pottenger Nutrition Foundation, 2009.

31 Dan Buettner, *The Blue Zones Solution: Eating and Living like the World's Healthiest People.* (Washington, DC: National Geographic, 2015).

Dr. Francis Marion Pottenger, Jr., a physician known for his work on "Pottenger's Cats," conducted research from 1932 to 1942. His most notable findings emerged when he observed the effects of diet across multiple generations of cats. Those cats fed an inferior diet exhibited a decline in health that worsened with each successive generation. This included evidence of skeletal deformities, allergies, and reduced fertility, all identified as direct consequences of inadequate nutrition. Dr. Pottenger's work highlighted principles now recognized as epigenetics—the influence of environmental factors on gene expression and health outcomes across generations.

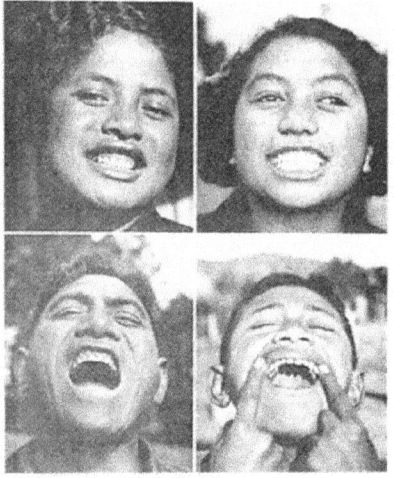

FIG. 69. Since the discovery of New Zealand the primitive natives, the Mann, have had the reputation of having the finest teeth and finest bodies of any race in the world. These faces are typical. Only about one tooth per thousand teeth had been attacked by tooth decay before they came under the influence of the white man

Figure 16

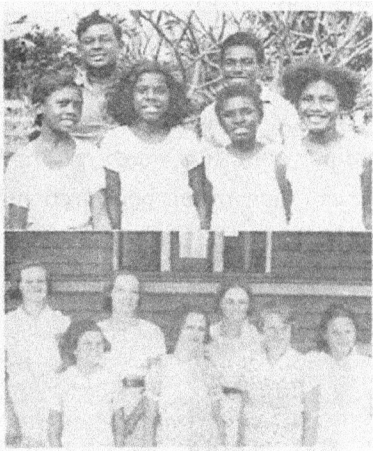

FIG. 62. School children from the two groups on Thursday Island. Note the beautifully proportioned faces of the natives, and the pinched nostrils and marked disturbance in proportions of the faces of the whites. The dental arches of the natives are broad, while many of the whites have very crowded teeth. The parents and children of the natives used native foods while the parents and children of the whites used the modern imported foods of commerce.

Figure 17

These images and text were printed with permission from Price Pottenger.[32]

---

32 Price Pottenger, accessed May 17, 2024, https://price-pottenger.org/.

Contributing Causes – The First Assault | 47

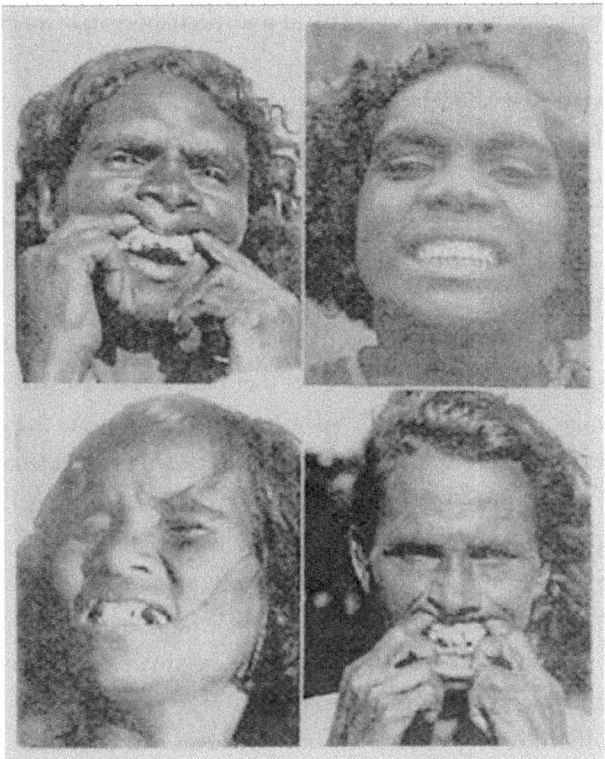

Figure 18: These are the aboriginal people of Australia.
The upper right is a woman with an indigenous diet, while the other three show rampant decay and deformation from Western diets.
This image was printed with permission from Price Pottenger[33]

Modern Diets:

Our diets are frequently characterized by an excess of inflammatory components. Mainly, they are seed fats and sugars.[34] Rather than incorporating beneficial saturated fats like olive oil or avocado, individuals often consume inflammatory seed oils, such as soybean oils, initially designed for industrial applications like machine lubrication. These oils are subjected to high-temperature processing and are now promoted as healthful despite

---

33 Price Pottenger, accessed May 17, 2024, https://price-pottenger.org/.

34 "The Truth about Fats: The Good, the Bad, and the In-between," *Harvard Health Publishing*. Harvard Medical School, April 12, 2022, accessed April 8, 2024, https://www.health.harvard.edu/staying-healthy/the-truth-about-fats-bad-and-good].

their susceptibility to becoming rancid and their potential for provoking inflammation.[35]

Inflammation within the body can trigger a cascading series of adverse effects, including the onset of conditions like arthritis, cancer, heart disease, fatigue, weight gain, weakened immune function, and other health concerns.[36] This chronic state of inflammation can also contribute to altering facial structure.[37] We will talk about inflammation in more detail later and many related inflammatory triggers.

Another problem with the contemporary diet is that it is too soft. Several studies suggest that consuming a softer diet may elevate the risk of malocclusion or misalignment of teeth.[38] The best way to promote the growth of jaws requires continual stimulation with appropriate forces. Inadequate forces and uses of the jaws can inhibit optimal growth patterns in the craniofacial region (Gupta et al., 2019; Lione et al., 2018; Zheng et al., 2020).[39] Weston A. Price, DDS, and Francis M. Pottenger Jr, MD conducted pioneering studies on this subject, and many later advanced their nutritional research.[40] This soft diet has caused us to be less able to digest plants. We will explain that further in the microbiome section to follow.

Other inflammatory foods, such as sugar and carbohydrates, have garnered attention for their adverse health effects. The industries responsible for producing these products have faced criticism for practices involving financial influence over significant institutions and scientists, ultimately

---

35 C. E. Ramsden, et al., "Re-evaluation of the traditional diet-heart hypothesis: analysis of recovered data from Minnesota Coronary Experiment (1968-73)." *BMJ*, 353, i1246 (2016), doi: 10.1136/bmj.i1246.

36 P. C. Calder, et al. "Inflammatory disease processes and interactions with nutrition." *British Journal of Nutrition*, 101, Suppl 1 (2009), S1-S45. doi: 10.1017/S0007114509377867. PMID: 19586558.

37 Benoit Chassaing and Andrew T. Gewirtz. "Gut microbiota, low-grade inflammation, and metabolic syndrome," *Toxicologic Pathology* 42, no. 1 (2014): 49-53, doi:10.1177/0192623313508481. Epub 2013 Nov 27. PMID: 24285672.

38 D. Zheng, X Li, C. Wang, et al., "Soft diet feeding induces physiologic and histologic changes in the rat mandibular condyle," *Journal of Oral and Maxillofacial Surgery*, 78, 2 (2020), 209.e1-209.e10.

39 Valeria Paoloni, et al. "Evaluation of the Morphometric Covariation Between Palatal and Craniofacial Skeletal Morphology in Class III Malocclusion Growing Subjects." *BMC Oral Health*, 20, 1, (2020), 152. doi: 10.1186/s12903-020-01140-4. PMID: 32460800; PMCID: PMC7251885.

40 Joan Grinzi, RN, and David Getoff, CCN, "Preserving and Advancing the Nutrition Research of Weston A. Price, DDS, and Francis M. Pottenger, Jr., MD." *Integrative Medicine* (Encinitas) 13, no. 1 (February 2014): 48-54, https://pmc.ncbi.nlm.nih.gov/articles/PMC4684111/.

promoting sugar-laden products as healthy options.[41] A notable case was exposed by an article in the *New York Times* on the sugar industry shifting the blame on fats in our diet as the cause of heart disease instead of sugar as the cause at Harvard University.[42] These biased recommendations came from respectable scientific papers, making them even more damaging.

The magnitude of soft drink use is a modern phenomenon that has exploded. When I was a child, a soft drink was a rare treat. Today, it is not only a substitute for water during a meal but has also become a standard hydration substitute that it was never designed to be. Just one 24-oz. fructose-sweetened soft drink can increase blood pressure by fifteen points systolic and nine points diastolic![43]

Worse yet are the energy drinks that have become a remedy for daytime low energy and sleepiness. The vicious cycle is evident. These drinks, even one energy drink per month, increase insomnia by 12 percent in males and 19 percent in females.

A study done in Norway links the association. I will paraphrase the results.

> Last week, researchers urged a prohibition on selling energy drinks to young people due to their association with anxiety, stress, and suicidal thoughts. The government is contemplating a proposal to cease the sale of energy drinks to children under sixteen in England.[44]
>
> A recent study published in *BMJ* (a leading medical journal) examined the impact of energy drink consumption on sleep patterns in young people. The findings revealed that any level of energy drink consumption heightened sleep problems. Men who consumed one to three drinks a month had a 12 percent higher risk of insomnia, while women had a 19 percent higher risk.

---

41 Robert H. Lustig, Laura A. Schmidt, and Claire D. Brindis, "The Toxic Truth About Sugar," *Nature* 482 (2012): 27–29, https://doi.org/10.1038/482027a.

42 Anahad O'Connor, "How the Sugar Industry Shifted Blame to Fat," *New York Times,* September 12, 2016, https://www.nytimes.com/2016/09/13/well/eat/how-the-sugar-industry-shifted-blame-to-fat.html.

43 Paul Frysh, "Surprising Things That Raise Your Blood Pressure," Hypertension/High Blood Pressure Guide. Medically reviewed by Carol DerSarkissian, MD. Last modified August 30, 2022. This doesn't have a citation number.

44 "Proposal to End the Sale of Energy Drinks to Children Under 16." GOV.WALES, accessed April 22, 2024, https://www.gov.wales/proposal-end-sale-energy-drinks-children-under-16.

For men having two to three drinks per week, the likelihood of bedtime after midnight increased by 35 percent, a 52 percent higher chance of sleeping less than six hours, and a 60 percent higher likelihood of waking during the night compared to those who rarely or did not consume them. Women with the same consumption frequency were 20 percent more likely to have a bedtime after midnight, 58 percent more likely to sleep less than six hours, and 24 percent more likely to wake at night.[45]

Lately, there is a politicized refrain about "believing in science." I agree with believing in science, but this does not mean we should accept any science study placed in front of us just because it comes from a supposedly reputable or peer-reviewed source. The sugar industry perverted science studies from reputable sources for its own purposes. This marketing strategy from the sugar industry has not only contributed to health problems but has also raised concerns regarding the addictive nature of these foods.[46]

The rise of the obesity epidemic in the United States is often cited as a sobering testament to the success of reshaping dietary habits in an unfavorable manner by the food industry. The obesity epidemic in America is a grim testament to their success at changing our eating habits from what was once good to pathetic.[47]

Pregnancy-induced obstructive sleep apnea (PISA) is a condition where a pregnant woman experiences obstructive sleep apnea (OSA), often due to weight gain, hormonal changes, and increased abdominal girth. While PISA is associated with several maternal complications, including hypertension, preeclampsia, and gestational diabetes, its direct impact on causing fetal deformities is not well-established. However, untreated severe OSA can lead to reduced oxygen levels and poor sleep quality, which may affect fetal

---

45 Joe Davis, "FIZZ ALERT Just One Energy Drink a Month Is Enough to Destroy Your Sleep, Scientists Find," *The Sun* (UK Edition), January 22, 2024, https://www.thesun.co.uk/health/25447198/energy-drinks-insomnia-sleep-problems/.

46 "Obesity and Overweight," World Health Organization Newsroom, March 1, 2024. https://www.who.int/news-room/fact-sheets/detail/obesity-and-overweight.

47 R. E. Scammon, The First Anatomical Atlas: The Influence of a New Science on Medical and Dental Education, *Dental Cosmos*, 53, 7 (1911), 705-718.

development and growth.[48] Many doctors miss this connection and could help expectant mothers with CPAP or oral sleep appliances while pregnant. Some have speculated that PISA contributes to receded jaws in the fetuses.

Along with the obesity epidemic has been the staggering rise in type 2 diabetes in children and adults. It used to be called adult-onset diabetes, but now that children are getting it,[49] this terminology has been dropped and is now just called type 2 diabetes. There is also an alarming rise in type 1 (aka Juvenile Diabetes) in adults! Diabetes, or insulin resistance in the brain, is also believed to contribute to Alzheimer's disease and has been termed type 3 diabetes.[50]

In the last fifty years, obesity rates have skyrocketed, and experts have come up with various explanations for this. However, a recent study suggests a new idea: fructose, a type of sugar found in many foods, might be a big reason behind the rise in obesity. The researchers propose that fructose changes how cells work, making people hungrier and craving more high-calorie foods like fats and carbs, leading to weight gain. Globally, obesity rates have tripled since 1975, and now about 13 percent of adults are obese. Fructose is being added to numerous foods, even in sausages and brats. In the U.S., the number of obese adults went from 34.3 percent in 2008 to 41.9 percent in 2020. This study highlights the potential link between fructose and the growing obesity problem.[51]

Fructose also contributes to non-alcoholic fatty liver disease and steatohepatitis (scarring, inflammation, and fat buildup). Dr. Robert Lufkin writes in an online LinkedIn post on March 3, 2024, that it drives several negative health outcomes, including fatty liver, insulin resistance (without increasing insulin levels), elevated urate levels, reduced nitric oxide availability, and 10 times more glycation damage compared to glucose.[52] Glycation

---

[48] Simone Marie, "Obstructive Sleep Apnea During Pregnancy: What's the Connection?" *Healthline*, last modified June 15, 2022, https://www.healthline.com/health/pregnancy/sleep-apnea-during-pregnancy.

[49] M. V. Stack, and D. R. James, The human infant as a dynamic interactive system. *Journal of the Royal Society of Medicine* 95, 9 (2002), 433-436.

[50] Guojun Bu, et al., "APOE4 and Insulin Resistance in Alzheimer's Disease," *Neuron*, Mayo Clinic, 2024.

[51] R. N. Helsley, et al., "Tissue-Specific Fructose Metabolism in Obesity and Diabetes." *Current Diabetes Reports*, 20, 11 (2020), 64. doi: 10.1007/s11892-020-01342-8.

[52] Robert Lufkin, "Lies I Taught in Medical School," a LinkedIn post March 2024, covered in his book, 2024 www.robertlufkinmd.com.

damage means, in simple terms, that you will age faster. Glycation damage creates age damage to your face. If you want to look younger and longer, stop eating fructose.[53]

Dr. Lufkin's post refers to an article in the *Journal of Hepatology* published in February 2018. To summarize, it implies that fructose can lead to the development of non-alcoholic fatty liver disease (NAFLD). This condition affects around 25 percent of the global population. It is characterized by the excessive buildup of fat in the liver, potentially resulting in inflammation and scarring, known as non-alcoholic steatohepatitis (NASH).[54]

Since obesity is such an issue, I will mention a recent weight loss trend. We live in a society that wants a pill or injection to solve our health problems and lack of discipline. Although most overweight people are advised to eat less and exercise, some need help, and the drug Ozempic® is gaining popularity for that purpose. Ozempic®, or semaglutide, was initially approved as a diabetes medication in 2017 but has gained attention for its potential weight loss effects. While not officially labeled as a weight loss drug, it's often prescribed off-label for obesity treatment. Studies show it can help reduce food intake and aid in weight loss.

Semaglutide, the active ingredient in Ozempic®, is closely related to another medication called Wegovy®, which gained FDA approval in 2021 as an anti-obesity drug. Semaglutide targets pathways linked to obesity and associated conditions like heart disease and sleep apnea. It works by making you feel full, but it does have side effects to consider.[55]

Please be aware that this approach to weight loss has come with reported experiences of negative results to the face. Ozempic® face is not a scientific term but is a subject discussed on social media.[56] This term, called the Ozempic® face, is likely only a condition of losing weight quickly.

---

53 Thomas Jensen, et al., "Fructose and Sugar: A Major Mediator of Non-Alcoholic Fatty Liver Disease." *Journal of Hepatology*, 68, 5 (2018), 1063-1075. doi: 10.1016/j.jhep.2018.01.019. PMID: 29408694; PMCID: PMC5893377.

54 Ibid.

55 Alyssa Northrop, "Ozempic For Weight Loss: Cost, Side Effects And Efficacy," *Forbes Health*. February 13, 2024.

56 Eleanor Noyce, "How 'Ozempic Face' Is Altering the Way People Look." *Metro*, May 2, 2024, accessed May 3, 2024, https://metro.co.uk/2024/05/02/ozempic-face-altering-way-people-look-2-20760591/.

Novel Newer Peptide Weight Loss Treatments Related to Ozempic®

This book introduces the knowledge that the modern airway needs to be optimally developed for many of us due to many contributing factors. Another reason for having a smaller airway is if lining airway tissues become too large. Tongue enlargement during weight gain is related to a "marbling effect," causing the airway tissues to become more crowded in the confined space. For a visualization, think of the tongue starting off as a lean filet mignon and, with marbling, becomes more like a ribeye steak. Some clinicians are now referring to the condition as "fatty" tongue syndrome.

Two decades ago, prospective observational studies reported that a 10 percent weight gain over four years was associated with a 32 percent increase in the apnea-hypopnea index (AHI) (suffocation events). Conversely, a 10 percent weight loss predicts a 26 percent decrease in AHI.[57]

Weight loss is a challenge in this modern day and age of hyper-palatable, low-nutrient value foods, decreased physical activity, and longer life spans. We are in an age of high-calorie, low-nutrition, highly processed foods/non-foods. As sleep quality declines, the survival response is to increase appetite to obtain more calories to compensate for the loss of restoration from naturally good sleep. If a person is sleep deprived voluntarily, which is common in this modern age, that person will, as a biological response, become hungrier and find it harder to become satiated.

This problem can be helped with treatment modalities that enhance the cue of feeling full and reduce the elevated hunger signal. Some of the effects of semaglutide come from its action on the hypothalamus. Semaglutide is like a peptide. It is a synthetic 31-amino-acid polypeptide analog of the glucagon-like peptide-1 (GLP-1) that is in our bodies. It is a Glucagon-like peptide-1 receptor agonist (GLP-1 RAs). Its action of the hippocampus can improve brain function.[58]

GLP-1 (glucagon-like peptide-1) boosts insulin secretion and stabilizes blood sugar levels after eating. It is different from Ozempic®-like drugs, as it naturally exists in our bodies.

---

[57] M. P. St-Onge and E. Tasali, "Diet Composition and Objectively Assessed Sleep Quality: A Narrative Review," *Journal of the Academy of Nutrition and Dietetics*, 122, 6 (2021) 1182-1195.

[58] Enhance.MD Team. "How Does Semaglutide Affect the Brain?" Medically reviewed by Dr. Thomas Macsay, N. D., published June 11, 2024, accessed July 15, 2024, https://enhance.md/how-does-semaglutide-affect-the-brain.

Doctors are looking into GLP-1 receptor agonists (GLP-1RAs) to treat type 2 diabetes because they curb appetite, cut down on how much we eat, and help regulate glucose levels. An agonist combines with the GLP-1 receptor sites to produce the same action that GLP-1 would. You might recognize some of the medications in this group, like Ozempic® and Monjaro®, because they're quite popular. Usually, these treatments involve getting an injection under the skin once a week.

A 2024 phase 3 clinical trial report revealed that tirzepatide, the primary component of the type 2 diabetes medication Monjaro®, and the weight loss treatment Zepbound, significantly reduces symptom severity by nearly two-thirds in adults with obesity and obstructive sleep apnea. This study, titled "Obstructive Sleep Apnea Master Protocol GPIF: A Study of Tirzepatide (LY3298176) in Participants with Obstructive Sleep Apnea," can be found on ClinicalTrials.gov.[59]

Allergies and Intolerances to Foods. Another aspect of today's food that can cause inflammation is that many are allergic or intolerant to foods. Approximately 65 percent of the global population is estimated to have a reduced ability to digest lactose after infancy.[60] Allergies and intolerance are not the same thing. Lactose intolerance is often due to a missing lactase enzyme needed to digest it. It tends to affect Asian populations more often than other ethnic groups. This intolerance does lead to body inflammation when foods containing lactose are consumed.

One of the food allergies is wheat intolerance. The prevalence can vary based on different studies and regions. Wheat intolerance is a broad term that includes conditions such as non-celiac gluten sensitivity (NCGS) and wheat allergy. Wheat intolerance differs from celiac disease, an autoimmune disorder triggered by gluten, a protein in wheat and certain other grains.

Some new world grains have been grown with DNA modifications to increase gluten and shorten their growing season. There is no conclusive evidence that these modifications are responsible for wheat intolerance.

---

59 Forest and Ray, "Obstructive Sleep Apnea Master Protocol GPIF: A Study of Tirzepatide (LY3298176) in Participants With Obstructive Sleep Apnea," Retrieved from ClinicalTrials.gov.

60 "Lactose Intolerance," Microsoft Start, accessed March 1, 2024, https://www.msn.com/en-us/health/condition/Lactose-intolerance/hp-Lactose-intolerance?source=conditioncdx.

The scientific community has yet to agree on what causes wheat intolerance.[61]

That being said, some studies suggest that certain types of wheat may be more likely to cause wheat intolerance than others. For example, some research has shown that modern wheat varieties may be more likely to cause wheat intolerance than older varieties.[62] Here are three categories of wheat sensitivities.

Non-Celiac Gluten Sensitivity (NCGS):
- Estimates suggest that non-celiac gluten sensitivity may affect a relatively small percentage of the population. Studies have provided varying prevalence rates, ranging from around 0.5 percent to 13 percent of the population, depending on the study design and criteria used for diagnosis.[63]

Wheat Allergy:
- Wheat allergy, an immune response to proteins in wheat, is less common than gluten sensitivity. It affects a smaller percentage of the population, particularly children. Prevalence rates for wheat allergy vary but are generally lower than those for gluten sensitivity.[64]

Celiac Disease:
- Celiac disease, an autoimmune disorder triggered by gluten, affects a smaller percentage of the population than gluten sensitivity. In the United States, for example, it's estimated that approximately one in 100 people may have celiac disease.[65]

---

61 Atul M. Chander, Sanjay K. Bhadada, Devinder K. Dhawan, et al., "Genetically Modified Wheat, Wheat Intolerance, and Food Safety Concerns," *European Medical Journal* (2018), accessed March 1, 2024. [https://doi.org/10.33590/emjallergyimmunol/10312759].

62 Ibid.

63 Carlo Catassi, et al., "Non-Celiac Gluten Sensitivity: The New Frontier of Gluten Related Disorders," *Nutrients*, 5, 10 (2013), 3839-3853, doi: 10.3390/nu5103839. PMID: 24077239; PMCID: PMC3820047.

64 I. Aziz, et al., "A UK study assessing the population prevalence of self-reported gluten sensitivity and referral characteristics to secondary care," *European Journal of Gastroenterology & Hepatology*, 26, 1 (2014), 33-39.

65 D. A. Leffler, P. H. Green, and A. Fasano, "Extraintestinal manifestations of coeliac disease," *Nature Reviews Gastroenterology & Hepatology*, 12, 10 (2015), 561-57.

These figures are rough estimates, and the prevalence of wheat intolerance can be influenced by factors such as geographic location, genetics, and changes in dietary habits. Additionally, awareness and diagnosis of these conditions have increased over the years, potentially impacting prevalence estimates.

As of January 2022, there is limited evidence to suggest a direct link between the inclusion of folic acid in bread and an increase in tongue ties. Folic acid is a synthetic form of folate. This B vitamin is essential for fetal development, and it is often recommended to pregnant women to help prevent neural tube defects (spina bifida) in the developing fetus.[66]

Tongue tie, or ankyloglossia, is a condition in which the strip of skin beneath a baby's tongue (lingual frenulum) is shorter than usual, restricting the tongue's range of motion. The evidence for this weak folic acid link and the causes of tongue tie can be complex and may involve genetic factors. There is ongoing research to explore this, as well as other potential environmental influences.[67] We will explore the embryological development of the tongue later. It is puzzling to see children being born with tongue ties and receding jaws, even before they have experienced any environmental influences. Tongue tied fetuses cannot swallow correctly either and this is possibly a reason that when born, they are already behind in jaw development. It is important to catch up with interventions as soon as possible. The mother's exposure seems to cause these deficiencies, as Weston Price said was the cause over a century ago.

I mention food allergies because they are becoming more prevalent and also because we are seeing more of them in children than ever before. I mention a lot of unsettled hypotheses just to make people aware of not merely each issue but the sheer volume of modern changes that may all interact to produce growth interferences. I also mention that they are inconclusive because it is extremely difficult to isolate a single cause from all the others to make a conclusive statement. We know allergies interfere with breathing, and in children, the airway development is impacted, forcing oral breathing.

---

66 "Vitamin B complex: functions, foods, deficiency and supplements"| Holland & Barrett," accessed July 24, 2024. https://www.hollandandbarrett.ie/the-health-hub/vitamins-and-supplements/vitamins/vitamin-b/what-does-vitamin-b-do/.

67 Elizabeth Caughey, DDS, "Tongue Tie and MTHFR Mutation," accessed March 1, 2024, https://caugheydds.com/2019/09/07/tongue-tie-mthfr-mutation/

Some allergies are easy to identify as causative agents, while food allergies can be challenging to identify.

Evidence suggests that food allergies, particularly in Western countries, are becoming more prevalent. This increase in food allergies has been noted in both children and adults. Some key points regarding the prevalence of food allergies include:

- Studies have reported an increase in the prevalence of food allergies among children. For example, a study published in *JAMA Pediatrics* found that the prevalence of food allergies in children increased from 3.4 percent in 1997-1999 to 5.1 percent in 2009-2011 in the United States.[68]

- Certain foods are more commonly associated with allergies. These include milk, eggs, peanuts, tree nuts, soy, wheat, fish, and shellfish. The prevalence of allergies to specific foods can vary by region and population. The prevalence of food allergies can vary globally, with higher rates often observed in Western countries. However, there is evidence of an increase in some non-Western regions.[69]

- Various factors, including changes in diet, environmental exposures, and hygiene practices, have been proposed as potential contributors to the increased prevalence of food allergies. A hygiene hypothesis suggests that reduced exposure to certain microbes in early childhood may influence the development of allergies.[70] Children need to play in the dirt and often are advised to take fewer baths. We are keeping our children too clean! You are your microbiome and your body.

- The increased prevalence of food allergies is complex and likely involves genetic, environmental, and lifestyle factors.

---

68 Ruchi S. Gupta, Elizabeth E. Springston, Manoj R. Warrier, et al., "The Prevalence, Severity, and Distribution of Childhood Food Allergy in the United States," *Pediatrics* 131, 1 (2013): e9-e17,-doi:10.1542/peds.2011-0204.

69 S. L. Prescott, and K. J. Allen, "Food allergy: riding the second wave of the allergy epidemic," *Pediatric Allergy and Immunology*, 22, 2 (2011), 155-160.

70 D. P. Strachan, "Hay fever, hygiene, and household size," *BMJ*, 299,6710 (1989), 1259-1260.

2. FOOD PROCESSING AND LAZY EATING

Not only is food refined, often removing nutrients, but it has been made so we don't have to chew. We are juicing our fruits and vegetables, losing the benefits of their fiber. We chop and blend our vegetables so that we can drink them and fluff up our bread. What that does is prevent us from chewing. Chewing is helpful for the development of our jaws, widening them and creating more airway space, especially in children.

The loss of fiber in our diets, among other losses, also contributes to changes in our gut microbiome to our detriment. I will cite this issue separately.

> Adam Hadhazy, in a paper published by Stanford University, expands on a collaborative effort. This includes contributions from Ehrlich and orthodontist Sandra Kahn, who co-authored the book *Jaws: The Story of a Hidden Epidemic*, published by Stanford University Press in 2018. Additionally, Robert Sapolsky, Marcus Feldman, and Seng-Mun "Simon" Wong authored a separate study at Stanford University (Hadhazy, 2020).[71]

Here is a summary of that article on food processing and chewing.

> Changes in human behavior, particularly with the shift towards agriculture, sedentism, and industrialization, have contributed to what some refer to as the "shrinking jaw epidemic." Factors such as softer diets, mainly due to the prevalence of processed foods, have led to reduced chewing activity compared to our ancestors, who consumed more fibrous and tough foods. This reduction in chewing can impact jaw development and size. Additionally, modern conveniences like protein shakes further minimize the need for chewing, potentially exacerbating the issue.[72]

---

71 Adam Hadhazy, "A hidden epidemic of shrinking jaws is behind many orthodontic and health issues, Stanford researchers say," *Stanford News*, July 21, 2020.

72 Ibid.

Anthropological Perspective of Facial and Jaw Development

In pre-Western Civilization, the jaws grew more effectively due to breast-feeding, and early transition to natural hard foods as early as eight to twelve months of age. The dried foods (they did not have refrigeration to preserve foods) were "jerky-like," allowing for more chewing work and helping to form the jaw. This optimal jaw growth enables the mouth to stay closed while sleeping.

Innuit cultures had almost no prevalence of tooth decay since there was no exposure to sugar or even complex carbohydrates.[73] Native American populations had a similar diet with excellent jaw structure, straight teeth, and excellent nasal airflow.

One generation spans about twenty years. In just a few generations, access to processed foods dramatically changed these populations, and they now experience frequent dental tooth decay, crowding of teeth, and more frequent snoring and mouth breathing. The Western diet had dramatically impacted good facial growth in four to five generations to crowded infected and "bad" teeth.

One of the first things you should see in a small jaw is crowded bad teeth. Anthropologic researchers have noticed these impacts by splitting research animals into groups with soft diets in one group versus whole foods in the other. The results were as expected. The soft diet animals developed crowding of teeth, and the whole foods had no negative impacts.[74] Even though this study was on wild animals and weaker "head strength" results from soft diets, implications of soft diets on health were highlighted so that when wild animals are rehabilitated using a hard diet, it improves their chance of survival once released back into the wild.

Food consistency from zero to two years old needs to be harder, not mushy, to promote normal jaw development. Right behind the jaw is the airway. A nice wide jaw with straight teeth helps develop a larger airway tubing. Think garden hose size versus an underdeveloped bite can be represented as small tubing: Think coffee stir straw.

---

73 Forest and Ray, "Why The Inuit Do Not Suffer from Tooth Decay," https://forestray.dentist/news/why-the-inuit-do-not-suffer-from-tooth-decay/

74 Rex Mitchell, "Soft food diet increases risks for captive animals released in wild," *Science News*, November 22, 2021.

That small tube makes it much harder to breathe through the nose and is called nasal dyspnea. This dyspnea pushes our body toward more mouth breathing. If a child experiences nasal breathing difficulty or dyspnea (air hunger), the child will naturally switch to mouth breathing as a compensatory process.

Children with early signs of slow jaw growth will develop smaller oral and nasal airspaces, crowding the back throat and not allowing for adequate space for the tonsils. These children may start snoring (abnormal breathing in children), and the friction of the tongue and soft palate against the tonsils can cause them to enlarge and become inflamed.[75] By improving breathing, the tonsils may be less irritated and be able to shrink to a normal size. Left swollen too long, the tissue changes, becoming hypertrophic (abnormally enlarged), which will not change, and surgery is the only answer to opening up the airway in some cases.

If a child has a small airway, breathing at night when the airway muscles relax, it is a lot of work. This effort can cause symptoms of bed wetting, ADHD, sleepwalking anxiety, or asthma. Ear tubes may be needed, frequent nasal and throat infections occur, and allergies can develop.

Humans are made to breathe through the nose at rest while sleeping. If a sleeper starts to mouth breathe, it dramatically changes the volume of dry air exposed to the lung passages, potentially drying out those airway lung tubes and causing hyper-responsive lung passages. It also changes blood chemistry with less CO_2 to become more hyperventilated and alkaline. Mouth breathing in children can impact the development of their facial structure, resulting in a condition known as "mouth-breathing face." People with this condition often have narrowed faces with small chins or underdeveloped jaws.[76]

Nose breathing allows for a balance of proper gas exchange in the lungs, humidification of the air, and natural production of nitric oxide in the paranasal sinuses. The gas is a natural defense mechanism of the healthy respiratory system. It is not just nose breathing; it is nose functions we are talking about.

---

75 Rohan Thompson, MD and Mark Splaingard, MD, "Management of Snoring," *Pediatr Rev* 42, 8 (2021), 471–473, https://doi.org/10.1542/pir.2020-000950

76 Cleveland Clinic, "Mouth Breathing: What It Is, Complications & Treatments," *Health Library*, https://my.clevelandclinic.org/health/diseases/22734-mouth-breathing

3. ALCOHOL CONSUMPTION

Many will not like this section. Here is a statement that will generate some considerable pushback. Please consider this information. There is no level of safe consumption of alcohol.

Many of you will cite studies saying that light consumption of alcohol is good for heart health. Even the Mayo Clinic has said so. However, these studies minimize the risks associated with cancer promotion known to exist with alcohol.

Dr. Jürgen Rehm, a member of the WHO Regional Director for Europe's Advisory Council for Noncommunicable Diseases and senior scientist at the Institute for Mental Health Policy Research and the Campbell Family Mental Health Research Institute at the Centre for Addiction and Mental Health, Toronto, Canada, points out that the potential protective effects of alcohol consumption, as suggested by certain studies, are closely tied to the choice of comparison groups and the statistical methods employed, which may not adequately account for other relevant factors.[77]

They go on to say that no research has shown that the possible advantages of light and moderate alcohol intake in preventing cardiovascular diseases and type 2 diabetes are greater than the cancer risk linked to the same levels of alcohol consumption for individual consumers.

They also go on to say there isn't a designated safe threshold for alcohol consumption. The risk to an individual's health begins with the first sip of any alcoholic beverage, regardless of the quantity consumed. What's certain is that the more one drinks, the greater the harm.[78]

Alcohol consumption dates back to 6660 to 7000 B.C.[79] It likely occurred when farming became a way of life. It does affect facial aesthetics and the airway. It is well known to cause alcohol fetal syndrome. Alcohol consumption, particularly during pregnancy, is associated with Fetal Alcohol Spectrum Disorders (FASD), which can lead to a range of physical, mental, and developmental issues. Facial abnormalities, such as a smooth philtrum

---

77 "WHO: No level of alcohol consumption is safe for our health," accessed July 22, 2024, https://www.alcoholandcancer.eu/post/who-no-level-of-alcohol-consumption-is-safe-for-our-health.

78 Carina Ferreira-Borges, "No Level of Alcohol Consumption Is Safe for Our Health," World Health Organization, January 4, 2023. WHO News Release.

79 American Addiction Centers Editorial Staff, "The History of Alcohol Throughout The World," Edited by Kelly Doran. Last updated January 12, 2024. American Addiction Centers.

(the groove between the nose and upper lip), thin upper lip, small eye openings, and an underdeveloped jaw are standard features of FASD.[80] These facial characteristics may impact the airway and potentially contribute to complications like obstructive sleep apnea.

FASD is a well-documented condition, and numerous studies have explored its impact on facial development and associated health outcomes.[81] The fact that this is called a spectrum disorder implies that not all of these characteristics of the disorder can present in every case, and the facial impacts can be selectively presented as well as lightly or densely presented.

In 1981, the U.S. Surgeon General issued a public health advisory, cautioning that alcohol consumption by women during pregnancy could lead to both physical and mental birth defects in children. The CDC has said there is no safe level of alcohol consumption by a pregnant woman that will not possibly affect the health and development of the fetus.

A *Medical Press News* article says presently, medical professionals and researchers acknowledge that approximately one in twenty U.S. schoolchildren may display various manifestations of fetal alcohol spectrum disorders (FASD). FASD encompasses a broad spectrum of alcohol-related physical, developmental, and behavioral impairments, often resulting in lifelong challenges for individuals affected by it.[82]

In that *Medical Press News* article by Michael Golding, they cited forty-one documented cases of children born with fetal alcohol syndrome when the mothers had no alcohol while trying to conceive and no alcohol while pregnant. They attributed this to male alcohol consumption.

Indeed, they performed experiments on mice. Here are their results. The study revealed that chronic alcohol consumption by male mice leads to significant developmental issues in their offspring, including abnormalities in brain, skull, and facial formation. Additionally, small heads and lower birth weight were observed, with these conditions worsening in correlation with increased alcohol intake by the male parent.[83]

---

80 S. J. Astley, "Comparison of the 4-Digit Diagnostic Code and the Hoyme Diagnostic Guidelines for Fetal Alcohol Spectrum Disorders," *Pediatrics*, 125, 5 (2010), e1171–e1177.

81 P. A. May, et al., "Prevalence and Characteristics of Fetal Alcohol Spectrum Disorders. *Pediatrics*, 134, 5 (2014), 855–866.

82 Michael Golding, "New Research Points to Dad's Drinking as a Significant Factor in Fetal Alcohol Syndrome," *Medical Press News*, November 15, 2023.

83 Ibid.

The advice to abstain from alcohol is widely ignored, and the emphasis is on women drinking when the evidence says that both should be completely abstaining. Alcohol is a drug. You do not take drugs during pregnancy at all, if possible.

I would say these things. You can do a lot to prevent this epigenetic influence on human development. The first thing I would say is don't drink at all. Not only should you not drink alcohol for your health, regardless of being of childbearing age, but drinking by men or women is utterly irresponsible for those trying to conceive children.

Knowing that most who do drink alcohol will likely not opt to stop drinking altogether, I hope that at least those contemplating having children will discontinue all consumption at least a couple of weeks before any attempt at conception.

For those who likely will no longer conceive a child and want to consider limiting alcohol, please consider the cancer risk. Not only that, but those who have sleep apnea need to know that alcohol exerts considerable adverse effects on quality sleep, and as individuals age, sleep tends to decline naturally. Chronic alcohol use can exacerbate this issue, negatively impacting both sleep and obstructive sleep apnea.[84] Alcohol is a relaxant that can worsen airway obstruction in sleep apnea. It inhibits the nervous system and brain's response to breathing issues during sleep, which can lead to more and longer-lasting breathing disruptions.[85]

Since I am on the topic of alcohol, I will deviate a bit from the facial and airway development theme to address its effects on sleep apnea and insomnia. Drinking alcohol may also contribute to sleep apnea. Alcohol slows down the central nervous system, which can worsen breathing in people with obstructive sleep apnea and central sleep apnea. If you cannot eliminate consumption of alcohol, individuals with sleep apnea should at least limit alcohol intake in several different ways and consult with their doctor about breathing problems.[86]

Alcohol, often seen as a way to help with sleep, actually harms the quality of your rest.

---

84 Eric Suni and Anis Rehman, "Alcohol and Sleep Apnea," Sleep Foundation, January 5, 2024, https://www.sleepfoundation.org/sleep-apnea/alcohol-and-sleep-apnea.

85 Eric Suni and Gerard Meskill, "Alcohol and Sleep Apnea," SleepApnea.org, September 19, 2023.

86 Eric Suni and Anis Rehman, "Alcohol and Sleep Apnea."

It Messes Up Sleep Patterns: Alcohol messes with your normal sleep cycle. While it might make you fall asleep quicker at first, it disrupts the deeper stages of sleep, like REM sleep. So, you will likely wake up feeling groggy instead of refreshed.

More Nighttime Bathroom Trips: Alcohol is a diuretic, making you need to pee more often during the night. This can break up your sleep (fragmentation) and make it less restful.

Aggravates Snoring and Sleep Apnea: Alcohol relaxes the muscles in your throat, making snoring and sleep suffocation worse. These issues further disturb your sleep and cause health problems.

Night Sweats and Dehydration: Alcohol can make you sweat more at night and dehydrate, making it harder to sleep comfortably.

REM Rebound: Once the alcohol wears off, your body tries to make up for the lost REM sleep by increasing it later in the night. This might lead to vivid dreams or nightmares.

Builds Tolerance and Dependency: Using alcohol regularly to help you sleep can make you need more of it to get the same effect. Plus, relying on alcohol to sleep can create a cycle of dependency.

Linked to Sleep Disorders: Long-term alcohol use is connected to sleep issues like insomnia and restless legs syndrome.

While alcohol might seem like a quick fix for sleep problems, it does more harm than good. Instead, sticking to healthy sleep habits like a consistent bedtime routine, relaxation methods, and avoiding alcohol before bed is vital for getting quality rest.[87]

I should say a quick note about Cannabis as well. Many are touting it as a sleep aid. The science is not settled on this. Cannabis can impact sleep differently depending on how much you use, the type you choose, and your unique body. Using a little THC might make it easier to fall asleep faster, but too much THC could disrupt your sleep patterns.

---

[87] S. He, B. V. Taylor, N. P. Thakur, and S. Chakravorty, "Sleep and alcohol use," in M. A. Grandner (ed.), *Sleep and Health* (London: Elsevier Academic Press, 2019), pp. 269–281.

Scientists think that certain chemicals in Cannabis called cannabinoids, affect sleep by changing how your central nervous system and immune system work:

- THC, which makes you feel high, is the main one.
- CBD is another one found in Cannabis, but it doesn't get you high.
- CBN or CBG isn't as well studied, but it's thought to help you sleep better, especially when combined with THC. Some studies suggest it might be suitable for sleep.[88]

Smoking pot was recently associated with heart risks. I will summarize the conclusions of Jeffers, A. et al. (2024). In an article titled "Association of Cannabis use with cardiovascular outcomes among US adults."[89]

This study was backed by the National Institutes of Health (NIH) and suggests that regular Cannabis smoking may substantially elevate the risk of heart attack and stroke. Published in the *Journal of the American Heart Association* and based on data from nearly 435,000 American adults, this research is one of the most extensive investigations into the connection between Cannabis use and cardiovascular incidents.

The study was also supported by the National Heart, Lung, and Blood Institute (NHLBI), a component of the NIH, and revealed that individuals who consumed Cannabis daily, primarily through smoking, had a 25 percent higher chance of experiencing a heart attack and a 42 percent higher chance of suffering a stroke compared to those who did not use the drug. Even occasional users faced an elevated risk of cardiovascular events, with weekly users showing a 3 percent higher likelihood of heart attack and a 5 percent higher likelihood of stroke.[90]

We presently have little to no science on the effects of Cannabis on facial and airway development. However, some say it is similar to tobacco use. Let's discuss that now.

---

88 Michael Breus, "Does Marijuana Affect REM Sleep? Here's How Cannabis Impacts Slumber," Sleep Doctor, January 24, 2024, https://sleepdoctor.com/cannabis-and-sleep/does-marijuana-affect-rem-sleep/.

89 *Journal of the American Heart Association*.

90 A. Jeffers, et al., "Association of cannabis use with cardiovascular outcomes among US adults," *Journal of the American Heart Association*, 13, 5 (2024) https://doi.org/10.1161/JAHA.123.030178.

4. TOBACCO SMOKE:

Smoking and exposure to secondhand smoke while pregnant can harm the baby's development in several ways.

Tissue Damage: Smoking hurts the baby's lung and brain tissues by reducing their oxygen levels so that they grow healthy. This affects breathing, brain health, and the ability to learn.

Birth Defects: Studies suggest smoking during pregnancy might increase the risk of cleft lip in babies and raise the chances of miscarriage. Often, a cleft lip results in smaller upper jaws, which might decrease the airway.

Preterm Birth: Pregnant smokers are more likely to have their babies early, which can lead to serious health problems or even death for the newborn.[91] Premature lungs in LBW infants may lead to respiratory distress syndrome (RDS). Breathing difficulties can impact overall growth and development.

Low Birth Weight: About one in five babies born to smoking mothers are too small, which can cause health issues. LBW infants often struggle with feeding and gaining weight. Their small size and immature systems can hinder effective breastfeeding or bottle feeding.

Sudden Infant Death Syndrome (SIDS): Babies born to smoking moms have a higher risk of dying from SIDS, and their lungs might not be as strong, causing more health problems.[92]

Reduced Fertility: Smoking makes it harder for women to get pregnant.

Inflammation: We will have several sections on the effects of inflammation as we proceed through this book. Inflammation has significant effects on developing faces.

---

91 "The Impact of Smoking and Alcohol on Fertility," Healthy Pregnancy Guide, accessed April 24, 2024, https://www.babydreamers.net/pregnancy/the-impact-of-smoking-and-alcohol-on-fertility/.

92 Askari Jaffar, "How Smoking Affects Women's Reproductive Health and Pregnancy," Hans India, accessed July 22, 2024. https://www.thehansindia.com/life-style/health/how-smoking-affects-womens-reproductive-health-and-pregnancy-800103.

Overall, smoking while pregnant is very risky for both the mom and the baby. Pregnant women should avoid smoking and being around secondhand smoke to keep their babies healthy.[93, 94]

Nicotine

Here is something you may not know. Nicotine can benefit you in its pure form and proper micro levels. Nicotine attaches to specific receptors in the body, which causes the release of different chemicals like catecholamines and serotonin. There is some evidence regular use of nicotine can lead to (1) positive reinforcement, (2) negative reinforcement, (3) weight loss, (4) better performance, and protection against (5) Parkinson's disease, (6) Tourette's syndrome, (7) Alzheimer's disease, (8) ulcerative colitis, and (9) sleep apnea.[95] The reason I included this is the intriguing information on sleep apnea. Other studies on nicotine say it is not good for use in sleep apnea. As with most studies, this needs more research.

For any possible sleep benefits, this must be done in small doses and not in tobacco or vaping systems. It must be done away from nighttime sleep periods. In higher doses, it will interfere with sleep with rebound negative effects.[96] This last negative effect reference is smoking-derived nicotine. Nicotine is known to be addictive, yet it is sold over the counter and can be used for good if done prudently. Never use it during pregnancy in any form.

5. LACK OF BREASTFEEDING:

The impact of the dietary food industry's influences has been exacerbated by the shift away from human breastfeeding in favor of bottles and formula. This is an example of food industry lobbying. The mechanics of breastfeeding are as important as the milk. Unlike nursing, bottle-feeding does not require

---

[93] Cleveland Clinic, "Low Birth Weight," https://my.clevelandclinic.org/health/diseases/24980-low-birth-weight.

[94] Rinta M. Babu, "Smoking during pregnancy is extremely dangerous. It can lead to growth retardation, birth defects such as cleft lip and cleft palate, and even intrauterine death of the fetus," *Medical Insights*, March 1, 2024.

[95] M.E. Jarvik, "Beneficial Effects of Nicotine," *British Journal of Addiction* 86, 5 (1991), 571-575, https://doi.org/10.1111/j.1360-0443.1991.tb01810.x.

[96] Jackie Compton, "Nicotine, Smoking and Sleep Apnea," *Smoking and Sleep Apnea*, June 25, 2024.

the child to engage in the process actively. Nursing requires the infant's jaw muscles to move and exert effort, while nursing creates more jaw space for the tongue, consequently expanding the airway. In cases where the tongue lacks sufficient room, the nursing pains accumulate. The tongue then moves backward into the throat, obstructing the airways. Additionally, this may narrow the upper jaw, face, and nasal passages, restricting essential nasal breathing.

The swallowing mechanism and the forces applied during bottle feeding differ significantly from suckling at a mother's breast, as highlighted by Dr. Brian Palmer on his website, where he discusses the process and its potential negative consequences (Palmer, n.d.).[97] Numerous studies have demonstrated a notable increase in the risk of malocclusion (misaligned teeth) among bottle-fed infants. For instance, one article links bottle feeding to obstructive sleep apnea in infants (Delli et al., 2013),[98] while another study establishes a correlation between bottle feeding and the development of crooked teeth in babies (Kramer et al., 2015).[99]

This combination of breastfeeding and tongue tie interference will be addressed in more detail as there are important issues around this topic.

6. PACIFIERS AND THUMB SUCKING:

Pacifiers pose a challenge similar to bottle nipple use in impacting dental arch development. A study has demonstrated a correlation between pacifier use and an increased incidence of crooked teeth in children.[100]

Thumb sucking is associated with an elevated prevalence of misaligned teeth, as indicated by another study that highlights increased rates of dental

---

97 Brian G. Palmer, "The Uniqueness of the Human Airway," *Sleep Review*, March 4, 2003.

98 K. Delli, P. A. Reichart, M. M. Bornstein, et al., "Are there specific congenital malformations of the jaws predisposing to pediatric obstructive sleep apnoea? A systematic review" *Journal of Oral Rehabilitation*, 40, 2, 121-129.

99 P. F. Kramer, C. A. Feldens, S. Helena Ferreira, et al., "Exploring the Impact of Oral Diseases and Disorders on the Quality of Life of Preschool Children," *Community Dentistry and Oral Epidemiology*, 43, 4, 272-282.

100 O. P. Kharbanda, et al., "Oral habits in school-going children of Delhi: a prevalence study," *Journal of the Indian Society of Pedodontics and Preventive Dentistry*, 33, 2 (2015), 127–133. doi: 10.4103/0970-4388.155133.

misalignment in individuals who engage in thumb-sucking.[101] It cannot be stated strongly enough that dental alignment is a consequence of arch development.

The fact that the tongue cannot reach the palate is not addressed in the cases of pacifier or digit sucking, called non-nutritive sucking. A new hypothesis is that the neurological circuit between the tongue and the palate is closed when the digit or pacifier is in place.

7. PREMATURITY:

Insufficient time for facial development because of premature birth can impede full growth. A study reveals that preterm babies face a three to five times higher risk of experiencing sleep-disordered breathing problems between the ages of eight and eleven.[102]

One of the big problems with premature babies is undeveloped lungs, and the babies are often put on baby CPAP machines. While this saves the baby's life, CPAP use on children is discussed later, but it does deform the developing face of babies and children with mildly mineralized soft facial bones.

8. MOUTH BREATHING:

The face has three necessary occlusions (occlusion means contact between tissues); the most common is the occlusion between the upper and lower teeth. There is also occlusion between the tongue, palate, and upper and lower lips. The lips do not contain oil glands, making them very susceptible to drying, so the occlusion of the lips is just as important as the other occlusions.[103]

Nasal breathing plays a key role in overall health, including the production of nitric oxide, a molecule vital for various bodily functions.[104] Nitric oxide in

---

[101] J. J. Warren, S. E. Bishara, and K. L. Steinbock, "Your Child's Thumb-Sucking Habit," *General Dentistry*, 49, 5, 500-503.

[102] J. L. Goodwin, et al., "Feasibility of using unattended polysomnography in children for research—report of the Tucson Children's Assessment of Sleep Apnea study (TuCASA)," *Sleep*, 26, 7 (2003), 925-929.

[103] Shirley Gutkowski, Collaborative Discussion with the Authors.

[104] L. F. Haas, "Thomas Young, nitric oxide, and the bradykinin mechanism." *Journal of Neurology, Neurosurgery & Psychiatry*, 72, 4 (2002), 540-541.

the nose helps to kill bacteria, yeast, and viruses; it also helps to expand the alveoli and blood vessels in the lungs to allow for better oxygen exchange.[105]

Dr. Zelk explains in his own childhood experiences and observations of his patients that we inhabit a world where allergies and respiratory infections are prevalent, often observed in children with persistent runny noses, ear infections, and frequent illnesses. The contemporary practice of placing children in daycare, where they are closely congregated five days a week, exposes them to infections from their peers. This high frequency of illnesses, estimated at eight to twelve per year, suggests that these children likely use mouth breathing for at least 50 percent of the time. Oral breathing exposes the lungs to unfiltered, non-humidified, and unsterilized air. It also trains the developing child to avoid nasal breathing, which lowers the tongue's posture. A good tongue posture resting in the palate is essential for good facial development and the development of straight teeth.

Figure 19

A former Lysol® commercial showed a sleeping sick child with open mouth. The image is emblematic of a major lack of awareness in our country of improper breathing. This child is breathing open-mouthed. Many children sleep open-mouthed even though they do not have a respiratory infection. Healthy children are breathing via open mouths because they are trained to, in large part, by eight to twelve illnesses per year. Furthermore, the child had what appeared to be a remote TV device in his hand. This might be unusual for this child because he is ill. Children are bombarded with electrochromic devices and electromagnetic frequency energy waves at an alarming rate.

---

105 J. Martel, Yun-Fei Ko, J. Young, D. Ojicius, "Could nasal nitric oxide help to mitigate the severity of COVID-19?" *Microbes Infect.*, 22, 4 (2020), 168–171. Published online 2020 May 6. doi:10.1016/j.micinf.2020.05.002.

These infections also often result in multiple antibiotic prescriptions that upset our microbiome balance.[106] Mouth breathing distorts facial growth.

Once nasal airflow is obstructed, mouth breathing prevents the tongue from naturally resting against the roof of the mouth. People cannot breathe through the mouth when the tongue is up where it is supposed to be. Go ahead and try it. Consequently, this impediment leads to further collapse of the jaws. The consequence is the development of narrow, V-shaped dental arches and overcrowded teeth.

This mouth breathing also upsets the oral microbiome, resulting in increased tooth decay and gum diseases. This scenario contributes significantly to the pervasive presence of orthodontic care among teenagers, which is expected but not healthy nor predominately genetically caused, and the seemingly routine necessity for wisdom teeth removal. Your wisdom teeth are not vestigial organs left over from evolution, as many of us were told during our professional education. Instead, they are meant to erupt into a jaw large enough to accommodate them. That is not happening in our modern world.

Chronic nasal congestion has been identified as a significant factor hindering facial growth, supported by several studies. A pivotal study often referenced in this context is a monkey study, which demonstrated that complete nasal occlusion at birth led to significantly smaller facial structures (Moss & Salentijn, 1971).[107] In contemporary society, children with chronic nasal congestion often exhibit distinctive facial characteristics labeled as "adenoidal facies," characterized by a forward head posture, allergic shiner under the eyes, nasal crease just above the bulb of the nose, Dennie-Morgan lines in the lower eyelids, (prominent skin folds or creases) open-mouth posture, and recessed chins, dark circles or venous pooling under the eyes, accompanied by underdeveloped cheekbones. As these children progress into adulthood, they likely will develop the "long-face" syndrome.[108]

---

106 Sandra Kahn, and Paul R. Ehrlich. *Jaws: The Story of a Hidden Epidemic.* 1st ed. (Palo Alto, CA: Stanford University Press, 2018).

107 M. L. Moss, and L. Salentijn, "The primary role of functional matrices in facial growth," *American Journal of Orthodontics*, 60, 6 (1971), 703-718.

108 Ibid.

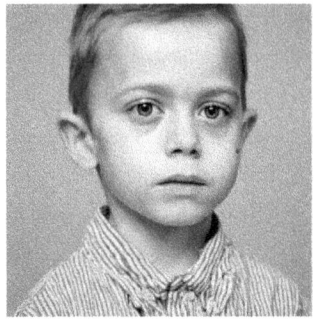 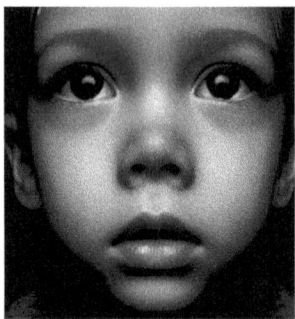

Figure 20 and 21: Adenoidal Facies
(Dall E 3® Bing® and Copilot®) images).
Venous pooling under the eyes, open mouth, receded chin, Receded cheekbones, forward head posture. Not all characteristics appear every time in those who suffer from this condition

A related subject concerning inadequate jaw development is the near-ubiquitous necessity of removing wisdom teeth. The skulls of early humans had enough room to grow wisdom teeth with space behind them. While the presence of impacted wisdom teeth is expected today, it is not normal. We are not growing to our genetic potential in the lower face! This book's primary emphasis is growing and redirecting facial tissues closer to our natural genetic potential of good functioning airways and developing our most esthetic genetic potential. Beauty and function go together! If your treatment for airway issues makes you less handsome or pretty, you might want to find out why. It's not always the case that a poor esthetic result is less healthy, but what's wrong with asking?

We are now being told by professionals that not only is there not enough jaw room for our wisdom teeth, but we commonly have our premolars removed to align teeth that are overcrowded into an uncrowded and stable state. This means we are supposed to believe that out of the normal thirty-two teeth we are supposed to have in our functioning dentition, we need to rid ourselves of eight teeth. That is a full 25 percent fewer teeth! Instead of trying to solve the problem of shrinking jaw sizes, we are to believe that just plucking out teeth is the answer and that by doing this, we cause no significant mouth and airway issues.

To emphasize this point, a new company is coming to the marketplace promoting a treatment called Zero3™ TBA. Zero3™ TBA is a technology created by TriAgenics, Inc., designed to prevent the development of wisdom teeth in children by applying gentle heat to the tooth buds using a probe. The procedure takes just sixty to ninety seconds and is promoted as being safe, effective, and straightforward. Zero3™ TBA stands for third molar Tooth Bud Ablation.[109] TriAgenics is currently seeking FDA approval for this technology and has successfully raised over $800,000 through crowdfunding.[110]

Their appeal is that removing third molars (wisdom teeth) is expensive and debilitating. That is true. Their solution is to just eliminate them from ever forming. I suspect this line of reasoning and treatment could also be used to stop the formation of premolars for those growing up with small jaws and, therefore, eliminate the need for those teeth to be removed for any orthodontic alignment in cases deemed advisable.

A problem might be that taking out teeth before they come out of the gums may stop the jaw from growing well or to its full genetic potential. Here are some articles that talk about these problems. Jaw growth without teeth: examining how the shape of the jaw changes in toothless mice and exploring the potential similarities in humans by K. L. Jones, and M. N. Brown.[111] It is known that missing teeth cause jaw atrophy, and although this article does not address anodontia (no teeth) in the development of jaws, the principle that teeth stimulate jaw growth is vital for readers to know. Another article from CDHP Dental Health is about different diseases that affect the face and teeth. This article discusses diseases that change the face and teeth, including missing teeth and jaw problems.[112] Another study by Smith and Doe, in the journal *Clinical and Radiographic Assessment of Craniofacial Morphology*, found that individuals with anodontia may have smaller jaw sizes or altered jaw shapes than those with a normal dentition.[113]

---

109 Retrieved from https://triagenics.com/3tba/, February, 2024.

110 Retrieved from https://www.facebook.com/TriAgenics/videos/triagenics-zero3-tba/6893596727372865/

111 K. L. Jones and M. N. Brown, "Effects of tooth loss on jaw growth in a rodent model." *Journal of Experimental Zoology*, 345, 2 (n.d.), 234-245.

112 CDHP Dental Health Project, "What Happens to the Jaws When You Lose Teeth?" Retrieved December, 2023, from https://www.cdhp.org/what-happens-to-jaw-when-you-lose-teeth/.

113 J. D. Smith and A. B. Doe, "Clinical and radiographic assessment of craniofacial morphology in individuals with congenital anodontia," *Journal of Dental Research*, 123, 4, 567-578.

We are not saying that this new tooth bud ablation causes jaws to be underdeveloped. We just do not know. The problem, as we see it, is that professionals, business-minded individuals, and companies are defaulting to easier and more profitable solutions. We believe they may have good intentions but inadvertently use science to provide a solution for some, but that does not address the root causes of a disease process and may make issues worse for many.

9. GENETICS:

Genetics plays a role in our facial and jaw development. Facial anatomy is primarily inherited from one's parents, and it's not uncommon for individuals to share similarities in mouth structure with their parents. This does result in a smaller mouth for some. However, the influence of genetics is not absolute. Epigenetics research indicates that environmental factors, habits, and the use of the mouth can substantially impact facial growth patterns, revealing the malleability of genetic predispositions.[114]

Claims suggest that we are evolving and that wisdom teeth are the vestigial organs of evolution are weak at best. Evolution has not had enough time to account for these sudden changes in human jaw sizes. Genetically, humans are designed to have expansive, well-developed jaws, broad smiles, and adequate room for all thirty-two teeth, including wisdom teeth. It is often our "epigenetic" influences that are perverting our genetic potential.

"Epigenetic" loosely means that there are influences on growth and development outside of our genetics that can overcome or subvert our genetic development. Unfortunately, there is evidence that epigenetic influences that change our genetic expression potential can be inherited along with our genetics.

Research in animals and humans has found evidence suggesting that things our grandparents experienced could affect our health. This happens through epigenetic inheritance, where environmental factors from previous generations can impact how our genes work and influence traits like metabolism, behavior, and disease risk.

---

[114] J. Jabbari, W. S. Oetting, and M. M. Lee, "A review of the genetics of human face morphology," *European Journal of Human Genetics*, 26, 3 (2018), 312-324. doi:10.1038/s41431-017-0011-6. F. Chédin, The nascent epigenetic landscape of RNA polymerase II. *Journal of Molecular Biology*, 428, 12 (2016), 2042-2050. doi:10.1016/j.jmb.2015.11.013.

However, scientists are still figuring out exactly how this works and how big of an effect it has. Some studies say these effects might fade, while others suggest they can stick around and affect future generations.

Epigenetics refers to changes in gene expression or cellular phenotypes (a cell's shape and functions) that occur without altering the underlying DNA sequence. Epigenetic modifications can be influenced by various environmental factors and lifestyle choices, impacting how genes are turned on or off.[115] If epigenetic changes are also inherited, these influences may become intractable if allowed to continue. Another possible epigenetic factor influencing our gene expression is domestication syndrome. On the other hand, with knowledge, we can influence these epigenetic influences in the right direction.

Overall, the rodent study by K. L. Jones and M. N. Brown, mentioned previously, highlights the complexity of mandible adaptation and the role of plastic bone remodeling in responding to environmental stimuli. It underscores the importance of considering genetic factors and environmental influences when studying skeletal morphology and function.[116] We want to manage this plasticity by using our knowledge of epigenetic influences, not just surrendering to some notion of cemented genetic fate.

10. DOMESTICATION SYNDROME:

In one sense, domestication syndrome refers to a set of physical changes that occur in animals as a result of their domestication. In the case of humans, the syndrome signifies alterations in physical appearance, particularly facial structure, brain size, and jaw size, that over time occur due to changes in diet, living environments, and social habits.

In evolutionary research, the transition from hunting and gathering to agrarian societies changed food types and preparation, impacting facial growth. Agricultural diets include softer, more processed foods, resulting in less mechanical stress on the jaw due to reduced chewing effort. Over

---

115 R. Mychasiuk, and G. A. S. Metz, "Epigenetic and Gene Expression Changes in the Adolescent Brain: What Have We Learned from Animal Models?" *Neuroscience & Biobehavioral Reviews* (2016), https://doi.org/10.1016/j.neubiorev.2016.07.013.

116 K. L. Jones, and M. N. Brown, M. N. "Effects of tooth loss on jaw growth in a rodent model," *Journal of Experimental Zoology*, 345, 2, 234-245.

generations, this dietary shift led to jaw size and facial appearance changes, manifesting in narrower dental arches, crowded teeth, and less prominent chin and cheekbones.[117]

In another sense, domestication syndrome can be considered this way: A recent *Psychology Today* article cites a Russian study on the domestication of foxes. In a very short time of breeding for more docile domestic behavior traits, they noted the foxes had shorter snouts, smaller teeth, smaller jaws, floppy ears, loss of pigment, and other changes in morphology. They assert we are, as humans, self-domesticating in several ways. The article ascribes these changes to unintended consequences of selecting for domesticity. They accompany this domestication as an intertwined bundle of interrelated traits. The article discussed many of their findings and also related them to autism in the sense that those with autism seem to adopt fewer of these domestication traits.[118] Some writing on this subject cites the influence of xenoestrogens (plastics that mimic female estrogen-like hormone influences in the body) in our diets as contributing factors to domestication syndrome.

11. POLLUTANTS:

Xenoestrogens, Like BPA (bisphenol A) molecules, may be the most significant disruptors of health and surround us daily. (We will cover PSAF xenoestrogens later.) These synthetic chemicals mimic estrogen, directly disrupting hormone signaling and action, ultimately elevating the body's estrogenic (female hormone) activity.

Disruption of the body's normal hormonal function poses various risks, including fertility issues, challenging menopausal transitions, alterations in uterine integrity, early puberty in children and teens, changes in cholesterol and blood vessel health, disruptions in sugar metabolism, thyroid function disturbances, weight gain, shifts in bone health, and imbalanced immune responses.

Critical developmental stages, particularly during in-utero and the first three years of a child's life, prove especially sensitive to xenoestrogens. While restrictions exist for some xenoestrogens in children's products, exposure

---

117 M. M. Lahr and R. Wright, "The question of robusticity and the relationship between cranial size and shape in Homo sapiens," *Journal of Human Evolution*, 30, 5 (1996), 411-428.

118 Christopher Badcock, "Autism and 'Domestication Syndrome in Humans: Signs of 'domestication syndrome' in humans are generally attenuated in autism," *Psychology Today*, August 24, 2016.

remains significant, with limited attention to pregnancy-related limits. Only France has wholly banned them.

Where do these xenoestrogens originate? Identified as over twenty human-made chemicals with estrogenic effects, they infiltrate numerous products, including plastics such as plastic water bottles, food storage containers, plastic wraps, and shower curtains.[119] They even line the inside of soft drink containers.

In addition to xenoestrogens, other pollutants exist in our food and environment. This section on pollutants talks about tongue ties with some negative influences on embryology-related jaw developments postulated to be caused by these pollutants. It is important in tongue and jaw development. The growth of the jaw and tongue are inseparably related.

Shirley Gutkowski cites these pollutants as part of the answer as to why sleep apnea is so prevalent.[120] She does recommend that the subject be researched for more definitive answers. The detrimental influence of pollutants to face development includes generations of epigenetic damage from food and pollution. We have many examples of pollution, including adding lead in gasoline and glyphosate in the soil. We could add to this list of pollutants, but for now, let's just say we have had many generations of damage.

The damage to reproductive cells of the human body is yet to be quantified. However, the hypothesis statements have yet to be clearly formulated to work toward a solid answer to why we see so much more sleep apnea today than in the past due to these pollutants. Therefore, we will leave it open-ended for the most part and focus on the decrease in the size of the human face over the last 150 years, which we must deal with now. This change includes a decrease in sinus volume and is where today's sleep apnea starts.[121]

These pollutants might be interfering with the embryological development of the tongue. This is a very important topic. Let us quickly go to oral anatomy embryology to understand how this works.

---

119 Tieraona Hudson, *Women's Encyclopedia of Natural Medicine* (New York: McGraw-Hill Education, 2010).

120 S. Gutkowski, "Primal Air." http://primalair.com.

121 Y. S. Huang and Christian Guilleminault, "Pediatric obstructive sleep apnea and the critical role of oral-facial growth: evidence," *Frontiers in neurology* 3 (2013), 184, https://doi.org/10.3389/fneur.2012.00184.

Certain aspects of the growth of the human body are nearly completely driven by DNA signals. Take, for instance, the size of the tongue. The size of the tongue grows due to information from the DNA. The top one-third of the head grows from DNA control. This produces massive amounts of synapses per hour in the growing newborn brain and head of the infant. However, the palate (or roof of the mouth) grows due to pressures. DNA dramatically influences the growth of the palate, but palatal growth is greatly influenced by tongue and cheek forces on its size and direction of growth.

In the growing fetus, the tongue forms before the heart. At week twelve of gestation, the tongue separates from the floor of the mouth. This separation is crucial and does not always completely occur.

Starting at week twelve of gestation, the tongue starts to separate from the floor of the mouth. This allows the tongue to press up against the palate. During swallowing and other activities of fetal growth, the tongue and palate interaction is also critical. The neurological circuit is left open without the interaction between the tongue and the palate.[122] Here is what we mean by this.

When the tongue is not on the palate, it can cause a sympathetic nervous system (SNS) response, which is responsible for the "fight-or-flight" response.[123] The sympathetic nervous system comprises a network of nerves responsible for initiating the body's "fight-or-flight" response. Activation of this system occurs during stress, danger, or physical activity. Its effects include heightened heart rate and breathing, enhanced eyesight, and suppression of processes such as digestion.

As a short aside on this subject of the sympathetic nervous system, the SNS response is triggered by the amygdala in the brain, which becomes hyperactive when people have symptoms like post-traumatic stress disorder.[124] When the brain detects a threat, the amygdala initiates a quick, automatic defense ("fight-or-flight") involving the release of adrenaline, norepineph-

---

[122] Leszek Kubin, et al., "Crossed motor innervation of the base of human tongue," *Journal of Neurophysiology* 113, 10 (2015), 3499-3510. doi:10.1152/jn.00051.2015.

[123] Bruno Bordoni, et al., "The Anatomical Relationships of the Tongue with the Body System," *Cureus* 10, 12 (2018), e3695. Published online December 5, 2018.

[124] Erin Maynard, Medically reviewed by Carly Snyder, MD, "How Trauma and PTSD Impact the Brain," Verywell Mind, February 13, 2020, https://www.verywellmind.com/what-exactly-does-ptsd-do-to-the-brain-2797210.

rine, and glucose, which energize both the brain and the body.[125] This fight-or-flight response can also occur in sleep apnea when oxygen levels from suffocation trigger a response to stay alive![126] If a person has multiple episodes per night of sleep apnea, they awake exhausted as though they fought for their life all night long. They did!

Now, back to embryology. This section on embryology comes in large part from Shirley Gutkowski, RDH.

The palate grows from competing tongue pressures from the inside and the lips and cheek muscles from the outside. This is what contributes to three-dimensional growth. After birth, if the tongue is completely functional, it continues to press against the roof of the mouth. The interference of this separation of the tongue from the floor of the mouth is where problems enter.

As was said, the palate grows from competing tongue pressures against the lips and cheek muscles. The palate is a grouping of bones called the maxilla, which holds the upper teeth and the anterior (front) portion of the orbit (eye socket). Without the tongue's pressure, the upper jaw becomes underdeveloped, affecting room for the teeth and the orbit's shape. So, how is it that the tongue is not reaching the palate? This is what we call a tongue tie. For most of us, we learned that a tongue tie meant that the tip of the tongue could not reach out past the lips.

Some restrictions interfere with the tongue's ability to reach the palate; one of those restrictions is a tongue tie. Other types of tongue ties are not visible, especially those at the back or middle of the tongue, and are referred to currently as posterior ties. Many healthcare professionals are not trained to see them. You need a professional, preferably an orofacial myologist, to help with this. Your general physician will likely not recognize it. Many, if not most, dentists don't either. The interference of this separation of the tongue from the floor of the mouth is where most problems enter.

This is needed for the neurological connection circuit between the cranial nerves V, VII, IX nerve X, and the nerves the Greater and Lesser Palatine,

---

125 Melanie Greenberg, Ph.D., "How PTSD and Trauma Affect Your Brain Functioning," *The Mindful Self-Express*, 29 Sep. 2018, https://www.psychologytoday.com/us/blog/the-mindful-self-express/201809/how-ptsd-and-trauma-affect-your-brain-functioning.

126 Fusion Sleep, "Fight or Flight Responses: The Link Between Sleep Disorders and Chronic Diseases." *Sleep Apnea Treatment - Sleep Apnea, Snoring, Sleeping Disorders*, 5 Oct. 2012, fusionsleep.com/blogs.

which branches from the trigeminal nerve V on the palate. This neurological connection may be the driving force for thumb-sucking. Nearly everyone knows of a newborn that was sucking his thumb immediately after birth and continued on for years. And other children take no interest in their thumbs whatsoever. The same can be said for pacifiers, categorically called non-nutritive sucking.[127] This may be a sign of the upcoming sleep-disordered breathing.

The underdeveloped maxilla is also known as the floor of the sinus. Now we get to see where idiopathic deviated septum and chronic sinus and/or ear infections may come from. Not everyone understands that ear infections are respiratory infections. The eustachian tube from the ear leads to the posterior segment of the human sinuses close to the throat. Without good volume in the sinuses, the mouth opens, putting pressure on the jaw joint, and the lymphatic tissue, known as the tonsils, is polluted with untreated air from the mouth.

The tonsils grow to accommodate their new job, further impeding the airway volume in a new location. Disuse of the sinuses, such as by mouth breathing, was shown to stunt the growth of the sinuses.[128] This begs the question: What will a forty-year-old man do with twelve-year-old-sized sinuses? No question that getting to the bottom of tongue mobility issues as early as possible, say in a few days, instead of waiting till years later, is the best prevention.

The best way to treat these conditions is with a complete team approach as the child gets further from their first birthday. Before age one, most dentists and ENTs can release a tongue. It most likely will need to be revised later, but simply addressing a tongue tie by stretching or modifying an infant hold for breastfeeding is often inadequate and detrimental to the growth and development of the child.

The child is challenging to manage between the ages of one and four. An optimal release is often only going to be possible in this age range if the child is put under general anesthesia, and no one wants that. Secondarily,

---

127 Irina A. Rubleva, et al., "Psycho-Neurological Status in Children with Malocclusions and Muscle Pressure Habits," *International Journal of Orthodontics*, 26,2 (2015), 21-4.

128 Lee, S.-Y., Guilleminault, C., & Chiu, H.-Y. (2015). Mouth breathing, nasal disuse, and pediatric sleep-disordered breathing. Sleep and Breathing, 19(4), 1257-1264. https://doi.org/10.1007/s11325-015-1154-6

we wait until the child is four or older. By that time, much damage will have occurred in the oral cavity and brain development.[129] [130]

Snoring is not inert: it is incredibly damaging to the growing child regarding facial development and the brain.[131] Children who snore or make any sound during sleep have a much more challenging time in school and can exhibit behavior problems throughout their lives.[132]

There is some controversy about the release of tongue ties. First, everyone must understand that surgery carries risk, even a "simple" tongue tie release. However, some accuse the professions of taking advantage of mothers' fears and insecurities for the sake of money. This accusation is misinformation far out of proportion to the benefits of this growing awareness of tongue tether release. We will cover this again later in more detail.

Water

We will touch on water—contaminated public water, too, even though I have no data to tie it directly to malformation of the face and jaws. It's just a note about good health and our environment. This is a summary from The Guardian and Consumer Reports at theguarian.com.

Consumer Reports and *The Guardian* collaborated to select 120 individuals from various regions of the United States, chosen from a pool of over 6,000 volunteers, to investigate contaminants such as arsenic, lead, and PFAS (per and poly-fluoroalkyl substances). These samples were sourced from water systems serving more than 19 million people.

Among the 120 samples analyzed, 118 revealed concerning levels of PFAS or arsenic surpassing the *Consumer Report's* recommended maximum or detectable amounts of lead. The findings in the article indicated:

---

[129] Amal Isaiah, et al., "Associations between frontal lobe structure, parent-reported obstructive sleep disordered breathing and childhood behavior in the ABCD dataset," *Nature communications* 12, 1, Article 2205 (13 Apr. 2021), 2205, doi:10.1038/s41467-021-22534

[130] Ibid.

[131] Lena Xiao, et al., "Neurocognition, Behavior, Socioeconomic, and Health Outcomes of Pediatric Obstructive Sleep Apnea," *American Journal of Respiratory and Critical Care Medicine*, 207, 7 (2023), pp. 936-938, doi:10.1164/rccm.202201-0051RR.

[132] B. Galland, et al., "Sleep Disordered Breathing and Academic Performance: A Meta-analysis," *Pediatrics*, 136, 4 (2015), e934–e946, https://publications.aap.org/pediatrics/article-abstract/136/4/e934/73873/Sleep-Disordered-Breathing-and-Academic?redirectedFrom=fulltext

- Over 35 percent of the samples contained PFAS, potentially hazardous "forever chemicals," exceeding CR's recommended threshold.
- Approximately 8 percent of samples exhibited elevated arsenic levels exceeding CR's recommended maximum.

Overall, 118 out of 120 samples showed detectable levels of lead. While the study's scope is limited by factors such as the single-day snapshot nature of the samples and their specific locations, which may not fully represent the overall water system's quality or variations over time, it offers valuable insights into the challenges facing America's drinking water infrastructure. The project, meticulously chosen by CR's statisticians to encompass a diverse range of community water systems nationwide, provides unique perspectives on this ongoing crisis.

The article said that every sample tested contained measurable levels of PFAS, a group of compounds commonly found in household products and linked to adverse health effects like learning delays in children and cancer. Over 35 percent of the samples exceeded safety thresholds established by CR scientists and health experts.

- Despite their prevalence, many consumers remain unaware of PFAS. A Florida, New York resident expressed surprise at discovering PFAS after having his water tested as part of the investigation. His water showed comparatively high levels of the chemicals, prompting him to seek out filters designed to remove PFAS.[133]

Per- and poly-fluoroalkyl substances (PFAS) are a group of extensively used, durable chemicals known for resisting grease, oil, water, and heat. They are a plastic product prevalent in consumer, commercial, and industrial products, including stain- and water-resistant fabrics, carpeting, cleaning products,

---

[133] Ryan Felton, Lisa Gill, and Lewis Kendall, "A nine-month investigation by the Guardian and Consumer Reports found alarming levels of forever chemicals, arsenic and lead in samples taken across the US," *The Guardian*, 31 March 2021.

paints, and fire-fighting foams.[134] Due to their enduring presence in the environment, PFAS are detectable in the blood of individuals and animals globally, existing at low levels in various food products and the environment. Scientific studies indicate that exposure to certain PFAS chemicals in the environment has been linked to negative health impacts in humans and animals.[135]

Some potential health effects related to PFAS exposure include developmental issues in children, immune system dysfunction, increased cholesterol levels, and an elevated risk of certain cancers.[136] Other tap water pollutants include nitrates, pesticides, herbicides, glyphosates, and bacteria.

Air

Outdoor air can be more polluted than indoor air for many homes. A recent article from Australia on magnetite possibly contributing to Alzheimer's disease adds to our list of pollutants.[137] However, many are polluting their indoor air with scented "air fresheners" and cleaning agents.

Our outdoor air is polluted, and what we do at home can be worse. Synthetic air fresheners often lack transparency in ingredient disclosure, with fewer than ten percent of ingredients typically listed on product labels. This lack of requirement to disclose fragrance ingredients means consumers often unknowingly expose themselves to potentially harmful substances.

Chemical analyses have revealed the presence of undisclosed compounds in air fresheners, adding to concerns about their safety.

A study by the NRDC (National Resources Defense Council et al.) tested fourteen common air fresheners, revealing that 86 percent of the products contained hazardous chemicals, even those marketed as "all-natural" or "unscented."[138]

---

134 US Environmental Protection Agency (EPA), "Basic Information on PFAS." *Per- and Polyfluoroalkyl Substances (PFAS)*, retrieved April 22, 2024, https://www.epa.gov/pfas/basic-information-pfas.

135 P. Grandjean, R., Clapp, P. Weihe, P., et al., "PFAS-contaminated drinking water and the association with child growth and development in a longitudinal study from the Faroe Islands," *Environmental Health*, 16, 1 (2017), 62, doi:10.1186/s12940-017-0278-x.

136 Ibid.

137 R. Haridy, "Magnetite pollution is damaging our brains and causing Alzheimer's," *Health & Wellbeing*, retrieved from *New Atlas* online, March 6, 2024.

138 Anne Steinemann, "Fragranced consumer products and undisclosed ingredients," *Environmental Impact Assessment Review*, 29 (2009), 32-38.

Unlisted chemicals found in air fresheners can encompass carcinogens such as benzene and formaldehyde, along with naphthalene, which is associated with adverse health effects, including cancer. Furthermore, hormone disruptors present in these products can provoke allergic reactions and other health complications.

The combination of these chemicals raises concerns as their synergistic effects may pose a greater risk than each chemical individually.[139]

Research indicates that the levels of chemicals emitted by air fresheners are often doubled in pets and humans, potentially impacting indoor air quality and contributing to respiratory problems, migraines, and asthma attacks.

These problematic products exist in other home products like laundry products.[140] Disinfectant wipes contain chemicals you breathe and get on your skin while using. Below are some of the common chemicals contained in them. These products are not very good at killing dangerous spores like C. difficile and merely push them around. Healthcare offices use these to clean countertops and operatory surfaces, unaware of their ineffectiveness and the healthcare toxic chemical risks to their staff using them.

In communal gyms and fitness centers, disinfectants containing quaternary (consisting of four) ammonium compounds are commonly used to sanitize equipment afterward. However, users may unknowingly expose themselves to these chemicals by applying them with bare hands and inhaling the fumes. With frequent exposure, these practices can pose risks, including respiratory health. There's a need for greater awareness and clearer guidelines to ensure safe handling and minimize exposure risks for gym patrons. There are safer options.

Dimethyl Ammonium Chloride:

Dimethyl ammonium chloride is a type of quaternary ammonium compound (QAC) used as an antimicrobial agent in disinfectants.

Recent studies have linked quats (an abbreviation for four), including dimethyl ammonium chloride, to serious health issues

---

139 A. L. Cohen and A. C. Steinemann, . "Exposure assessment of fragrance ingredients in personal care products in a US population: results from a pilot study." *Journal of Exposure Science & Environmental Epidemiology*, 17, 4 (2007), 331-338.

140 N. Nematollahi and A. C. Steinemann, "Fragranced consumer products: Chemicals emitted, ingredients unlisted," *Environmental Impact Assessment Review*, 74 (2019), 1-9.

such as infertility, birth defects, metabolic disruption, asthma, and skin disorders.

Quats are also associated with antimicrobial resistance and environmental pollution.

Dioctyl Dimethyl Ammonium Chloride:
This is a quaternary ammonium compound used as an antiseptic and disinfectant. It disrupts intermolecular interactions and causes the dissociation of lipid bilayers (disintegration of fat in microbes). The activity of DDAC—whether it prevents growth (bacteriostatic) or kills microorganisms (bactericide)—depends on its concentration and the microbial population's growth phase.

Recent studies conducted in mice have demonstrated that the combination of Dioctyl dimethyl ammonium chloride (DDAC) with Alkyl (60 percent C14, 25 percent C12, 15 percent C16) dimethyl benzyl ammonium chloride (ADBAC) can lead to infertility and birth defects. These findings starkly contrast previous toxicology data on quaternary ammonia compounds that were reviewed by regulatory agencies such as the U.S. Environmental Protection Agency (U.S. EPA) and the EU Commission.[141]

Alkyl Dimethyl Benzyl Ammonium Chloride:
Alkyl Dimethyl Benzyl Ammonium Chloride (ADBAC), also known as benzalkonium chloride (BZK), is a type of cationic surfactant. It falls under the category of quaternary ammonium compounds (QACs). A 0.1 percent concentration is the maximum that does not produce primary irritation on intact skin.

ADBAC can be harmful if ingested or inhaled.[142] As with any chemical, the concentration is important because this product is common and needed in low concentrations as a bacterial control product in many commercial solutions and lotions.

---

141 Keith A. Hostetler, Louan C. Fisher, and Benjamin L. Burruss, "Prenatal developmental toxicity of alkyl dimethyl benzyl ammonium chloride and didecyl dimethyl ammonium chloride in CD rats and New Zealand White rabbits," *Birth Defects Research,* 2021. *DOI: 10.1002/bdr2.1889.*

142 Ibid.

Products such as carpets, paints, lotions, soaps, plastics, and others should be examined and reduced or eliminated from your environment. Remember, there is a near-infinite variety and volume of pollutants and their interactions that we do not understand and should try to control.

Choosing natural alternatives or non-toxic air fresheners, laundry products, and disinfectant wipes can help promote a healthier indoor environment.

12. IATROGENIC CAUSES:

These transformations in jaw size are believed to be partly responsible for many modern orthodontic and dental issues. They contribute to the prevalence of malocclusion (how the teeth fit together when you bite down), smaller jaw size, airway restriction, and an increased need for orthodontic interventions in modern populations. They also lead to more tooth decay and gum diseases.

However, the inappropriate treatment of these modern conditions can also contribute to smaller jaw sizes, less attractive faces, and sleep apnea airway issues. When interventions to care for these problems make them worse or create new diseases, we call these iatrogenic causes. These causes and their science are often controversial in professional healthcare organizations and regulatory bodies. These iatrogenic causes are not just pointed at orthodontic care but also general dental care and physician care, including uses of CPAPs on developing faces, inappropriate use of certain medications for missed diagnosis of sleep issues, especially in children, lack of awareness of tongue tie, and much more. Some of these consequences are unavoidable, and some are avoidable. We will devote time to this subject.

13. MICROBIOME IMBALANCES:

In this section, we will cover both gut and mouth microbiomes.

I am limiting the list of factors interfering with our facial and airway development to those most likely to cause structural change rather than just physiology interferences in health and airway function. We cannot make a clear distinction, though; some factors overlap to larger or lesser degrees. Such is the case with our microbiome balance. Does this imbalance just impact how we sleep and the function of our airways, or does this issue directly impact bone and facial structures? There is enough evidence to include the position that it does affect the structures of our growth and is an epigenetic influence on growth and development.

Jaime Tartar, Ph.D., a professor and research director at NSU's College of Psychology and a member of the research team, suggests that the strong bidirectional communication between the gut and the brain implies they mutually affect each other. Regarding previous findings, Tartar notes that inadequate sleep likely significantly impacts gut health and microbiome diversity.[143]

Recent studies propose that the gut microbiome, composed of various microorganisms like bacteria, viruses, fungi, and other microbes inhabiting the digestive tract, holds considerable importance in various aspects of human health, including sleep quality and disorders like sleep apnea. The oral microbiome has recently been in the news for its effects on nitric oxide levels in our body. Here are some ways the gut and oral microbiome may affect our overall health and sleep apnea:

Microbiome Imbalance Factors:

Modern humans have less diversity in the gut microflora than in previous generations. Many factors play a role in this. In the findings listed below, John Timmer in Ars Technica reveals recent findings that every individual has their own combination of gut microbiota. The idea that we can identify the "optimal" microbiome balance for humans is likely unattainable. Our own microbiome is as individualized as a fingerprint, says Sarah Williams of Stanford University.[144] We cannot find that standard normal biome in all modern humans, let alone know what standard it should be based on. Should it be based on the present "normal" or past human microbiome normal? We don't even comprehend what we have lost.

Modern humans do not have the same microbiome as our ancient

---

143 J. Tartar and R. Smith, "New Study Points to Another Possible Correlation between Sleep and Overall Good Health," *ScienceDaily*, October 28, 2019, accessed March 2024, https://www.sciencedaily.com/releases/2019/10/191028164311.htm.

144 Sarah Williams, C.P., "Microbiomes are Personal," *Stanford Medicine News Center*, 12 March 2024, https://med.stanford.edu/news.

ancestors. We are not as able to digest plants as we used to be. In addition, urban dwellers have less cellulose-digesting bacteria in their guts than rural humans. Cellulose is the fiber in foods. The difference between the urban and rural dwellers is wide, with urban dwellers having only 5 percent compared to rural dwellers at 20 percent.[145] Our ancient ancestors had 40 percent. This is determined by examining the ancient feces of humans.

We didn't even know humans harbor cellulose-digesting bacteria in their guts, discovered as recently as 2003. Another study highlighted by *Ars Technica* sheds light on the role of gut bacteria in breaking down cellulose, a key component of plant cell walls, aka fiber. These cellulose-digesting genomes resulted in twenty-two findings in humans. These bacteria coexist with us symbiotically, with contributions from our primate ancestors and domesticated herbivores.[146]

Urban living has led to a decline in cellulose-digesting bacteria in the gut microbiome of humans. In contrast, rural populations, maintaining traditional diets and natural environments, retain a more diverse array of these bacteria.

The gut microbiome is crucial to our health; the findings surprise many in the medical community. Much more investigation is essential, but you can act based on your knowledge.

Antibiotics are mentioned in many places in this section about microbiome balance. Antibiotics are a major disruptor of the microbiome in every area of the body. These biomes exist. The gut biome also affects how one feels and one's learning ability. The biome is not just bacteria, either. It includes fungi and viruses. Most viruses are in the form of phages, which means they infect the bacteria in the gut. Dan Robitzski reported on this in the publication *The Scientist*. The article found that specific phages could increase our cognition while others could reduce cognition. So, even your ability to think is linked to the microbiome.[147]

---

145 John Timmer, "FEEDING TIME — Urban humans have lost much of their ability to digest plants; Rural populations still have lots of the gut bacteria that break down cellulose," *Ars Technica*, 14 March 2024, https://arstechnica.com/science/2024/03/human-gut-bacteria-that-can-digest-plant-matter-probably-came-from-cows/.

146 Ibid.

147 Dan Robitzski, "Bacteria-Infecting Viruses in Gut Microbiome Linked to Cognition." *The Scientist*, 16 Feb. 2022, retrieved April 2024, https://pubmed.ncbi.nlm.nih.gov/2360451/.

You will not see probiotics for phages on the store shelves. They are all bacteria probiotics; the makers assume they know what we need in a microbiome mix. We all have unique microbiomes. Mine and yours do not match anyone else's. The microbes help us digest our food and extract its nutrients. They can fight diseases for us, too. They partner with our immune system.

In many ways, who you are is not just your cells and your unique DNA but also your microbiome. You are a combination of your own cells and your microbiome. Without those microbiomes you could not be you. If you change that microbiome with antibiotics, it is affecting you and your "self."

Defining the self is extremely difficult. It is particularly so if you believe, as I do, that the self is more than just the material you. That is the turf of theologians and philosophers, so let's just say that in the material world, we are our microbiome and physical body.

This microbiome interference by antibiotics is highlighted in a new way by a study on, curiously, kidney stones. Here is an abbreviated summary of that study. Certain bacteria in this study stopped kidney stones, but antibiotics prompted the unlucky to get them. Please note that the author includes the oral cavity in the microbiome discussion.

In individuals with kidney stones, the microbial network that typically exists and functions well in healthy individuals becomes disrupted. This breakdown affects the production of essential vitamins and metabolites in various body areas, including the gut, urinary tract, and oral cavity.

The study observed that those who had developed kidney stones had previously been exposed to antimicrobial substances, such as antibiotics, antivirals, and antifungals, resulting in a higher prevalence of antibiotic-resistant genes in those microbes.

Dr. Burton, an associate professor in the Department of Microbiology and Immunology at Schulich Medicine & Dentistry, explained that individuals with kidney stones exhibited an unhealthy microbiome, particularly in the gut, which showed a tendency to release toxins into the kidneys. Furthermore, they displayed antibiotic resistance.

To maintain a healthy microbiome in the oral cavity, urinary tract, and gut, consuming a balanced diet rich in prebiotic and probiotic foods that support these regions is recommended. Examples include yogurt and fermented foods for gut health and nitrogen-rich, high-fiber vegetables like chard, beets, and celery for oral health. Additionally, minimizing the use of antimicrobial agents whenever possible is advised.[148]

I am sure by now you can see why antibiotics are so disruptive to your microbiome and even your "self" and how important that is. Let's look into how this relates to sleep apnea.

Inflammation: Disruptions in the balance of the gut microbiome may result in chronic low-grade inflammation extending to the airways. This inflammatory response could potentially contribute to the onset or exacerbation of sleep apnea. Intermittent hypoxia associated with obstructive sleep apnea induces alterations in the gut microbiota, disturbing the gut-brain axis and worsening symptoms of irritable bowel syndrome (IBS). This dynamic could be viewed as a cyclical process, where OSA contributes significantly to the deterioration of gastrointestinal symptoms, subsequently impacting sleep negatively.[149]

In children and adults, excess fat around the abdomen organs causes sleep-related breathing disorders. An article from J. Grains et al. in *PubMed* says their initial observations, based on a longitudinal study of children not diagnosed with clinical OSA, indicate that inflammation originating from visceral fat may precede the onset of the disorder, hinting at a possible causal pathway.[150]

While there is no direct link of inflammation from any source to improper development of facial structures, we know that a dysfunctional and chronic activation of immune systems can increase the risk of respiratory illnesses. This leads to chronic mouth-breathing and less healthy nasal breathing. If a child is constantly sick with a stuffy nose, the tongue does not support and widen the palate. The mandible or lower jaw development is affected when the maxilla or upper jaw narrows. We will discuss this further in another section.

---

148 Bronwyn Thompson, "Healthy oral, gut and urinary bug network can smash kidney stones," *New Atlas*, December 21, 2023.

149 Ellen M. S. Xerfan, et al., "The relationship between irritable bowel syndrome, the gut microbiome, and obstructive sleep apnea: the role of the gut-brain axis," Springer Link, August 15, 2023. https://link.springer.com/article/10.1007/s11325-023-02898-x.

150 J. Gaines, et al., "Increased inflammation from childhood to adolescence predicts sleep apnea in boys: A preliminary study," *Brain Behav Immun* 64 (2017), 259-265, doi:10.1016/j.bbi.2017.04.011.

The gut microbiome has been assaulted in modern times by antibiotics. They are overused and are incredibly detrimental to the gut and oral microbiome. Some of these changes are permanently stuck in our bodies. The development of C. difficile is a dangerous dysbiosis (an imbalance in the different types of microorganisms) of the intestines often associated with any antibiotic treatment. Some are worse than others, like clindamycin. Many people pick this C. difficile bacteria up at a healthcare facility.

As we said, a bidirectional relationship was found in a study of gut microbiota on sleep apnea. Some bacteria were associated with promoting sleep apnea, and others were associated with decreasing the incidence of sleep apnea.[151]

They further said that the metabolites derived from gut microbiota, specifically 3-dihydro carnitine, epiandrosterone sulfate, and leucine, were recognized as potential risk factors for obstructive sleep apnea. This article suggested that probiotics to support gut microbiome health and even fecal transplants could help rebalance a dysbiotic gut microbiome.

As with almost every article you read in peer-reviewed publications, they end by saying further research is needed to verify these findings. More research is required to ascertain whether interventions targeting microbial activity to lower leucine levels and supplement betaine could effectively manage OSA. They also found that bacteria that secrete short-chain fatty acids (SCFA) may be protective of OSA. However, currently, there are no clinical trials that have outlined the positive impacts of probiotic supplementation in preventing OSA. Therefore, additional research is necessary to assess whether probiotics and short-chain fatty acids (SCFAs) offer promising new approaches to combat dysbiosis associated with OSA.[152]

I looked but could find no mechanism by which these bacteria and their by-products worsen or help sleep apnea other than increasing inflammation.

---

151 Weiheng Yan, et al., "Causality Investigation between Gut Microbiota, Derived Metabolites, and Obstructive Sleep Apnea: A Bidirectional Mendelian Randomization Study," *Nutrients* 15, 21 (2023), 4544, https://doi.org/10.3390/nu15214544.

152 Ibid.

Inflammation?

As a quick aside comment on science studies, I would say this because this information on inflammation brought it to light for me and maybe for the readers, too.

I cannot find a concrete reason why inflammation causes OSA. It may cause throat tissue to be more collapsible. Authors in the scientific realm often refrain from definitively stating the causes of a disease, and understandably so. Establishing direct cause and effect is challenging, and it's rare to encounter articles that unequivocally declare such relationships.

While it would be beneficial if they speculated on how inflammation exacerbates OSA, such hypotheses are typically reserved for the conclusion of papers, suggesting potential avenues for future studies. The written ponderings of how inflammation affects the cells and organs of our bodies are interesting to me. However, the safer approach is to state associations or links with a disease process rather than cause and effect. The inferences of these links or associations can be strong or weak and yet still tell you very little, even if substantial, if they don't tell you why.

The authors of this book adhere to a similar methodology. As we navigate through this information, I encourage you to recognize these associations, and collectively, we can work toward enlightened actions to provide assistance. There are numerous factors to consider in this endeavor, and you will see actionable tactics.

Obesity:

There is a strong link between obesity and sleep apnea. Certain gut bacteria can affect metabolism, appetite regulation, and the absorption of nutrients. Dysbiosis, or an imbalance in the gut microbiome, can lead to weight gain and obesity,[153] risk factors for sleep apnea. Obesity itself is inflammatory and, therefore, can affect all organs of the body for a lifetime, even if—and likely more so—with developing children. These microbiota changes also cause us to crave sugars, fats, and starches.[154]

---

153 P. J. Turnbaugh, R. E. Ley, M. A. Mahowald, et al., "An Obesity-Associated Gut Microbiome with Increased Capacity for Energy Harvest," *Nature* 444, 7122 (2006), 1027-1031. https://doi.org/10.1038/nature05414.

154 P. D. Cani, R. Bibiloni, C. Knauf, et al., "Changes in gut microbiota control metabolic

Another study published in the journal *Frontiers in Endocrinology* found that the gut microbiome can influence the levels of leptin and ghrelin, which are hormones in the body, affecting appetite and energy metabolism. Leptin and ghrelin influence our hunger levels. Leptin is suppressed and ghrelin is increased by the gut microbiome.[155] This is the opposite of what you want if you are to lose weight.

Sleep-wake cycle regulation: Research indicates that the gut microbiome plays a role in modulating the formation and regulation of neurotransmitters such as serotonin and GABA, both of which are implicated in regulating the sleep-wake cycle. Imbalances in these neurotransmitters can disrupt sleep patterns and potentially worsen sleep apnea symptoms.

Disrupting your normal sleep-wake cycle can also disturb eating habits, leading to further disruptions in the behavior of your gut microbiome. Given that the microbiome regulates various bodily processes, this research has established a connection between the rhythmic activity of gut bacteria and the internal clocks of the body.[156] It has an influence on your circadian rhythm, directly influencing sleep. Again, eating affects our growth and development.

Intestinal permeability:

A well-balanced gut microbiome supports the integrity of the intestinal lining, thus preventing the leakage of toxins and detrimental substances into the bloodstream. On the other hand, dysbiosis can result in heightened intestinal permeability, commonly known as leaky gut, which permits harmful substances to pass into the bloodstream. This can trigger systemic inflammation and potentially worsen sleep apnea. Inflammation is again activated.[157]

---

endotoxemia-induced inflammation in high-fat diet-induced obesity and diabetes in mice," *Diabetes* 57, 6, June 2008, 1470-81, DOI: 10.2337/db07-1403.

155 Jochen Seitz, et al., "The Impact of Starvation on the Microbiome and Gut-Brain Interaction in Anorexia Nervosa," *Frontiers of Endocrinology* 10, Feb 19, 2019, doi: 10.3389/fendo.2019.00041.

156 Rita Steyn, "Gut Microbiome Can Affect Circadian Sleep-Wake Cycle," *Pacific Northwest National Laboratory*, June 26, 2023.

157 Monica Levy Andersen, et al., "Exploring the potential relationships among obstructive sleep apnea, erectile dysfunction, and gut microbiota: a narrative review," *Sexual Medicine Reviews*, 12, 1, Dec 2023, 76-86, doi: 10.1093/sxmrev/qead026.

Immune modulation:

The gut microbiome regulates the immune system. Imbalances in the gut microbiome can lead to an overactive or weakened immune response, which may contribute to the development or severity of sleep apnea. As we said, it also lowers our ability to resist respiratory illness and creates open-mouth breathing.[158]

Research in this area is ongoing, and the precise mechanisms through which the gut microbiome affects sleep apnea are not fully understood. However, maintaining a healthy gut microbiome through a balanced diet, regular exercise, and probiotic supplementation may benefit sleep quality and sleep apnea management. Intermittent fasting can also positively affect the gut microbiome.[159] In turn, it can affect growth and development, especially in children. Don't go overboard in probiotic consumption. You can get too much of it and cause an imbalance in the microbiome instead of a better balance.[160]

Adults, don't be dismayed by our constant references to children, as if it is too late for you. While some damage caused by sleep suffocation is not reversible, there is much we can do for adults. Stay with us, and we will cover the options for adults, too. You will see amazing things. It is also always advisable to consult a healthcare professional for personalized advice and treatment options.

Microbiome of the mouth:

Before we leave the microbiome subject, I must address the microbiome of the mouth. It is important that this microbiome be balanced as well. I am particularly interested in this subject because I co-founded an oral mouth rinse company. Of course, this means I have some self-interest in this subject, and Dr. Zelk encouraged me to write about it because he believes my study and research on it are accurate and meaningful.

---

158 Angela Betsaida B. Laguipo, BSN, "Dysbiosis and the Microbiome," *New Medical Life Sciences*, news-medical.net.

159 I. Paukkonen, et al., "The impact of intermittent fasting on gut microbiota: a systematic review of human studies," *Frontiers in Nutrition* 11 (2024), 1342787.

160 Cynthia Sass, MPH, RD, "Can You Overdose on Probiotics? Risks and Side Effects," *Health*, updated on August 11, 2022. Medically reviewed by Jay N. Yepuri, MD.

In the news cycles, some subjects are picked up, blown out of proportion, and even reported incorrectly. This is the case with antimicrobial mouth rinses. Most of this discussion revolves around nitric oxide. This molecule in the body helps relax blood vessels and serves as a signaling molecule for many body functions. Also, it helps us utilize oxygen in the lungs better; therefore, it is an appropriate subject in airway and oxygen health.

This molecule is made primarily in the inner lining of blood vessels and body tissues. Some is made in the sinuses.

In the case of mouth rinses, key opinion leaders, bloggers, and celebrities have seized the little information that has come out. The bandwagon slogans and talking points use words to describe mouth rinses as "scorched earth" treatments of the oral microbiome or unbalancing the oral microbiome. I hear these statements frequently: "I don't believe in killing all the bacteria." "The balance of the microbiome should be preserved." "I don't believe in the scorched earth approach to therapy." "Antimicrobial rinses raise your blood pressure." (Please also get this distinction. Antimicrobials are not the same thing as antibiotics.)

These commentators often assert that there are hundreds of articles to support what they are saying. These commentators nearly always include all antimicrobial mouth rinses in the same boat. No distinction is made as to brand or kind of rinse, even though this is not true if you read the studies.

This subject was even mentioned on the Dr. Oz show I watched a few years ago. It was mentioned that antimicrobial mouth rinses in a study done in Houston raised systolic blood pressure by three points on average. That article was on tongue cleaning, and a prescription mouth rinse called chlorhexidine.

Others mention that the reason for this effect on blood pressure is that the bacteria in the mouth that help convert nitrate-rich foods to compounds that can be used to make nitric oxide are destroyed. These bacteria are called nitrate to nitrite-reducing bacteria.

So, let's start with some of my statements. 1. No mouth rinse I know of creates a "Scorched Earth" environment in the mouth. 2. I don't believe in killing all the bacteria in the mouth. 3. The oral microbiome balance should be preserved and enhanced if possible. 4. Most importantly, antimicrobial mouth rinses balance and can enhance the oral microbiome.

Please realize that oral microbiome dysfunction is causing tooth decay and gum diseases. These are called dysbiosis. Many studies are now showing that periodontal (gum) disease contributes to the initiation and worsening of diabetes, dementia, heart disease, high blood pressure,[161] general inflammation, and the reduction of nitric oxide[162] in the blood vessels, and much more. So, in this regard, mouth rinsing could be the restorer of nitric oxide levels rather than reducing the levels.

Cleaning the mouth with toothbrushes and mouth rinses can balance this dysbiosis. Antibiotics, however, are much more likely to create an imbalance in the oral microbiome and the gut. Not all antimicrobials are created equal, but most do not create resistant bacteria like antibiotics, and the best rinses create no resistant microbes.

Support for this stand on antimicrobial mouth rinses balancing the oral microbiome comes from this article by Philip D. Marsh et al. 2014, entitled, "Prospects of oral disease control in the future–an opinion." I will paraphrase their statements.

He says that antimicrobial mouth rinses might operate more precisely, primarily hindering the growth and activity of organisms associated with oral diseases while sparing those linked to oral health. Using any antimicrobial substance carries the risk of bacterial resistance development, mainly when used at concentrations below those that cause cell death. Nonetheless, there is no indication of a change in Minimum Inhibitory Concentration (MIC) for agents found in oral care products after prolonged clinical usage. Unlike antibiotic treatment, antimicrobial oral care products could preventively stabilize the natural oral microbiota under circumstances that might otherwise predispose a site to tooth decay or gum inflammation, thereby preserving the advantages derived from the resident microbiome.[163]

In addition to that, a few rinses remove toxins produced by the microbes in addition to the microbes themselves.[164]

---

[161] Rbert Preidt, "Gum Disease Linked to High Blood Pressure," *HealthDay Reporter*, Health Day News, March 29, 2021.

[162] Ibid.

[163] Philip D. Marsh, David A. Head, and Deirdre A. Devine, "Prospects of Oral Disease Control in the Future – An Opinion," *Journal of Oral Microbiology* 6 (2014), 26176.

[164] R. D Downs, J. A. Banas, and M. Zhu, M, "An In Vitro Study Comparing a New Two-Part Activated Chlorine Dioxide Oral Rinse to Chlorhexidine and Commercial Rinses," Perio Implant Advisory

The most negatively implicating rinse is chlorhexidine. Other rinses and pastes with many issues are those with triclosan. In all the studies I read, chlorhexidine was the one rinse somewhat implicated in nitric oxide reduction or small elevations of systolic blood pressure.

Triclosan rinses and toothpaste were quietly removed from the market just one month before the writing of a study with the lead author, Tribble et al. I do not know if any of the study participants were using triclosan rinses and pastes before being placed on the chlorhexidine rinse in that study.[165]

If you read the studies, you will realize there are fewer than we have been told that explore mouth rinses' impact on microbiomes and blood pressure.[166]

One popular dental blogger states that bacteria in the nose create nitric oxide; he also states that 25 percent of your body's nitric oxide comes from the mouth bacteria and that all antimicrobial mouth rinses are bad for you. He is wrong on all three points. He is confusing oral bacteria and nasal bacteria. There are currently no known bacteria in the nose producing nitric oxide. The mouth is not the source of 25 percent of your nitric oxide.

On the contrary, about 75 percent of ingested nitrate is cleared through the kidneys, while 25 percent of ingested nitrate is circulated in the blood and subsequently excreted in saliva. In saliva, approximately 20 percent of that nitrate (equivalent to around 5–8 percent of the nitrate intake) undergoes conversion to nitrite through the action of commensal bacteria present on the tongue. Then nitrite (NO_2) is absorbed in the intestines.[167] Some nitrite you swallow is converted in the stomach to nitric oxide.

Of those studies, many are cited as saying something they never said in that study. For example, in the study "Frequency of Tongue Cleaning Impacts the Human Microbiome Composition and Enterosalivary

---

(2015), accessed May 25, 2024, https://www.perioimplantadvisory.com/clinical-tips/hygiene-techniques/article/16411500/an-in-vitro-study-comparing-a-two-part-activated-chlorine-dioxide-oral-rinse-to-chlorhexidine.

165 Gena D. Tribble, et al., "Frequency of Tongue Cleaning Impacts the Human Microbiome Composition and Enterosalivary Circulation of Nitrate," *Frontiers of Cellular Microbiology*, March 1, 2019.

166 Khrystyna Zhurakivska, et al., "Do Changes in Oral Microbiota Correlate With Plasma Nitrite Response? A Systematic Review," *Frontiers in Nutrition* 11 (2024), 1342787.

167 Norman G. Hord, Yaoping Tang, and Nathan S. Bryan, "Food Sources of Nitrates and Nitrites: The Physiologic Context for Potential Health Benefits," *The American Journal of Clinical Nutrition* 90, 1 (July 2009), 1–1.

Circulation of Nitrate,"[168] the authors only studied chlorhexidine in its nitric oxide-reducing and blood pressure-increasing properties, and they also emphasized the role of tongue cleaning used in conjunction with the mouth rinse. This study had only twenty-six participants. Yet this article is cited as condemning all mouth rinses. It is an interesting article, but it does not comment on any other type of rinse.

It is also noteworthy in this same *Frontiers* article, just mentioned by the lead author Tribble, that all of the participants in the study were using another antimicrobial mouth rinse before the study and then told to stop using that mouth rinse and to begin using chlorhexidine. I am unaware of how long they waited after discontinuing their old mouth rinse before starting on the chlorhexidine or when baseline readings were done. However, even though I don't know these things, this study would seem to me to imply that the other antimicrobial mouth rinses the participants were using before going on chlorhexidine did not affect the nitric oxide levels and blood pressure, especially if they began the new study rinse immediately after discontinuing the rinse they were using. Notably, many subjects in this study also cleaned their tongues before the study.

Contrary to the widely held beliefs championed by advocates, especially those I consider "scorched earth evangelists," this study presents findings that challenge the conventional wisdom about the effects of all mouth rinses. Importantly, the study reveals intriguing and significant insights. Let me explain.

In this same *Frontiers* article, they noted that six hours after chlorhexidine mouth rinse and tongue scraping, the oral microflora grew richer and enhanced in its nitrate-reducing properties. It grew back balanced. The fact that it grew back balanced in the Tribble study supports the assertion that antimicrobial rinses may balance the oral microbiome, as stated in the article by Philip D. Marsh mentioned previously.

Everyone involved in this study maintained good oral health. Consequently, one might infer from these participants' positive oral health status in the Tribble study that mouth rinsing benefits not only those in a diseased state of oral health but also individuals with healthy mouths.

---

168 Gena D. Tribble, et al., "Frequency of Tongue Cleaning Impacts the Human Microbiome Composition and Enterosalivary Circulation of Nitrate."

This enrichment of the oral flora by chlorhexidine needs further exploration because if other studies support it, the idea of mouth rinses improving and maintaining our oral microbiome could be significant.

An application of this finding is that you might conclude from this study that even using chlorhexidine once per week with tongue scraping may help you maintain a healthy nitric oxide-promoting and balanced oral microbiome. I am not necessarily advocating that. I am no fan of chlorhexidine, a prescription-only oral mouth rinse approved for only two weeks of use and only for gingivitis.

Chlorhexidine is frequently used off-label, including use in the more severe form of gum disease called periodontitis. Even worse, it is used in post-surgery cases to help heal wounds, even though it impairs fibroblast (the most common cell type represented in connective tissue) cell function. It is prescribed for many other uses, in large part due to its FDA clearance. That clearance provides excuses to use it nearly everywhere. That clearance is only for gingivitis and is only FDA-cleared for two weeks.

Not all over-the-counter mouth rinses on the market harm your health, nor do they affect blood pressure or reduce nitric oxide production. Indeed, two studies I read showed other antimicrobial rinses did not affect nitric oxide levels or blood pressure, the most notable of which is Listerine™. Listerine™ had no more effect on the tongue microbiome than water.[169]

Good oral hygiene, including antimicrobial mouth rinses, has been shown in numerous studies to be good for you. Just as showering and washing your hands removes some good bacteria, so does cleaning your mouth. Let's keep the hundreds of years of good hygiene science and not throw it out based on ambiguous conclusions that all antimicrobial rinses are bad for your oral microbiome and blood pressure.

People who sleep in dentures have a double chance of getting pneumonia in the elderly.[170] Those who wear dentures should rinse their mouths with antimicrobial rinses.

A prospective study noted an association between snoring and chronic

---

[169] Mary Woessner, et al., "A Stepwise Reduction in Plasma and Salivary Nitrite with Increasing Strengths of Mouthwash Following a Dietary Nitrate Load," *Nitric Oxide* 57 (2016), 1-9, https://doi.org/10.1016/j.niox.2016.01.002.

[170] T. Iinuma, et al., "Denture Wearing during Sleep Doubles the Risk of Pneumonia in the Very Elderly," *Journal of Dental Research*, October 2014, DOI: 10.1177/0022034514552493.

bronchitis, which increases the risk of chronic bronchitis. These findings lend credence to the theory that snoring plays a role in the onset of chronic bronchitis. Why is this important?

Their conclusion on this chronic bronchitis finding is that they do not know the mechanism of the inflammation and that they thought vibrations may cause the inflammation.[171] However, a study is needed to see if the aspiration of snore-vibrated loosened oral and nasal bacteria is a cause of this inflammation and even COPD. Those who snore should be mouth rinsing.

HAP and VAP also are related to the aspiration of oral bacteria. This stands for hospital-acquired pneumonia and ventilator-associated pneumonia. In studies done with these patients, toothbrushing by nurses did lower pneumonia numbers and deaths from that pneumonia. They did some studies on chlorhexidine without significant results. Chlorhexidine is not a good bacterial biofilm remover. (Kalil 1966)[172]

It wouldn't be surprising if future studies reveal some potential trade-off risks associated with additional antimicrobial mouthwashes besides chlorhexidine. All therapies have benefits and risks, but the benefits of antimicrobial rinses far outweigh the risks. I agree some rinses are better than others.

Before we move on, there are also nitrate and nitrite supplements you can look into to help with this nitric oxide support. One of the ways to get the benefits of nitric oxide is to use sodium nitrite supplements when using chlorhexidine mouth rinses. A study on nitrite supplementation vs. nitrate supplementation showed that sodium nitrite supplements can overcome mouth rinse blunting of the enterosalivary pathway and were able to reduce blood pressure, while nitrate supplements could not improve blood pressure in antimicrobial rinsing subjects.[173] Oral probiotics are also made to introduce good oral bacteria to the oral microflora and other bacteria in the gut. Some foods help with nitric oxide production for our bodies, too, including green leafy vegetables, spinach, kale, beets, and Swiss chard, which are rich

---

[171] Inkyung Baik, et al., "Association of Snoring With Chronic Bronchitis," *JAMA*, January 28, 2008.

[172] Andre C. Kalil, Mark L. Metersky, Michael Klompas, et al., "Management of Adults With Hospital-Acquired and Ventilator-Associated Pneumonia: 2016 Clinical Practice Guidelines by the Infectious Diseases Society of America and the American Thoracic Society," *Clinical Infectious Diseases* 63, 5 (2016), e61-e111, https://doi.org/10.1093/cid/ciw353.https://pubmed.ncbi.nlm.nih.gov/27418577/.

[173] Pinheiro, Lucas C., et al. "Oral Nitrite Circumvents Antiseptic Mouthwash-Induced Disruption of Enterosalivary Circuit of Nitrate and Promotes Nitrosation and Blood Pressure Lowering Effect." Free Radical Biology and Medicine 101 (2016): 226-235

in nitrates, which can be converted to nitric oxide[174] with the help of oral bacteria. Garlic contains allicin, which can contribute to increased nitric oxide production. Citrus fruits: oranges and grapefruits are high in vitamin C, which supports nitric oxide synthesis. Pomegranates and pomegranate juice have been linked to improved nitric oxide function. Nuts and seeds: walnuts and sunflower seeds contain L arginine, an amino acid converted in nitric oxide production. Watermelon contains citrulline, a precursor to arginine, which can boost nitric oxide levels. Finally, omega-3 fatty acids may help as well.

14. EMF RADIATION:

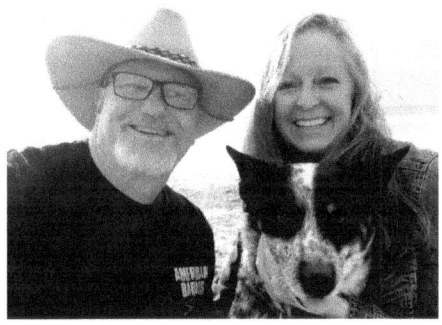

Figure 22: This photo is a personal one sent to me by them Russel Kort, DC, Joanette Biebesheimer, MS, and Kaizen, the world's only EMF service dog.

We are swimming in higher and higher doses of electromagnetic field (EMF) radiation. It is non-ionizing radiation as opposed to ionizing radiation that is present in an X-ray. Since the advent of the everyday use of cell phones in the mid-1980s, extremely low frequency (ELF) EMF levels have exceeded levels before that time by more than exponential jumps. Ole Johannson, PhD, says the number has exceeded a quintillion times in the last ten years.[175] That number is one, followed by eighteen zeros, was published in 2014. This is

---

174 "5 Foods for Improved Blood Circulation!" Accessed March 22,2024, https://www.goodluck-gourmetga.com/stories/5-foods-for-imrpoved-blood-circulation/.

175 Olle Johansson, and Einar Flydal, "Health Risk from Wireless? The Debate Is Over," *Electromagnetic Health Blog*, November 1, 2014, accessed July 22, 2024, https://www.electromagnetichealth.org/.

the radiation from your microwave ovens, cell phones, cell towers, routers, and any electrical current.

In September of 2023, France banned the sale of the iPhone 12 due to excess radiation from that phone.[176]

Even though this subject does not necessarily directly tie into the deformation of our faces and narrower airways, we include this in the mix of modern and very foreign environments we live in. It does affect our sleep and brain inflammation. Many of these modern environmental influences have a bidirectional effect on us, in which structural development is compromised, which creates sleep disorders with their own inflammatory microbiome and growth abnormalities. As we mentioned at the beginning of this book, once the environmental assault damages our bodies, then these structural malformations and chemical abnormalities in our bodies also become contributors to more health assaults.

How does it affect our sleep health?

Research has explored the impact of EMF radiation on sleep and health, suggesting that it can affect both. Here is a breakdown of the information:

- EMF radiation has been found to lower melatonin levels, which regulate our sleep-wake cycle.
- Studies from the University of Melbourne indicate that EMFs trick the pineal gland, responsible for melatonin production, into thinking it's daytime, reducing melatonin levels.[177]
- Adequate melatonin is vital for restful sleep, and disruptions can cause sleep problems. Melatonin is also a powerful antioxidant. Melatonin can neutralize free radicals and reduce oxidative stress in cells, which helps protect against damage caused by reactive oxygen species. Additionally, melatonin has been found to enhance the activity of other antioxidants in the body and the brain.[178] We believe melatonin is a very beneficial supplement for everyone. You must be aware that

---

176 Anders Hagstrom, "France Orders Apple to Pull iPhone 12 from Market over High Radiation Emission," *Fox Business*, September 13, 2023.

177 "Effects of Electromagnetic Fields on Melatonin Production and Sleep," *University of Melbourne Research Report* (2018).

178 Lucien C. Manchester, et al., "Melatonin: Buffering the Immune System." *International Journal of Molecular Sciences* 16, 4 (2015), 7396-7427. doi: 10.3390/ijms16047396.

many on the market are of poor quality, and those made into tablets are likely heat-damaged melatonin.

- Lack of sleep due to EMF exposure can lead to brain inflammation, which is linked to various health issues like neurodegenerative diseases.[179]
- Sleep is crucial for cell regeneration, detoxification, and repair. When sleep is compromised, these processes are affected, impacting overall cell quality.
- Healthy cells are essential for organ function and overall health, and EMF protection products often claim to improve cell health.
- EMF radiation may disrupt our circadian rhythm, which regulates our sleep patterns.
- The pineal gland interprets EMFs as light, leading to imbalances in melatonin levels and potentially affecting sleep quality.[180] This is similar to the effect of artificial light. We are also living in a time when there is too much artificial light, which also suppresses melatonin production.[181] The two together have resulted in much lower melatonin levels in our modern lifestyle bodies. The only light that should be allowed in the sleeping area is red. A complete lack of light is better. Eye masks can help with light exposure, and some eye masks are made for EMF shielding for the eyes, but our skin contains specialized cells called melanopsin-containing photoreceptors that react to that light.[182] It is important to have a dark room. Ear plugs help, too.

---

179 "Impact of EMF Radiation on Cell Quality and Repair," *Journal of Cellular Health* 25, 3 (2022), 123-140.

180 J. Martel, S. H. Chang, G. Chevalier, D. M. Ojcius, and J. D. Young, "Influence of electromagnetic fields on the circadian rhythm: Implications for human health and disease," *Biomed J*, 46, 1 (2023), 48-59.

181 Rob Newsom and Dr. Abhinav Singh, "Blue Light: What It Is and How It Affects Sleep," *Sleep Foundation*, updated January 12, 2024, https://www.sleepfoundation.org/bedroom-environment/blue-light.

182 Debbie Moon, "Melanopsin: Light Response, Circadian Rhythm, and Blue Light Exposure," *Genetic Lifehacks*, April 5, 2024, https://www.geneticlifehacks.com/melanopsin-light-response-circadian-rhythm-and-blue-light-exposure/.

Another study, among many, is one showing suppression of sperm counts even with one hour of EMF exposure.[183]

The World Health Organization has reviewed the literature on the many effects of this environmental condition. You can look up their information.

Here is a link to Ryan's story, or go to www.beautifulfacesbook.com and find the QR code page. He was an electrician who suffered from electromagnetic hypersensitivity (EHS), and his story of how he overcame the debilitation is quite a remarkable story.

Figure 23: Scan this QR Code to access the Resource folder and the link to Ryan's story.

Not all the information is clear regarding EMF implications, but we do believe that EMF radiation should be minimized as much as possible. We have some advice from Dr. Russel Kort, DC, an expert in this subject. Dr. Kort and Joanette Biebesheimer,[184] a biochemist, revealed that EMF damage such as that from the Havannah Syndrome is similar to concussion injury.[185]

We do not know why some people are more sensitive to EMF than others. Dr. Kort and Ms. Biebesheimer believe that sleep health is a key to their approach to care, and it may be that non-restorative pathological sleep affects certain unlucky individuals more than most.

Here are some EMF hygiene practices suggested by Dr. Kort.

---

[183] Ashok Agarwal, et al., "Effects of radiofrequency electromagnetic waves (RF-EMW) from cellular phones on human ejaculated semen: an in vitro pilot study," *Fertility and Sterility* 92, 4, October 2009, 1318-1325.

[184] Russel Kort, DC and Joanette Beibeshiemer, MS at DoctorEMF website, https://doctoremf.com/.

[185] R. Blank, "EMF & Brain Damage – What 'Concussion' Tells Us About EMF Science," *SYB Blog*, last updated January 23, 2024, originally published March 9, 2020

Contributing Causes – The First Assault | 105

1. Keep your cell phone three feet away from your head while sleeping.
2. Turn off your router in the house at night. Keep the router far from your bedroom.
3. Do not put your laptop computer in your lap while using it.
4. Turn off your cell phone while sleeping.
5. Use wired earphones instead of Bluetooth earbuds. Use these when speaking on the phone to keep the phone away from your head.
6. Stop using smartphones at least one hour before bedtime.
7. Take cell phones away from children while they sleep. EMF radiation penetrates their brains much more deeply than adults.
8. Use EMF radiation barriers for eyes using eye masks made for that and cell phone shields.
9. Take antioxidants such as good-quality melatonin and EMF micronutrients designed to attenuate the inflammation caused by EMF. Research the best ones.
10. Don't put the phones in your pocket.

Rebecca's Case

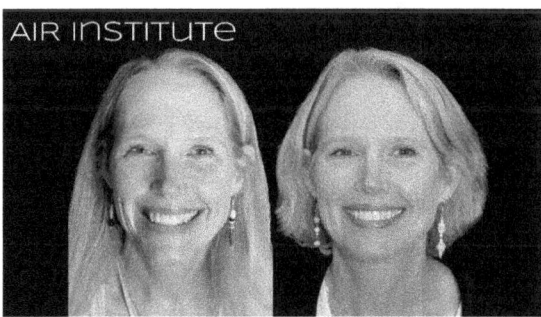

Figure 24

When Rebecca started her care, she came with these signs and symptoms: Bruxism (grinding her teeth), jaw pain, and headaches. In her words, "I get headaches all the time and often wake up with a sore jaw and headaches.

I feel tired all the time." Her sleep study showed she was experiencing suffocating events at an average rate of 17.6 times per hour. She was diagnosed with moderate obstructive sleep apnea.[186] In the two photos (Figure 24), you can see the treatment enhanced airway volume and also enhanced Rebecca's appearance in the right photo.

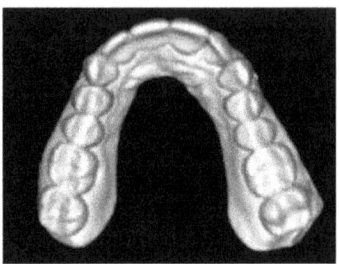

Figure 25: Pre-treatment upper arch form [187]

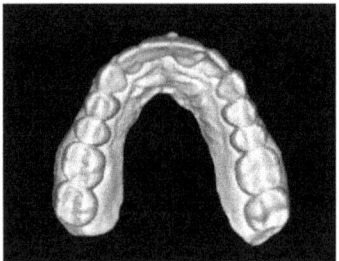

Figure 26: Post-treatment upper arch form [188]

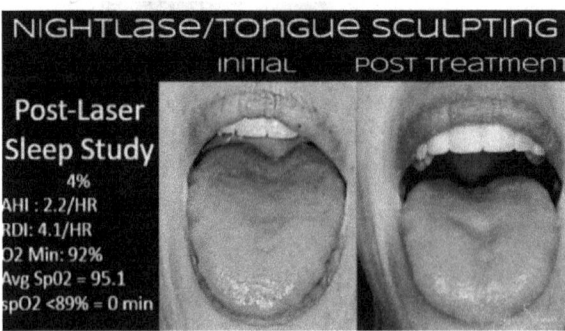

Figure 27

---

186 Geoffrey Skinner, "Meet Dr. Geoffrey Skinner - Hillsboro Dentist." *Hillsboro Dental Excellence*.
187 Ibid.
188 Ibid.

Notice the lateral scalloping of the tongue has also decreased (Figure 27). Nightlase® is a non-cutting laser application. You do not need to know the meaning of all these numbers right now. Just note that the tongue is lower and smaller. This is a midway treatment for Rebecca.[189]

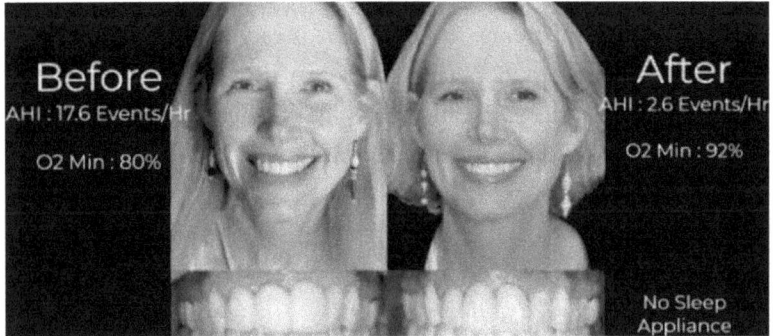

Figure 28

This is a midway status for Rebecca. Those unfamiliar with sleep metrics need to know that a smaller number on the AHI is better, and an increased number on O2 is better.[190]

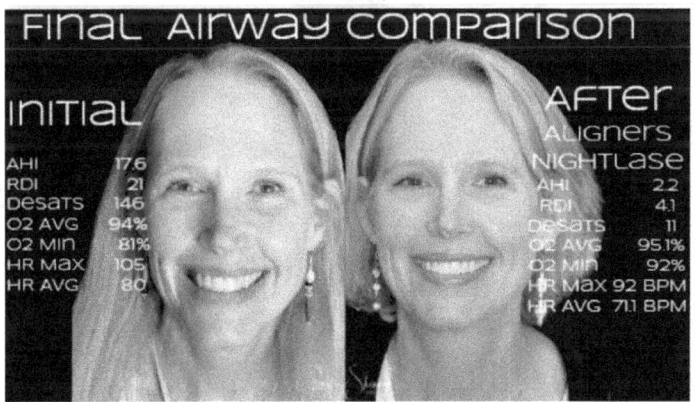

Figure 29

---

189 Ibid.
190 Ibid..

Figure 29 shows the final reading on Rebecca after clear aligner treatment by Dr. Skinner, who widened her dental arch, giving her tongue more room. This, combined with NightLase® treatment, daily xylitol, and HOCL nasal rinsing, gave a nice result. No CPAP, oral sleep appliance, or nightly airway management are needed now. AHI went from 17.6 to 2.6 events per hour sleeping, which is better and, in simple terms, means she has less than three suffocation events per hour. The lowest blood oxygen sleep score went from 80 percent to 92 percent. This increase in blood oxygen is also better. Note the broader smile and lack of dark space corridors at the place where the teeth meet the corners of her smile. This results in better health and better beauty.[191]

Raymond's story

This case with Raymond is presented by Dr. Skinner and will be detailed much more near the end of this book. In that section, you will begin to understand the orthodontic concept of intrusion with autorotation, the potential and limitations of orthodontic airway care, and the Portland Protocol of the Air Institute, which Dr. Zelk and I endorse.

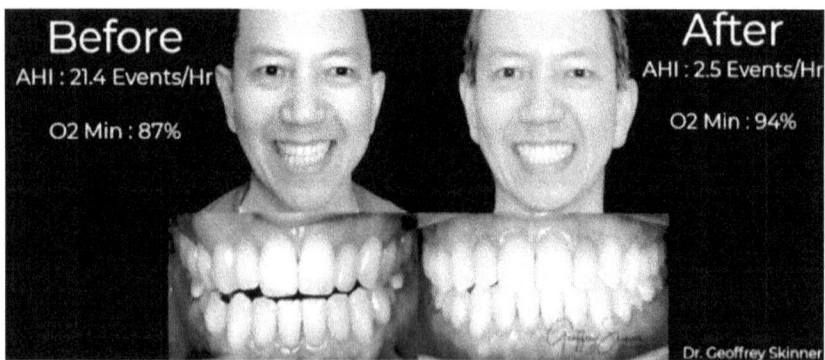

Figure 30

With Raymond, no CPAP was needed (see Figure 30). Clear aligner orthodontics was used, and NightLase®. AHI went from 21.4 to 2.5 events per hour. (This is the number of suffocation events per hour.)

---

191 Ibid.

The lowest blood oxygen sleep score went from 87 percent to 94 percent. Note the broader smile and lack of dark space corridors where the teeth meet the corners of his smile, and note the closed open bite area of the front teeth. Note that the posterior or back teeth are less sloped into the mouth, which broadens the arches and creates space for the tongue.[192]

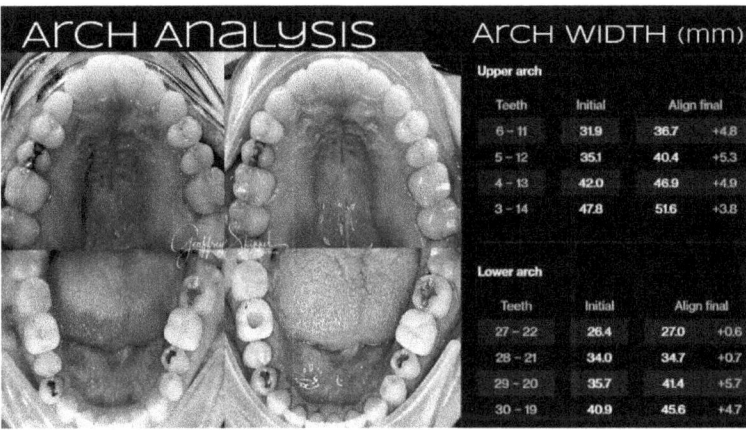

Figure 31

Please note with Raymond that the width of the teeth from one side of the mouth to the opposite side on the upper arch (maxillary arch) has increased by four to five millimeters from near the front of the mouth to the back part of the mouth after treatment. The lower (mandibular) teeth show minimal width improvement in the front area but good width improvement near to the molar and at the molar areas. This has created much more room for the tongue.

Raymond had this to say about his care with Dr. Skinner:

> "Having the clear aligner treatment has absolutely changed my health and my life. Changing the vertical position of my teeth and wearing a clear aligner appliance in the evening to keep my mouth and jaw positioned in a certain way has stopped me from snoring, much to the appreciation of my spouse! I've also been participating

---
192 Ibid.

in annual NightLase® treatments to keep the airway open as much as possible, again helping with the apnea. The doctors I worked with have all the technical data showing the improvements in my oxygenation levels and other metrics, but to me, how it translates is I am again remembering vivid dreams and no longer waking up tired and wanting to yawn all day.

CHAPTER 4

The Concept of Facial Beauty

Recap of Rebecca's and Raymond's stories

Are you equally amazed by the real-life cases you've just witnessed here? The traditional treatment of the above two example patients' sleep apnea would have been a CPAP for the rest of their lives with no improvement of facial beauty. Not only have these patients' health spans improved and now more closely matched their life span, but the person's facial appearance has also shown a remarkable transformation.

Note also that Rebecca does not need any oral sleep appliance or CPAP. Raymond wears an Invisasleep[193] that does not advance the lower jaw forward but merely keeps his lower jaw from falling back into his throat while sleeping. Can we promise this result for everyone? No, but we can give many hope for a better future. Rebecca and Raymond will need a once-per-year maintenance laser treatment for their tongues and palates and continued daily nasal hygiene. This laser treatment is a no-anesthesia and no-cutting type of laser. It is called Nightlase® [194] from Fotona Lasers, and essentially, it is a procedure done by dentists and other healthcare professionals to shrink

---

193 This is a device invented by Joseph Zelk, Portland Oregon.

194 Shiffman HS, Khorsandi J, Cauwels NM. Minimally-invasive combined Nd: YAG and Er: YAG laser-assisted uvulopalatoplasty. *Photobiomod Photomed Laser Surg* 2021; 39: 1-8.

the size of the tongue, reduce snoring and tighten up the soft palate and throat tissues. This FDA-cleared laser treatment helps open the airway with minimally invasive laser-assisted uvulopalatoplasty (LAUP).[195]

The Fotona NightLase® laser procedure is a researched method that significantly reduces the intensity and duration of snoring. This non-invasive treatment uses laser energy to heat the tissue at the back of the throat, creating more space between the soft palate and tongue. This widening helps alleviate snoring. The FDA clears the procedure for snoring, and it is safe, painless, and effective. We will explain NightLase® in more detail throughout the book.

Although Fotona® has FDA clearance for various ENT surgery and soft tissue treatment applications, including non-surgical uvulopalatoplasty,[196] its specific approval for treating sleep apnea and breathing disorders is not explicitly stated. Nevertheless, extensive research supports its effectiveness in reducing snoring; we know snoring disrupts health. Studies are being done for sleep apnea with promising results. More information about this laser is available at Fotona.com. We will show some supporting clinical cases in the book. Ongoing study of its use in obstructive sleep apnea is a continuing priority.

We will also discuss the adaptation of Nightlase therapy for use on the nose, now referred to as NaseLase. This approach holds promise for reinforcing the collapsible nasal opening in certain patients. It's worth noting that this procedure is still in the developmental phase and undergoing early-stage studies.

A Vision for Health and Beauty

What if we could raise our children to reach their genetic potential, growing into the best versions of themselves physically and mentally? What if we could mitigate the negative modern epigenetic factors that affect our blood

---

[195] Harvey S Shiffman, Jay Khorsandi, Nichole M Cauwels." Minimally Invasive Combined Nd:YAG and Er:YAG Laser-Assisted Uvulopalatoplasty for Treatment of Obstructive Sleep Apnea" *Photobiomodul Photomed Laser Surg*, 2021 Aug;39(8):550-557. doi: 10.1089/photob.2020.4947. Epub 2021 Feb 25. PMID: 33635143 DOI: 10.1089/photob.2020.4947

[196] Kakkar, Mayank et al. "Use of Laser in Sleep Disorders: A Review on Low Laser Uvulopalatoplasty." *Volume 2021*, Article ID 8821073, DOI: 10.1155/2021/8821073. Published on February 28, 2021. Academic Editor: Yuan-Yang Lai. Received on September 14, 2020; revised on January 13, 2021; accepted on February 11, 2021.

oxygen levels, impact our facial aesthetics, and lead us toward deteriorating health and appearance?

What if this goal of improved appearance could be achieved with minimal reliance on plastic surgery, Botox and collagen fillers, pharmaceuticals, cosmetics products, or strict regimens of self-discipline? What if, instead, we could embrace enjoyable, inspiring, and natural solutions that most people would readily adopt? And what if, in the process, we could also reduce our national healthcare expenditures by as much as 50 percent while improving the quality of care?

Let's pose a straightforward yet fundamental question. What constitutes the most crucial vitamin for our health? Before I give you that answer, let's look at these numbers. In the United States, annual spending on supplements and alternative health approaches amounts to a staggering $30 billion,[197] a testament to our growing interest in health and wellness. Additionally, according to statistics from legal cases and also according to AEDIT.com (Aesthetic Edit), over 7 million people had Botox treatments in 2016, making it the most popular cosmetic procedure nationwide. Over $4 billion is expended on Botox facial aesthetic treatments in the U.S., with over half a billion allocated to collagen fillers.[198]

Our way forward is to dive deeply into the past. What nutrients have our bodies always needed? A well-balanced diet with all the essential proteins, fats, amino acids, micronutrients, fiber, proper water, and vitamins has always been the standard answer.

Dr. Joseph Zelk, a sleep specialist, answers this question. When he meets patients, he asks, "What is the most important supplement we can take? Vitamin "O"! Oxygen!" Although it is not an actual vitamin, there is nothing more urgently needed and also nothing so widely ignored in our quest for health. It's not even mentioned in the same category as water.

We often address a wide range of health issues, including high blood pressure, mental illness, insomnia, strokes, cancers, dementia, heart disease, kidney failure, weight gain, ADHD in our children, diabetes, postural

---

[197] National Center for Complementary and Integrative Health (NCCIH). "Americans Spent $30.2 Billion Out-Of-Pocket On Complementary Health Approaches." *For Immediate Release: Wednesday, June 22, 2016.* Accessed April 10, 2024.

[198] "Botox: Cosmetic and Medical Uses, Procedures, and Side Effects." *Medical News Today.* Accessed April 10, 2024.

problems, back pain, headaches, autoimmune diseases, arthritis, chronic fatigue, sleep disturbances, dental problems such as tooth decay and periodontal disease, tooth grinding, vision impairments, and numerous other common diseases without looking for a root cause. These conditions are typically managed with medications, surgical procedures, radiation therapy, and chemotherapy, incurring substantial costs. However, we frequently overlook a crucial foundation of our well-being, the first and most critical foundation of our health: developing and maintaining a healthy airway, the craniofacial respiratory complex.

You might ask what I mean when I say we ignore it. Airway and sleep health should be pivotal screening tools for optimal health. The CDC labeled sleep deprivation a public health epidemic in 2014, with over 70 million adults suffering from a sleep disorder. They mentioned it was an unrecognized epidemic.[199]

In several real-life cases presented within this book, a recurring pattern emerges: many patients did not receive a sleep disorder diagnosis until they sought care from an airway-focused health practitioner who comprehends the fundamental significance of airway health. Many of these cases involve individuals who underwent extended conventional treatments, with outcomes ranging from no improvement to deteriorating health. In extreme cases, the desperation prompted contemplation of suicide.

As Dr. Zelk explains, in some cases, a lifetime of damage from sleep suffocation has resulted in permanent damage to the brain, such that people have residual anxiety and PTSD-like symptoms. We may stop the progression of this damage but be unable to regain this permanent loss of health and well-being. It is similar to a long-time smoker who quits smoking; some of the damage is not reversible, but not all damage is permanent.

Dr Zelk explains: Untreated sleep apnea is linked to a higher risk of developing Alzheimer's disease.[200] A 2020 study discovered that brain damage related to sleep apnea begins in a similar location and spreads in a manner akin to Alzheimer's disease.[201] Recent research has explored the

---

199 Centers for Disease Control and Prevention. "CDC Labeled Sleep Deprivation a Public Health Epidemic in 2014." *CDC Newsroom*, 2014.

200 Jackson, Melinda. "Sleep Apnea and Alzheimer's Disease: A Troubling Link." Turner Institute for Brain and Mental Health, Monash University. Last modified January 15, 2020. https://www.monash.edu/turner-institute/sleep-apnea-and-alzheimers-disease.

201 Ibid.

overlap between Alzheimer's disease and sleep apnea, shedding light on potential shared mechanisms or pathways between the two conditions.[202]

Gray matter and white matter are both affected. Gray matter is composed of cell bodies and synapses, while white matter consists of myelinated nerve fibers that facilitate communication between different brain regions. Earlier research primarily focused on OSA and gray matter volume, but a 2014 study revealed that untreated severe OSA is also associated with the breakdown of white matter in the brain.[203]

Effective treatment for sleep apnea, such as (CPAP) therapy, can reverse brain damage caused by oxygen deprivation during sleep.[204] Additionally, lifestyle changes, weight management, and positional therapy can help manage sleep apnea. Seeking medical advice and treatment is crucial if sleep apnea is suspected, as early intervention can prevent further damage and improve overall health.[205]

Unfortunately, the significance of sleep health is frequently not targeted earlier in developing disordered sleep breathing in comprehensive medical examinations and evaluations. This neglect largely stems from a failure of systems within large groups to allow physicians time to explore their professional curiosity. It also stems from the insufficient inclusion of sleep-breathing health education in medical and dental school curricula, compounded by misinformation in the limited content they were given.

This may also be due to OSA's bad "brand" in the public domain. OSA is associated with CPAP treatment, which many patients are not open to using, especially early OSA progression. CPAP treatment alternatives should be introduced to the public so that awareness of all treatment options improves informed consent. We do that in this book.

This book showcases many life transformations and enhanced facial

---

[202] Jackson, Melinda, and Thornton, Simon. "The Overlap Between Alzheimer's and Sleep Apnea." Brain and Mental Health Research. Last modified March 2020. https://www.brainresearchinstitute.org/alzheimers-sleep-apnea-overlap.

[203] O'Driscoll, DM, Horne, RS, and Davey, MJ. "Impact of Sleep Disordered Breathing on Cognitive Function in Children." *Journal of Paediatrics and Child Health* 46, no. 5 (2010): 279-286. doi:10.1111/j.1440-1754.2010.01725.x.

[204] Shapiro, Colin M., MD, FRCPC, and Fung, Maury. "Sleep Apnea and Brain Damage: Untangling Cause and Effect." National Sleep Foundation. Last modified April 15, 2022. https://www.sleepfoundation.org/sleep-apnea/sleep-apnea-and-brain-damage.

[205] Ibid.

beauty resulting from the guidance of these airway-focused healthcare professionals, emphasizing the attainment of a more accurate representation of each individual's genetic potential.

While the book provides general guidelines on how these experts facilitate individualized growth and development based on body types, it's important to note that defining beauty is subjective and varies greatly among individuals. Beauty encompasses multifaceted factors influencing our perceptions of facial aesthetics.

In general, beauty is often associated with good health. Somehow, the cosmetics industry has separated the two. The growth of cosmetic medicine and dentistry has also contributed to this separation. What I mean by that is that it is now possible to have cosmetic surgery or cosmetic dentistry performed that allows a person to look healthy when they are not.

The natural combination of health and beauty makes intuitive sense, though. This is why beauty is sought out by so many and is closely tied to health; however, beauty cannot be applied rigidly as always equal to health.

The Concept of Golden Proportion in Beauty

The Golden Proportion, also known as the Golden Ratio or Phi (φ), is a mathematical concept that has been recognized for its aesthetic appeal and has been associated with principles of beauty in various fields, including art, architecture, and even facial aesthetics. The Golden Proportion is represented by a ratio of approximately 1.618 and is often found in naturally occurring patterns.[206]

The Golden Proportion in Facial Aesthetics:

Facial Features:
In facial aesthetics, the Golden Proportion is thought to play a role in the harmony and balance of facial features. Specific ratios, such as the relationship between the width of the mouth and the distance between the eyes, are considered to approximate the Golden Ratio.[207]

---

206 Livio, Mario. *The Golden Ratio: The Story of Phi, the World's Most Astonishing Number.* Broadway Books, 2002.

207 Lombardi, A. V., and Reeve, J. P. "Do Facial Esthetics Influence Treatment Demand?" *American Journal of Orthodontics and Dentofacial Orthopedics* 103, no. 3 (1993): 242-252.

Artistic Representation:
Artists and sculptors have employed the Golden Proportion in their work, seeking to create visually pleasing and harmonious compositions. The use of these proportions in facial representations is believed to contribute to perceptions of beauty. Leonardo da Vinci used the golden ratio. It is also known as the Divine Proportion in his paintings and drawings.[208]

Dentistry and Smile Design:
The Golden Proportion is often applied to smile design in dentistry. The proportion of tooth widths from one tooth to another and the relationship between teeth and other facial features is considered when designing aesthetically pleasing smiles. Teeth size in proportion to face size, the distance between eyes, the width and shape of the nose, the distance from chin to nose, and the tip of the nose to eye level are all assessed in facial esthetics.[209] These ratios vary, and while some consider the golden ratio not applicable, they can be used as a tool for guidance in proportion aesthetics.

For example, a tooth with a square shape is less beautiful than a rectangular one. A six-millimeter wide and six-millimeter tall tooth is square, and the ratio of width to length on a square tooth is 1.000, but a tooth that is six mm wide and ten mm long has a ratio of the length to width of the tooth of 1.6667 (ten divided by six), or quite close to the Golden ratio and it looks much better. This strict application of the Golden Ratio to tooth size is impossible unless adjusted to account for ethnic differences.[210] It can be done if this is considered and the proportions modified. This is true for all the Golden Proportion conversations on beauty; however, the general principle of aesthetic proportion is valid in beauty and health.

Oral health and facial beauty are closely interconnected. A healthy and attractive smile is often considered a significant aspect of facial beauty. Here are a few ways in which oral health can impact facial beauty:

---

208 Meisner, Gary. "Da Vinci and the Divine Proportion in Art Composition." *Golden Number.* July 7, 2014. Accessed April 10, 2024.

209 Proffit, William R., Henry W. Fields, and Larry J. Moray. "Prevalence of Malocclusion and Orthodontic Treatment Needed in the United States: Estimates from the NHANES III Survey." *International Journal of Adult Orthodontics and Orthognathic Surgery* 13, no. 2 (1998): 97-106.

210 Murthy, B. V. Sreenivasan, and Niketa Ramani. "Evaluation of Natural Smile: Golden Proportion, RED or Golden Percentage." *J Conserv Dent.* 11, no. 1 (2008): 16–21.

1. Straight and aligned teeth: Crooked or misaligned teeth can affect the appearance of the face, particularly the smile. Orthodontic treatments like braces or clear aligners can help straighten teeth, improving facial aesthetics. However, the reverse is also true. If a tooth is lost early, even so-called baby teeth, the jaws may not fully develop in size and may be misshaped. The jaws may shift from one side to the other or be abnormally shifted forward or backward, causing an improper proportion of the facial aesthetic.

Tooth loss and loss of the space it maintains can also happen. If the tooth is not lost but merely so decayed that the teeth around it tip into the space created by the loss of the volume and shape of the tooth, shortening the dental arch size in that area can happen.

Another ratio called Bolton determines the width of the upper teeth and the width of the lower teeth. The analysis was developed by Wayne Bolton and is primarily used to measure the front teeth.

This Bolton ratio showing up in a negative or positive direction must be accounted for in orthodontic planning and care. If not, it looks terrible, and the teeth will not fit together correctly. Having a ratio that is different from usual is called a Bolton Discrepancy. A standard deviation of more than two is considered a significant discrepancy. One of the problems of this standard is that the people that Bolton measured in his paper in 1958 consisted of only Caucasians.

2. Gum health: Healthy periodontal tissues are essential for an attractive smile. Gum disease, characterized by redness, swelling, or bleeding gums, can impact the smile's appearance and overall facial beauty. Swollen gums can make a tooth appear shorter. The early forms of the disease can advance to longer-looking teeth, eventually progressing to bone loss and tooth loss, again causing jaw shortening and crookedness. Maintaining good oral hygiene and seeking timely dental care can help prevent gum disease.

3. Although this is not a structural issue, teeth color: Stained or discolored teeth can significantly impact facial beauty. Regular dental cleanings, avoiding tobacco and excessive consumption of staining substances (such as coffee or red wine), and practicing good oral hygiene can help maintain a bright and attractive smile.

4. Facial structure is mentioned above: The development of the jaws and proper alignment of teeth can influence the facial structure. Malocclusion or improper bite can affect the overall facial aesthetics. There are many other influences on the jaw's facial structures, which we will address.

5. Breath odor is not a direct jaw structure issue, but many don't know that bad breath molecules are toxic to gum tissues. Covering up the odors does not help. Breath odor, bad breath, or halitosis can result from poor oral hygiene, gum disease, or other dental issues. It can negatively impact facial beauty and social interactions.

We have already discussed the microbiome of the mouth and gut. The mouth and gut microbiomes can contribute to generalized body inflammation and affect the growth and development of the facial bones and tissues.

Maintaining good oral health through regular dental care, proper oral hygiene, and a healthy lifestyle can contribute to facial beauty and a confident smile. Consulting with a dentist can provide personalized guidance on maintaining oral health and enhancing facial aesthetics. These issues can interfere with proper genetically programmed growth potential and the jaws' and airways' balanced proportion potential.

Nature and Beauty

The presence of the Golden Proportion in natural structures, such as flowers and seashells, has led to the belief that these proportions are inherently attractive (Figure 32). Our perception of beauty may be influenced by patterns found in the natural world.[211]

The Fibonacci sequence and the Golden Ratio, represented by the Greek letter φ (phi), are closely interconnected. The Golden Ratio, approximately 1.618, arises when you add two consecutive numbers in the Fibonacci sequence as the sequence extends toward infinity.[212] As the Fibonacci numbers grow, their ratio approaches the value of the Golden Ratio.

---

211 Al-Rudainy, D., and Khedkar, S. "Golden Proportion as a Predictor of Perceived Smile Esthetics." *Journal of International Society of Preventive & Community Dentistry* 5, no. 5 (2015): 358-363.

212 "God's Handiwork -- Fibonacci Numbers." Accessed . July 23, 2024, http://www.british-israel.us/34.html.

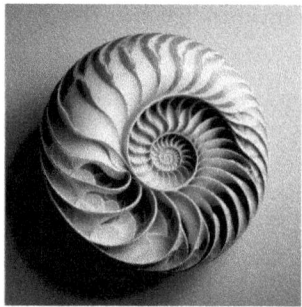

Figure 32: This is a DALL-E 3 generated image from Dall E 3® Bing® and Copilot® of a nautilus shell. It is not anatomically accurate in minor details, but the overall spiral structure is proper in its natural proportion and demonstrates a Fibonacci sequence (in which each number is equal to the sum of the preceding two numbers).

While the Golden Proportion has been celebrated as a guide for beauty, we acknowledge that perceptions of beauty can be highly subjective and influenced by cultural, individual, and societal factors. Beauty standards and preferences can vary across cultures, challenging the Golden Proportion as the sole determinant of beauty. Some argue that contemporary views on beauty have evolved, and there is a broader acceptance of diverse facial features and proportions that may not strictly adhere to the Golden Ratio.

The Golden Proportion has historically influenced perceptions of beauty, particularly in art and aesthetics. While it continues to be considered in various fields, it is essential to approach discussions of beauty with an understanding of the subjectivity and cultural nuances that shape our perceptions.

There is another ratio used in dentistry that seems to correlate with the Golden Proportion, called the Shimbashi. I could not find any direct relationship between the Golden Shimbashi and the golden ratio. However, the Golden Shimbashi is a rule of proportion, and the Golden Ratio is a proportion. Please hold on because I do have a point to all these ratios.

The Golden Shimbashi is a golden rule of proportion used to assess the vertical dimension of occlusion (VDO) in dentistry. It was developed by Dr. Henry "Hank" Shimbashi from Edmonton, Alberta.[213] VDO is the

---

213 Stonisch, Mary Sue. "Biomimetically Driven Dentistry." *Dentistry Today.* Accessed September 13, 2022.

distance between the upper and lower jaw when the teeth are together. It is referred to as the vertical dimension of occlusion. It just means the distance of the lower jaw to the upper jaw when the teeth are together (occlusion).

If a person grinds their teeth at night or during the day, they can wear the teeth down so much that the VOD is short. It also does not look right and can violate the Golden Proportion of the size of the lower face. When you look at the person, their lower face height is short in proportion to their upper face height. This moves them out of the Golden Ratio. It also moves them out of the Shimbashi standard ratio.

Also, when the lower jaw moves up because the teeth are short, the lower chin and jaw protrude forward, causing a protruding chin. They have the "Wicked Witch of the West" look with the chin and nose closer together.

We see this very frequently in complete denture patients. The jawbone under the denture shrinks so that the lower jaw and chin rotate forward, and sometimes, it looks like the chin will touch the nose. It is called an underbite by the lay public. It makes a person look older than they are. It can inflame and hurt the jaw joints, which are called the TMJs.

We will come back to the Golden Ratio in a moment, but let's address teeth grinding or what dentists call bruxism for a moment. What many do not know is that grinding of the teeth (bruxism) is a recognized association with sleep apnea. People clench and grind at night to tighten muscles in the neck and tongue, which helps them keep the airway open. The jaw moves around because they unconsciously look for a jaw position to open the airway.[214] This is another big reason dentists are in the sleep airway field.

Some healthcare workers are injecting Botox into jaw muscles to stop the grinding. This is not a good thing to do unless the person is tested for sleep apnea and has been ruled out as having obstructive sleep apnea as the cause of the tooth grinding. If that is not done, stopping the grinding with Botox could impede the airway even more. Dr. Mark Montgomery, a chronic pain and TMJ expert, says Botox use on patients' jaw muscles is almost never recommended for any reason because it impedes normal neuromuscular feedback and function.[215]

---

214 Manfredini, D., et al. "Epidemiology of Bruxism in Adults: A Systematic Review of the Literature." *Journal of Orofacial Pain* 27, no. 2 (2013): 99-110.

215 Montgomery, Mark, DMD, Montgomery Dental, P.C., Albany, OR.

Bruxism is classified into "awake bruxism" and "sleep-related bruxism." Sleep-related bruxism, in particular, is more strongly associated with sleep apnea.[216] Both bruxism and sleep apnea share common risk factors, such as stress, anxiety, and sleep disturbances. Individuals with sleep apnea may be more prone to bruxism.[217] This tooth grinding is often seen in children and is not recognized as a sign of sleep apnea. Here are some of the causes of bruxism in sleep apnea.

Sleep apnea involves repeated episodes of interrupted breathing during sleep, leading to brief awakenings and activation of the central nervous system. These arousals may contribute to bruxism episodes during the night.[218]

CPAP therapy has been found to reduce the severity of bruxism in individuals.[219] This suggests a relationship between the resolution of sleep apnea and the reduction of bruxism.

Nighttime arousals are unconscious awakenings while asleep, which are associated with sleep apnea and may trigger bruxism episodes. These arousals shift a person's sleep from deeper to lighter stages of sleep and can result in muscle activities, including teeth grinding.[220]

The Connection of Golden Ratio to Better Health and Airways

We will now connect the principle of the Golden Ratio to beauty and then to better health. As you can see in what I have written so far, artists and healthcare workers consciously or unconsciously strive to put people into more naturally beautiful states for that beauty and health. Orthodontics uses cephalometric X-ray tracings of the side of the head, measuring the angles and distances for multiple bone landmarks and teeth positions. Every one of these measurements has a normal range for health and beauty. Not all

---

216 Lavigne, G. J., et al. "Neurobiological Mechanisms Involved in Sleep Bruxism." *Critical Reviews in Oral Biology & Medicine* 14, no. 1 (2003): 30-46.

217 Khoury, S., et al. "Sleep Bruxism-Associated Factors in Children with Primary and Mixed Dentition." *Pediatric Dentistry* 38, no. 3 (2016): 228-233.

218 Lobbezoo, F., et al. "Bruxism Defined and Graded: An International Consensus." *Journal of Oral Rehabilitation* 40, no. 1 (2013): 2-4.

219 Villa, M. P., et al. "Effect of Rapid Maxillary Expansion on Sleep and Respiratory Quality." *Sleep Medicine* 15, no. 5 (2014): 536-542.

220 White, D. P., and Younes, M. K. "Obstructive Sleep Apnea." *Comprehensive Physiology* 2, no. 4 (2012): 2541-2594.

are explicitly related to the Golden Ratio, but they are built around form and function.

For example, we mentioned that tooth grinding can reduce the size of the lower face below the value of the Shimbashi Ratio and that it also affects the Golden Ratio of the entire face. Not only is this less attractive, but it is also less healthy. We also mentioned that the shape of teeth can become square, and that is not within the Golden Proportion of 1.62. Square-shaped teeth happen when ground down by bruxism far enough to upset this ratio. Restoring teeth to their proper size and ratio is better-looking and healthier. It is healthier for the teeth and the jaw joint and for the balance and relaxation of the muscles in the jaws, spine, and neck, which often reduces headaches and creates healthier airways.

Unrecognized by Everyone

The correlation between disease and compromised airways is intricate. Some individuals may exhibit typical signs linked to airway compromise starting in early childhood, yet it looks normal to most people. The condition termed Early Childhood Malocclusion (ECM) means the primary (baby) teeth lack "primary spacing" (Figures 33 and 34). Studies from the early 1900s found that there should be approximately enough space between the lower front teeth to put a nickel coin between a child's teeth at age five. That's not happening for most children and is often not recognized by dentists as important. ECM can be the first overt sign that the airway is compromised.

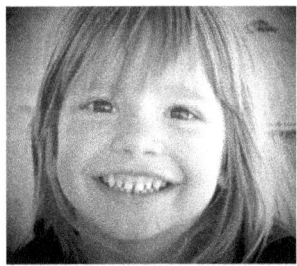
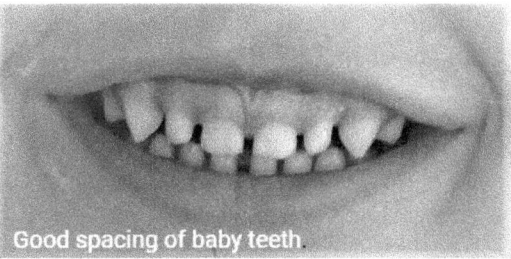

Good spacing of baby teeth

Figures 33 and 34: Photo Courtesy Shirley Gutkowski with permission. This child's teeth show good primary spacing. Some may consider this spacing less attractive but it is important to realized this is the desired look.

Even at an earlier age, a child born with a receded chin should sound an alert for a parent or health professional. As the child grows, other anatomical signs will present, such as narrow jaws, adenoidal facies with venous pooling causing dark circles under the eyes, deviated septums, crooked teeth, enlarged tonsils and adenoids, chronic ear infections, snoring, poor decision making, attention deficit disorder, bed wetting, headaches, migraines, high blood pressure, and forward head posture. Without investigating the root causes for any of these signs, you might miss the chance to intercept an airway issue or signs of sleep apnea that have not yet manifested clinically. These need to be recognized by more healthcare professionals.

Conversely, adults may look attractive and possess good signs like wider dental arches, ideal posture, open nasal passages, low weight, and youthfulness while still experiencing severe sleep apnea and airway collapse necessitating treatment. This complexity underscores airway health's diverse and multifactorial nature and its relationship to enormous variations in health conditions.

I, for example, noted in the last two years on my yearly physical that there is now one question on the preliminary questionnaire that was not there previously and that I must answer before coming into my clinic for the exam. The question is, "Do you snore?" Now, that is a very important question for an annual physical, and it should also be included in all healthcare screening questionnaires for every healthcare profession. I was glad to see it. It may be the most critical question to ask any patient presenting for care. I checked it as a "Yes" on the form. Even though this is a small start, it is not enough.

Other questions should be asked about daytime sleepiness, too. This example is typical of the lack of sleep health awareness in all health professions. It is also important that even if this question is addressed by your doctor one particular year, it should be addressed every year because sleep disorders generally get worse with age.

I did not ask my doctor about this question. I knew enough about my condition and was getting treated, so I did not need to ask. Most should ask their medical doctor about their sleep health. To be fair, this question should also be brought up in your dental or chiropractic exams, but most dentists and chiropractors do not do this either.

Having these screening questions for all DOT (Department of Transportation) examinations would be extremely valuable. Many DOT medical examiners are now chiropractors. Dr. Hannah will explain this a bit later.

During your next dental and physical examinations, bring up the topic—it's beneficial for you, your dentist, and your physician. Just bringing up the issue of snoring is important. Snoring is a significant indicator strongly associated with sleep apnea. Estimates suggest that 80 percent and close to 100 percent of individuals who snore have obstructive sleep apnea. You should openly discuss and thoroughly assess this with your health professional. Dr. Zelk says, "Consider snoring as the smoke indicative of the fire of sleep apnea, or, more accurately, 'sleep suffocation.'"

It's regrettable that most individuals experiencing sleep apnea are unaware of the problem for many years, leading to a gradual decline in their health and lifespans. They are usually only aware if a sleep partner or family member tells them they snore. Some apps can help you become aware of and manage your snoring. Dr. Zelk says the average time from initial symptoms to diagnosis is fifteen to twenty years.[221] This is unacceptable. Much accumulated health damage could have been avoided if treated earlier.

It took more than fifty years after a paper showing hemodynamic changes with OSA[222] and multiple studies on sleep health since that time for the American Heart Association to add sleep to their list as a pillar of heart health. It has taken decades for oral sleep appliances to be considered a mainstream option for adult OSA. Let's all pray the future comes faster for helping the kids.[223]

Another noteworthy example regarding the limited awareness of airway health pertains to the routines healthcare workers become accustomed to and why airway issues, particularly during nighttime sleep, receive relatively little attention in mainstream medicine. For example, the University

---

221 Reddy, E. V., et al. "Prevalence and Risk Factors of Snoring and Obstructive Sleep Apnea Among Middle-Aged Urban Indians." *Sleep Medicine*, vol. 43, June 2018, pp. 74-84. DOI: 10.1007/s11325-999-0119-z.

222 Khatri, I. M., et al. "Hemodynamic Changes During Sleep in Hypertensive Patients." *Sleep Medicine*, vol. 43, June 2018, pp. 74-84. DOI: 10.1007/s11325-999-0119-z.

223 Lloyd-Jones, D. M., "American Heart Association Adds Sleep to Cardiovascular Health Checklist." *American Heart Association Newsroom*, June 29, 2022

of Wisconsin studied sleep apnea patients. It revealed that even ten years after being released from the study, some patients remained undiagnosed by their medical practitioners.[224] This fact is perplexing because you would think that these individuals would tell the medical primary care providers that they had been diagnosed with sleep apnea in this study, and it may be that they did.

A reference to the problems of unrecognized and undertreatment by healthcare professionals comes from a lack of sleep specialists and a lack of those who understand and treat or refer for sleep disorders. Here is a summary from the *Journal of Clinical Sleep Medicine*, which is the most insightful on the lack of sleep diagnosis, referral, and management in centralized medicine. These insights could easily describe dentists as well.

> The field of sleep medicine faces an overlooked challenge in addressing healthcare disparities and providing adequate care despite the American Academy of Sleep Medicine's advocacy efforts. A critical aspect of this issue is the limited availability of healthcare providers with the expertise to accurately diagnose and manage sleep-related problems and disorders. This gap in provider availability is particularly concerning, given that access to healthcare services plays a crucial role in determining overall health outcomes.
>
> Primary care providers often bear the responsibility of managing patients with sleep problems due to the shortage of trained specialists in sleep medicine. However, many of these providers feel ill-equipped to effectively diagnose and treat sleep disorders due to a lack of sufficient clinical training and knowledge in this area. As a result, a significant portion of patients with symptoms suggestive of conditions like obstructive sleep apnea do not discuss these concerns with their primary care providers.
>
> This issue is compounded for marginalized racial and ethnic groups as well as other socially disadvantaged populations. The shortage of sleep specialists, especially in federally qualified health centers that cater to individuals from lower socioeconomic

---

[224] Flemons, W. W., et al. "Home Diagnosis of Sleep Apnea: A Systematic Review of the Literature." *Sleep Medicine*, 43, 74-84. DOI: 10.1007/s11325-999-0119-z.

backgrounds, further exacerbates disparities in access to adequate sleep healthcare for these vulnerable populations.[225]

What We Are Going to Show Next—The "A" Team

We will talk about the anatomy of the airway, airway disease, and sleep disorders caused by that disease, including dental diseases. At the same time, we will show how airway issues also impact our look, our facial symmetry, and our concept of beauty, and why proper size airways often lead to beautiful faces, fewer car accidents, better athletic performance, and fewer chronic and acute diseases. In doing so, this awareness might also just save our healthcare system.

More importantly, we will introduce you to a new approach from allied health professionals to treating these airway issues that improve our faces beautifully!

We re-introduce your dentist, orthodontist, staff members, and other dental health professionals as your new airway health management team led by the dentist! This dental healthcare team is a big part of your A-Team (Airway Team). This book provides information that the public can rally behind to help fix the lack of awareness regarding this epidemic.

We have made great strides in the area from recent *New York Times* bestsellers like *Breath* by James Nestor and *Why We Sleep* by Mathew Walker, MD. A newer book, *Is Your Tongue Killing You?* was written by Joy Moeller, a myofunctional therapist and it included contributions from noteworthy names in the dental and medical industry.[226] *Your Child's Best Face* by Dr. Felix Liau contains great photos and excellent information on impaired mouth syndrome.[227] Our book you are reading is an evolution of these important books into "What Do We Do?" about this epidemic. The following chapters tell you how.

---

225 Singh, R., Juarez, P. D., Redline, S., & Jackson, C. L. "Shortage of sleep medicine specialists in federally qualified health centers: an illustrative example of differential access to care." *Journal of Clinical Sleep Medicine*, 19(10), 1849–1850. DOI: 10.5664/jcsm.10688.

226 Moeller, Joy L. *Is Your Tongue Killing You?* Independently published, August 20, 2023. ISBN-13: 979-8858186953.

227 Liao, Felix. "*Your Child's Best Face: How to Nurture Top Health & Natural Glow.*" Whole Health Dental Center, Pllc, October 24, 2022. ISBN-13: 979-8986426808.

This book explores a promising new direction in healthcare, driven by a visionary A-team of dentists, other allied healthcare professionals, and a growing awareness within the medical community. It is still a relatively small group of early adopters of this new information in the dental and orthodontic professions, but it is increasing. It addresses a recently identified issue in modern society: airway insufficiency and the pervasive problem of sleep disorders.

Remarkably, it's only within the last seventy years that the medical community began recognizing the existence of sleep disorders, thanks to the pioneering work of psychologists in the field of sleep science. This field of study has now become dominated by medical professionals and specialists in sleep medicine.

According to the CDC, several U.S. surveillance systems assess short sleep duration or insufficient sleep duration among the U.S. population. Sleep deprivation often results from obstructive sleep apnea or its lesser-known and devastating cousin, Upper Airway Resistance Syndrome. Understanding how short sleep duration and sleep insufficiency vary by demographic and geographic characteristics can help programs prioritize efforts to improve sleep health.[228] In fact, the CDC labeled sleep deprivation a public health epidemic in 2014, with over 70 million adults suffering from a sleep disorder.[229]

The rising prevalence of sleep apnea in the U.S. is also a cause for concern. Sleep apnea is the blockage or partial blockage of breathing passages while sleeping. Often, it is designated based on the apnea hypopnea index (AHI). Some believe this measuring method is deficient; however, it is the most common. Apnea is a blocked airway, and hypopnea is a restricted airway. The severity is classified by how many times per hour you have these two airway events. So, for adults, fewer than five events per hour is considered a normal range. Five to fourteen per hour is considered mild sleep apnea. Fifteen to twenty-nine AHI per hour is considered moderate sleep apnea, and anything thirty or more is considered severe.

For children, these readings do not hold. The pediatric scale determines that an AHI greater than one per hour is considered abnormal, with an AHI

---

[228] Centers for Disease Control and Prevention. 2022. "Data and Statistics | Sleep and Sleep Disorders." CDC Sleep Data and Statistics.

[229] Howe, Neil. "America the Sleep-Deprived." *Forbes*, August 18, 2017.

between one and five considered mild, an AHI greater than five and up to ten considered moderate, and an AHI more significant than ten per hour considered severe OSA.[230] More than the AHI number is involved with a diagnosis, but for this book, it is a helpful rule of thumb for our readers.

Data previously published in the *American Journal of Epidemiology* show that the estimated prevalence rates of obstructive sleep apnea have increased substantially over the last three decades, most likely due to the obesity epidemic.[231] I will maintain the position that weight gain is not the only cause of sleep apnea, and instead, many times, sleep apnea is the cause of weight gain. Dr. Zelk mentions that 30 percent of OSA patients have no obesity contributing to the problem but have craniofacial respiratory complex development deficiencies. It can and does create a vicious cycle because weight gain makes sleep apnea worse, and sleep apnea makes weight gain worse.

Support for this view of pediatric obstructive sleep apnea in non-obese children comes from Huang YS, et. al. in *Frontiers in Neurology*. They say that sleep apnea in children who are not obese is not only linked to issues with oral-facial growth, but they also declared it a disorder of oral-facial growth. [232]

It is now estimated that 26 percent of adults between the ages of thirty and seventy years have sleep apnea.[233] How is obesity connected to OSA? Two main ways: The tongue becomes overladen with fat cells, too. As Dr. Zelk has explained, a simplified illustration would describe the tongue at a normal as resembling a "lean filet mignon." As the person gains weight, all the fat cells in their body enlarge, including those in and around the tongue. So now, the tongue resembles more of a "marbled rib eye steak," which is larger and heavier and takes up much more room in the mouth cavity.

Secondarily, adipose tissue (human fat) is deposited around the airway in the neck, squeezing the breathing tube, making it easier to collapse and

---

230 Hady, Kelly K., and Caroline U. A. Okorie. "Positive Airway Pressure Therapy for Pediatric Obstructive Sleep Apnea." *Children (Basel)*, vol. 8, no. 11, 2021, p. 979. DOI: 10.3390/children8110979.

231 "Rising Prevalence of Sleep Apnea in US Threatens Public Health." Accessed [April 24, 2024]. https://rtmagazine.com/disorders-diseases/chronic-pulmonary-disorders/asthma/rising-prevalence-of-sleep-apnea-threatens-public-health/.

232 Huang YS, Guilleminault C. Pediatric obstructive sleep apnea and the critical role of oral-facial growth: evidences. *Front Neurol*. 2013 Jan 22;3:184. doi: 10.3389/fneur.2012.00184. PMID: 23346072; PMCID: PMC3551039.

233 Howe, Neil. "America the Sleep-Deprived." *Forbes*, August 18, 2017.

harder to spring back. The ease of collapsibility of those throat muscles is measured by an index called PCRIT, and that particular collapsibility is not mainly caused by fat deposits. Those fat cells are shrinkable! This is not to minimize the impact of shrinking faces over the last several generations, contributing to a higher prevalence of sleep-breathing disorders.

CHAPTER 5

What are Sleep-Related Breathing Disorders? The Second Assault

Dr. Zelk can answer this question best. His own childhood story is all too common.

My own story begins at birth. Like 10 percent of annual births in the USA each year, I was born with a significant tongue tie. The tongue made breastfeeding challenging, and the breastfeeding didn't last long for me.

In children born with tongue ties, swallowing patterns are likely abnormal, even in utero. One consideration for tongue tie and its negative impact on jaw development is the potential insufficient swallowing pattern in the gestating baby. A baby swallows amniotic fluid which also contributes to jaw development and dental arch development. This may receive more attention as this consideration becomes more part of the discussion.

As you can see from the following picture (Figure 35), the mouth-breathing habit is evident even as an infant. In the first few years of life, there were several visits to the pediatrician for pharyngitis and bronchitis. By the age of three, an ENT recommended adenoid and tonsils removal surgery noting, on X-ray imaging very large adenoids and tonsils (kissing tonsils). The surgery improved respiratory health for a short time. Unfortunately, my mouth-breathing habit was established by this time and not successfully corrected (with a great deal of effort) until I was in my 40s.

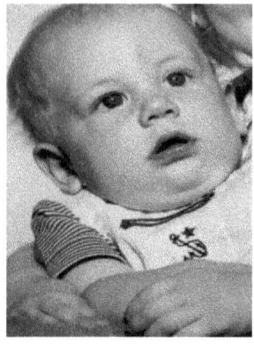 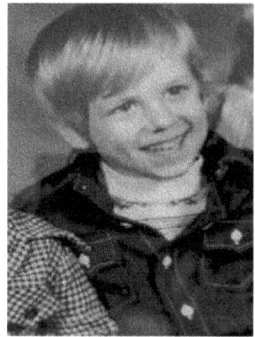 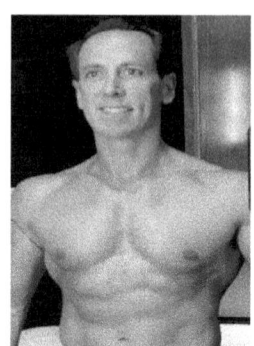

Figures 35, 36, 37

With chronic mouth breathing and narrowing of the midface, environmental allergies continued to cement obligate mouth breathing, resulting in chronic nasal restriction (Figure 36). Growing up in low-income housing, it is a good possibility I was exposed to mold mycotoxins and poor indoor air quality. These factors contributed to several X-rays of ear infections annually, resulting in three separate rounds of ear tube placements to help the ears drain. Getting water in the ear with ear tubes can be excruciating for the child. This led to a delayed interest in learning to swim and even a hysterical fear of pools and beaches for some time.

During the 1970s and 1980s, I was prescribed an average of four to six rounds of antibiotics, prednisone, and albuterol nebulizers each year. Now we know side effects can negatively impact growth and development. My father was six feet tall, and my uncle was six feet five inches. I stopped at five feet seven inches and felt these chronic medications were significant contributors to the difference in height. By increasing awareness of these considerations for parents, I hope to save their children from these frustrating experiences and improve their potential optimal health.

Frequent ear infections, nasal congestion, tongue tie, poor breastfeeding, leading to oral breathing, and chronic antibiotic exposure provide a strong case for sleep-disordered breathing if reported in a child's medical history, which was my presenting issue. I had to undergo adenotonsillectomy (removal of adenoids and tonsils) due to recurrent throat infections, bronchitis, and pneumonia. This only mildly reduced the frequency of these issues; I was already a trained mouth breather. Any of these issues in your child should prompt investigation.

Despite all these issues, I was not a snoring child. I breathed loudly and heavily at times but did not snore. A child can struggle to breathe and still not snore. This is why regular snoring in children is considered abnormal by the American Academy of Sleep Medicine and the American Academy of Pediatrics since the guidelines were published in 2005.

Regardless of the child's weight, many children may be unhealthy with obstructive sleep apnea. I am now part of the deficient airway adult cohort suffering from Upper Airway Resistance and deficient nasal volumetric anatomy due to my compromised childhood health and narrow facial dimensions. These epigenetic factors have essentially altered my facial shape. The influence of the environment can change the form factor of modern faces. I have a dolichocephalic head and face structure. This is medical speak for longer face height (Figure 37). This facial type is becoming relatively standard even though it wasn't necessarily their genetic programming but epigenetic influences on the facial profile.

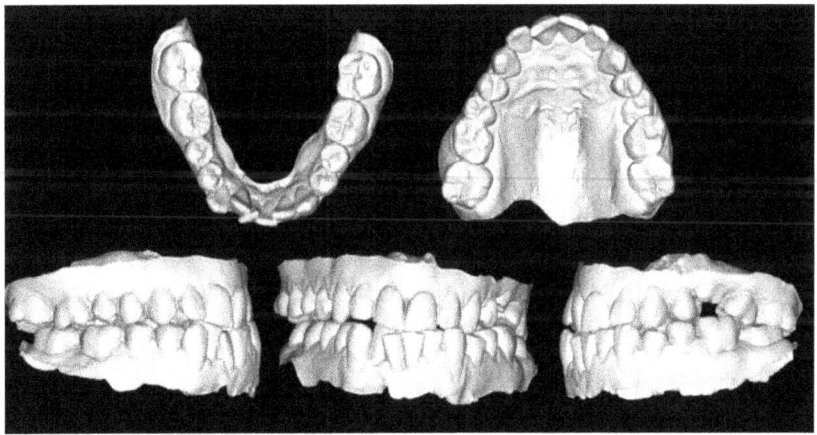

Figure 38

Figure 38 shows pre-treatment models for Joseph Zelk (age forty-eight). As you can see, there is severe crowding and jaw shifts. Joe is being treated with clear orthodontic aligners.

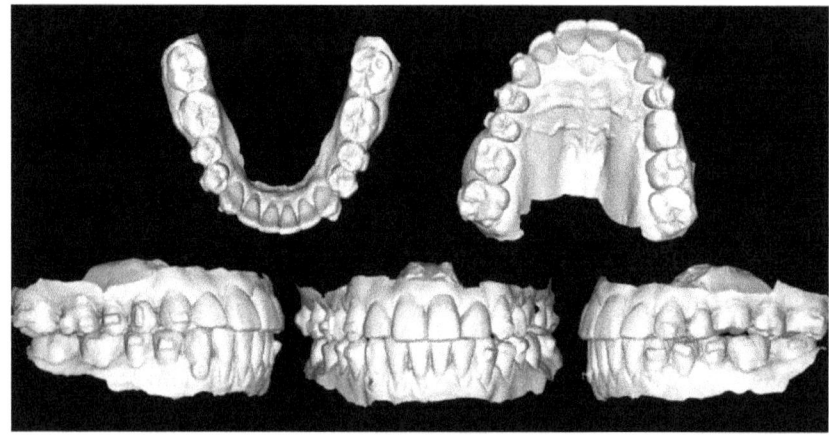

Figure 39

This is a mid-progress set of models in figure 39. He is still in clear aligners at the time of writing. Note the lack of crowding; the jaw shift is also now corrected. Dr. Geoffrey Skinner, DDS, Portland, Oregon, is doing this treatment.

Today, at age fifty-one, I am 9 percent body fat, focused on exercise, intermittent fasting, and functional nutrition (since 2013), putting me into the larger category of underdiagnosed thin people. So, many people put all their effort into optimal performance and are walking around with only half of the results they could get from their exercise and nutritional efforts since the doctors aren't asking the questions covering sleep-breathing health. Remember, the person suffering from the problem is unconscious; they can't tell you they have a problem. The bed partner needs to see the issue with snoring. This is a significant reason why at least 80 percent of OSA is undiagnosed today.

I work diligently to stay healthy, but without treatment for my sleep-breathing restriction, it is like I am in a boxing match with one hand tied behind my back. No matter how hard I fight back, I lose every minute of the fight until that hand is freed. Since my airway is narrow, any increase in my weight can dramatically increase the severity of sleep apnea when the tongue grows in size with each pound gained. But at this weight, fat tissue is not the issue, and for many of us weight gain has simply made the sleep breathing problem more obvious, but not the primary cause of the sleep apnea in the first place.

Due to my poor sleep as a child, I was unable to gain weight without great effort. Medical health was not the only negative impact. Like 10 percent of the current pediatric population, I was also diagnosed with ADHD and was a wild kid, bouncing off the walls and hard to tame. The distraction was so great that until the second grade, I was placed in special education. This is likely a major cause for the placement of many of our children today into special education due to the almost 90 percent of undiagnosed sleep in our children.

Thinking back, some of my behavior improved when I began playing trumpet in the band in fifth grade. This music habit continued into college, where I received a music scholarship. This habit of playing a brass instrument likely strengthened much of my upper airway muscles and diaphragm and mildly improved my nasal breathing. The realization of these airway deficiencies was not stumbled upon till I started to work in sleep medicine. Interestingly, a paper on improved human sleep apnea by playing a didgeridoo instrument supports this idea of alternative airway health therapy in the *British Medical Journal*.[234]

Due to my poor health and frequent hospitalizations throughout my childhood, I became obsessed with taking control of my health. From my teenage years, I focused on good nutrition, exercise, and prioritizing my sleep time. Many of my health issues improved with these interventions, and my respiratory and general health improved significantly. I felt I had done as much for my health as was possible. Little did I know that the most significant impact on my long-term health promotion had yet to be discovered. Until my thirties, I just made excuses that I have allergies, and since I didn't snore, I didn't even put the dots together until I volunteered to take a sleep study to check the calibration of some new sleep testing equipment. When the test came back abnormal, I didn't believe it. When I took another test six months later, the same result came back, and at that point, I figured I would run an experiment.

I tried an auto-titrating CPAP and failed miserably. I couldn't keep the CPAP on for more than a few hours, and if I managed to use it the whole night, I was exhausted in the morning from the disruption to my sleep caused by the air pressure.

---

[234] Puhan, M. A., et al. "Didgeridoo playing as alternative treatment for obstructive sleep apnoea syndrome: randomized controlled trial." *BMJ*, 332, 266. DOI: 10.1136/bmj.38705.470590.55.

After the CPAP attempt, I went to a local dental sleep medicine provider and had him fit me with an oral sleep appliance. The first night I stopped getting up to pee twice a night (which I thought was related to high water intake), I woke up an hour earlier without the alarm, feeling alert and ready to go on with my day. A week later, the heartburn I had been struggling with for the last six months went away completely without changing my diet. A year later, I noticed I hadn't had a cold sore and usually would have had three to four episodes by then, seeing that my immune system was more robust. My average night of sleep went from a compulsory nine hours a night to seven and a half hours a night. I felt better than I did with nine hours of sleep before wearing the oral appliance. My personal experience launched my quest to look into CPAP alternatives for my sleep apnea and upper airway resistance patients.

From that point forward, I took mild sleep apnea more seriously, realizing that even mild cases of sleep apnea can dramatically deprive a patient of a well-rested, healthy quality of life. Unfortunately, many clinicians still don't consider mild sleep apnea worth treating.

For the general state of the unaware public, relating to OSA or Obstructive Sleep Apnea Hypopnea Syndrome, a frame of reference may need to be formed to identify this issue better. As mentioned before, picture a more accurate description, "sleep suffocation." It is a more precise way of presenting the problem, and people understand its importance better when said this way. In addition to an unaware public, compromised sleep breathing of most any severity is largely ignored by primary care physicians and pediatricians.

Thirty percent of OSA patients have no obesity contributing to the problem but have craniofacial respiratory complex development deficiencies. The other 70 percent or so end up developing "sleep suffocation" as obesity sets in and unmeasured numbers of people gain weight due to sleep breathing disorder or SBD. [235]

Nearly 80 percent of moderate and severe OSA cases are undiagnosed[236] still today. This constitutes the majority of what sleep specialists encounter on a daily basis. Insomnia cases, advanced sleep phase disorders, circadian

---

235 "A Hidden Sleep Killer." Accessed April 22, 2024. https://bengreenfieldlife.com/podcast/sleep-podcasts/a-hidden-sleep-killer/.

236 Ibid.

rhythm disorders, delayed sleep phase syndrome, jet lag, restless leg syndrome, periodic limb movement, narcolepsy, and around one hundred other sleep disorders often receive less attention compared to obstructive sleep apnea (OSA). A comprehensive understanding of sleep issues requires careful consideration of OSA.[237]

Modern Perception of Sleep and Breathing

I jest with most of my patients on the initial consultation and ask them, "What is the most important vitamin?" I have logged an extensive list of answers over the years. The most critical vitamin is vitamin O. Most folks are confused when they hear this comment. Then a light bulb goes off, and they realize I am referring to oxygen. For all aspects of metabolism, the central vitamin is, in fact, one we do not ingest but instead breathe. But, of course, oxygen is not a vitamin because it is inorganic. By all other criteria, it is the central player in the need for essential nutrients. Thus, it is the ultra-vitamin. To obtain sufficient quantities of this crucial nutrient, we must be good nasal breathers while awake and asleep. We may be falling short in both of these states of consciousness with predominantly stress-driven unconscious breathing during the day and likely sleep suffocation at night.

The phenomenon of sleep is both loved and hated by the modern American. Look at many typical catchphrases indelibly etched in the contemporary psyche, including . . .

"Sleep is a symptom of caffeine deprivation."

"I can sleep when I am dead."

"Sleep is a luxury I can't afford."

The CDC reports that 30 percent of adults admit to less than six hours of sleep a night. Most of this is not insomnia but chosen lifestyles. The myth of getting by with less sleep to get ahead has been around for only a short time, though, since the early 1900s. The graveyard shift was invented to ramp up manufacturing during World War II. Thomas Edison, a notorious short sleeper, famously described his optimal day as working for eighteen hours a day and getting by with four to five hours of sleep per night.[238]

---

237 Ibid.

238 "The Terrifying Condition Of Sleep and Dying Earlier Without It." Accessed April 22, 2024.

The early 1900s showed the average American slept just over eight and a half hours a night. Our lack of sleep has resulted in a massive increase in deadly microsleep automobile accidents, among many other devastating physiological effects.

It's remarkable how rapidly our emphasis on prioritizing sleep has diminished. Certain medical researchers have identified a correlation between the rise in autoimmune disorders and the insufficient opportunity to rejuvenate one's health through adequate sleep.

Sleep apnea results in the same conditions as inadequate sleep time. However, like autoimmune disorders, insufficient sleep is not considered a disease; instead, the body is "short-circuiting" and initiating some self-inflicted problems. Remember the two-phase assault we mentioned at the start of this book? This is another example of the second leg of the attack in which the body itself is destroying people's health, beauty, and vitality.

The definition of insufficient sleep is concise: a neurological condition characterized by individuals consistently failing to acquire adequate sleep necessary to maintain normal wakefulness. Perhaps one day, it may include in the definition that failing to get enough "restorative" sleep optimally supports the immune system.

This fact is reiterated elsewhere in this book. A few years ago, I discovered that epidemiologists had illustrated a significant decrease in the average nightly sleep duration among Americans over the past few generations. In 1950, the average was eight and a half hours, which declined to seven and a half hours by 1970 and further decreased to six and a quarter hours by 2000, continuing to diminish over subsequent years.[239] If you combine this alarming statistic with the fact that many of these same individuals will also have sleep apnea, even the sleep they do get is fragmented, suffocating, non-restorative sleep.

So, what does this mean to someone who wants to stay in optimal health? What are the negative impacts revealed by research when individuals don't obtain sufficient sleep? And what amount of sleep is necessary for optimal performance, particularly for a healthy individual or an athlete aiming to reach their peak?

---

https://bengreenfieldlife.com/article/sleep-articles/the-terrifying-condition-of-sleep-and-why-youll-die-earlier-if-you-dont-experience-it/.

239 Pacheco, Danielle, and Dr. Anis Rehman. "Pain and Sleep." *Sleep Foundation*, May 23, 2023.

What is sleep Apnea? Why we appreciate sleep health now

UNDERSTANDING SLEEP APNEA

In 2014, when the U.S. Centers for Disease Control and Prevention (CDC) labeled sleep deprivation a "public health epidemic," they did not distinguish between sleep deprivation and sleep apnea. While sleep deprivation is distinct from sleep apnea, both conditions often yield similar effects. The bed partner usually suffers sleep deprivation when they sleep with a person who has sleep apnea, and they know why, while the person with sleep apnea, robbing other individuals of deep restorative sleep in the bedroom, has no idea why. The person with sleep apnea does not hear their snoring noise or choking episodes.

Sleep deprivation can arise from various sources, including sleep apnea, insomnia, or simply not allowing oneself sufficient sleep time. Both sleep deprivation and sleep apnea are linked to a myriad of health issues, such as hypertension, diabetes, kidney damage, teeth grinding, GERD, depression, obesity, and more. Despite affecting millions globally, many cases of sleep apnea go undiagnosed, leading to serious long-term consequences.

When you experience sleep apnea, your body enters the sympathetic mode. This is the fight-or-flight state we have all heard so much about, and regular sleep is reserved for REM stages of sleep and REM's dream activity.[240] Heart rate variability decreases (HRV). We want heart rate variability increased in non-REM sleep and more parasympathetic mode. We need to get the body back into the parasympathetic mode while sleeping. In simple terms, this is the relaxed mode of sleep.

Joseph Zelk, a sleep specialist, explains this best. I will jump in at specific points to define the terms he uses for the reader.

1. Sleep-disordered breathing (SDB) encompasses a spectrum of conditions ranging from mild sleep disturbances like sighing to serious conditions like obstructive sleep apnea and central sleep apnea. Initial studies suggest that the disruption or fragmentation of nightly sleep caused by SDB accelerates aging. This common

---

[240] Breus, Michael J., Ph.D. "Why Heart Rate Variability Matters for Sleep." *Psychology Today*, April 8, 2022.

disorder leads to oxidative stress and inflammation and is linked to various age-related health conditions. Recent research has associated sleep-disordered breathing with accelerated aging, which in turn contributes to the deterioration of youthful appearance.

2. Obstructive sleep apnea is a prevalent yet often undiagnosed condition linked to significant morbidity and mortality. It involves intermittent blockage of the upper airway during sleep, leading to reductions or pauses in airflow and subsequent drops in blood oxygen levels. This triggers sympathetic neural activation, resulting in nighttime hypertension and cortical arousal, leading to sleep fragmentation and limited time spent in deeper sleep stages. Common symptoms include snoring, restless sleep, daytime fatigue, generalized pains, and morning headaches. Left untreated, OSA increases the risk of various health issues, including hypertension, stroke, congestive heart failure, and sudden death, regardless of age.

3. The prevalence of OSA, as defined in large part by an apnea-hypopnea index (AHI). (A) stands for complete stopping of breathing, (H) stands for restriction of airflow, and (I) stands for number of times per hour) of an AHI of five or higher for adults. The prevalence of Obstructive Sleep is often underestimated. It affects up to 24 percent of adult males and 9 percent of adult females. Most of these patients experience snoring. Surprisingly, 80–90 percent of OSA cases remain undiagnosed. Alongside OSA, insomnia is another prevalent sleep disorder. It is estimated that 12 percent of adults suffer from OSA and that 80 percent of this patient population is undiagnosed. A recent European study found the prevalence in a middle-aged general population of 43.1 percent for moderate and 19 percent for severe OSA. Young children should be under one AHI.

4. Sleep is essential for maintaining the brain's white matter. Sleep promotes cleaning out brain metabolism byproducts and replacing them with fresh nutritional products. It also promotes myelination (the coating cells around nerves) and the proliferation of oligodendrocyte precursor cells in the central nervous system. (These cells support the production of myelination protection of nerve cells.)

5. Sleep-disordered breathing (SDB) and poor sleep quality have also been linked to changes in gray matter, as previously mentioned. Simply put, the difference between the brain's white matter and gray matter is that white is the more automatic, emotional portion and the more primitive part of our brain. In contrast, gray is the more rational and deliberative part. The negative impact of SDB on white matter microstructure changes has recently been connected. Recent research has shown that older and middle-aged individuals experiencing insufficient sleep and increased daytime sleepiness, as opposed to those who are cognitively healthy, exhibit associations with spinal fluid biomarkers indicating amyloid deposition, tau pathology, axonal (nerve) degeneration, and neuroinflammation. Beta-amyloid deposition, in combination with tau pathology, is the protein strongly associated with Alzheimer's disease, and it causes inflammation.

DEFINITIONS

- **High-sensitivity C-reactive protein:** This is a marker of inflammation in the body.
- **Homocysteine:** An amino acid linked to inflammation; high levels may indicate health issues.
- **Hematocrit:** The proportion of cellular elements of blood; an elevated level may suggest inflammation or dehydration.
- **Intermittent hypoxia:** Periodic blood oxygen levels drop, often occurring in OSA.
- **Nuclear factor kappa B:** A protein that plays a role in inflammation and immune responses.
- **Hypoxia-inducible factor-1:** A protein that responds to low oxygen levels, influencing various cellular processes.
- **Tumor necrosis factor-alpha and interleukin-8:** Substances involved in inflammation.
- **Myeloid cells:** White blood cells responsible for participating in immune responses.

- **Dyslipidemia:** An abnormal level of lipids (fats) in the blood.
- **Oxidative stress:** Occurs when there is an imbalance between free radicals and antioxidants, potentially leading to cellular damage.
- **High-density lipoproteins (HDL):** Referred to as "good cholesterol," high-density lipoprotein (HDL) aids in removing other forms of cholesterol from the bloodstream.
- **Low-density lipoprotein:** Known as "bad cholesterol," has the propensity to accumulate on the walls of blood vessels, consequently contributing to the development of atherosclerosis.
- **Metabolic syndrome:** Encompasses a group of conditions that increase the chances of heart disease, stroke, and type 2 diabetes.
- **Sympathetic activity:** The part of the nervous system responsible for the fight-or-flight response.
- **Insulin resistance:** A condition where the body's cells don't respond effectively to insulin, increasing blood sugar levels.
- **Endothelial dysfunction:** Impaired functioning of the inner lining of blood vessels.

Sleep apnea primarily consists of obstructive (OSA) and central (CSA) types. The obstructive form accounts for about 84 percent of diagnosed sleep disorders, often involving breathing interruptions during sleep ranging in time from ten to sixty-plus seconds multiple times per hour, which, stated plainly, equates to suffocation while sleeping. This may result in anxiety disorders with an unknown cause.

As Dr. Zelk has said, "The term 'apnea' fails to convey the severity of the experience; individuals are essentially suffocating." These interruptions, known as apneas (no breathing) and hypopneas (restricted breathing), are measured during sleep studies and typically recorded if lasting ten seconds or longer. If they are shorter, they are not recorded, even though some may consider them significant. These alterations in breathing also alter the chemistry of the blood. I'll spare you the math and physics and focus on blood oxygen levels. In simple terms, the oxygen levels dip.

During a sleep study, the apneas are partly measured by oxygen reduction in the blood. The percentage of oxygen drop events is recorded using pulse oximetry when levels drop 3 percent and 4 percent on the scoring device. Most of the time, OSA occurs due to airway blockages, either partial (hypopneas) or complete (apneas), hindering oxygen flow to the lungs during sleep. Anatomical abnormalities, excess weight, insufficient room behind the tongue, constricted nasal openings, or relaxed throat muscles can cause these suffocation events. Central sleep apnea arises from impaired brain signals affecting the respiratory muscles.[241]

Less severe episodes of sleep interruptions can keep a person from getting into the deep restorative sleep stages. These arousals or partial awakenings from sleep are not noticed by the sleeper when they occur. They also interrupt and prevent entering stage 3, the deep sleep stage, and the fourth stage, called REM sleep. This interferes with physical and emotional restoration in the body. It interferes with learning, too. These arousals are destructive to health. They also prevent the brain's glymphatic system from cleansing the brain of toxins while sleeping. This has been linked to the progress of dementia.[242]

Undiagnosed sleep suffocation can have severe consequences, particularly in cardiovascular health, leading to increased stress on the heart and blood vessels due to decreased oxygen levels during apneas. Interruptions in sleep negatively impact daytime function, causing drowsiness, poor decision-making, and reduced productivity, not to mention mood disorders. The condition often progresses to severe health issues such as strokes, high blood pressure, depression, and diabetes, contributing to immense costs, both in well-being and financially.[243]

Sleep apnea is significantly underdiagnosed, with around 70 to 80 million Americans lacking a diagnosis of the disease, while those with traditional treatments such as CPAP often experience high failure rates. This book aims to showcase alternative therapies, emphasizing the need for raising awareness,

---

[241] Young, T., et al. "Research on Diagnosed Instances of Sleep Disorders." *Journal of Abnormal Psychology*, 127(3), 298-310. DOI: 10.1037/abn0000410.

[242] Kahn, Sandra, and Paul R. Ehrlich. *Jaws: The Story of a Hidden Epidemic*. Stanford University Press, April 10, 2018. ISBN-13: 978-1503604131.

[243] Benjafield, A., et al. "Estimation of the Global Prevalence and Burden of Obstructive Sleep Apnoea: A Literature-Based Analysis." *The Lancet Respiratory Medicine*, 7(8), 687-698. DOI: 10.1016/S2213-2600(19)30198-530198-5).

increasing screenings, and advocating for early intervention to provide appropriate treatment options and ultimately enhance individuals' quality of life.[244]

Two of the most significant contributors to sleep apnea, most often cited in articles, are age and excess weight. This may have been true generations ago, but today, thin little women and children also suffer. We go deeper into our modern lifestyle and show you there are profound causes that we believe are more important than this standard answer. These causes can be addressed with better outcomes than just telling people to lose weight and then placing them on a lifetime of CPAP ventilation.

Yes, age and weight do play into our susceptibility to sleep apnea. As we grow older, our throat muscles tend to lose tone and relax, which makes it easier for airway blockages to occur, and being overweight increases this likelihood even further. Fat cells in the tongue become larger, using up valuable airway space.[245] Other potential causes often cited in the literature are important, too, and include smoking habits, alcohol consumption, or personal history with certain medical conditions such as diabetes or hypothyroidism.

Upper Airway Resistance Syndrome

Before we get into the effects of sleep apnea on health, I have one more definition to review. UARS is challenging to diagnose, and some consider it unimportant. I do not. And, since it occurs about two and a half times more often in women than in men, it would be highly unethical not to highlight it and its importance.

Sleep-disordered breathing disorders (SDB) encompass chronic conditions like snoring, upper airway resistance syndrome (UARS), obstructive sleep apnea (OSA), and central sleep apnea (CSA) with its subtypes.[246] These conditions are characterized by abnormal breathing during sleep, historically described based on the recording technologies and knowledge of the time.[247]

---

244 CDC. "Declaration on Sleep Deprivation as a Public Health Epidemic." 2014.

245 Kahn, Sandra, and Paul R. Ehrlich. *Jaws: The Story of a Hidden Epidemic*. Stanford University Press, April 10, 2018. ISBN-13: 978-1503604131.

246 Sankri-Tarbichi, A. G. "Obstructive sleep apnea-hypopnea syndrome: Etiology and diagnosis." *Avicenna Journal of Medicine*, vol. 2, no. 1, 2012, pp. 3-8. [PMC free article] [PubMed]

247 Arnold WC, Guilleminault C. "Upper airway resistance syndrome 2018: non-hypoxic sleep-disordered breathing." *Expert Rev Respir Med*. 2019 Apr;13(4):317-326. [PubMed]

UARS has been studied for many years, but there still needs to be an explicit agreement on what diagnostic criteria should be used or whether UARS is a distinct syndrome from OSA.[248]

While OSA and CSA are defined by the number of apnea (stop breathing) and hypopnea (restricted breathing) episodes per hour of sleep (apnea-hypopnea index or AHI), UARS is defined as airflow limitation due to increased respiratory effort leading to arousals from sleep without significant desaturation (lower oxygen in the blood) (i.e., RERAs) associated with daytime symptoms.[249] The heart rate may go up so quickly in these restricted breathing events, especially in young people, that the oxygen levels that usually would go lower in older individuals do not happen in the young and, therefore, are not recorded as an event on a sleep test.[250] Heart rate variability (HRV) may also decrease, indicating a more sympathetic than parasympathetic state.[251]

UARS has also been more specifically defined as an apnea-hypopnea index of fewer than five events per hour, oxygen saturation of the blood greater than or equal to 92 percent, and respiratory effort—related arousal event index greater than or equal to five per hour. Another study used slightly different numbers but included daytime sleepiness and fatigue in the definition.

Upper airway resistance syndrome often occurs when the airway narrows partially, and there is heightened resistance in the back of the palate and tongue areas. This increased resistance makes breathing more challenging, leading to repeated awakenings during sleep and disturbing the normal sleep cycle.

Wrapping your head around this phenomenon is like struggling to pull air through a coffee stir straw. The effort associated with this struggle can cause the sleeper to have the shoulders hunched up, the jaw muscles sometimes clenched with grinding, and the neck tense. This can happen for minutes

---

248 Chervin RD, Guilleminault C. "Obstructive sleep apnea and related disorders." *Neurology Clinics, vol. 14, no. 3, 1996, pp. 583-609. [PubMed]*

249 Ogna, A., Tobback, N., Andries, D., et al. "Prevalence and Clinical Significance of Respiratory Effort-Related Arousals in the General Population." *Journal of Clinical Sleep Medicine*, vol. 14, no. 8, 2018, pp. 1339-1345. [PMC free article] [PubMed]

250 Julie Marks, Medically Reviewed by Sabrina Felson, MD, "What is Upper Airway Resistance Syndrome?" *WebMD,* July 16, 2023.

251 Draghici, Adina E., & Taylor, J. Andrew. "The Physiological Basis and Measurement of Heart Rate Variability in Humans." *Journal of Physiological Anthropology*, vol. 35, article number 22, 2016, 28 September 2016.

and hours throughout the night without the sleeper being aware of the issue until they wake up in the morning with a headache or tense shoulders.

These frequent respiratory-related arousals (RERA) cause non-refreshing sleep, excessive daytime sleepiness, or unexplained daytime tiredness. One of the main parameters of UARS is flow limitation during sleep, which is without significant oxygen desaturation in the blood and does not meet the definition of hypopnea. What is so challenging for diagnostic equipment is that these tests rely on oxygen dropping measurably in the bloodstream. In UARS, all this breathing effort can happen with normal oxygen levels. As I explained, heart rate may catch up to the restricted oxygen levels quickly and keep that oxygen level high enough that the sleep test machine does not record it.

UARS might be an early stage of OSA, shedding light on how sleep-disordered breathing progresses. It could also be its own sleep-breathing disorder. However, we don't have much data on how often non-apneic respiratory events happen. These events are mostly linked to extended periods of restricted airflow and arousal caused by extra effort in breathing. When airflow worsens during sleep, it can narrow the upper airway in people with less-than-ideal anatomy. For those who are vulnerable (remember one phenotype we mention is people who are more sensitive to restricted airflow), having a low arousal threshold during sleep may contribute to sleep problems, leading to disrupted and uneven sleep due to periods of restricted airflow and sleep-disordered breathing.

UARS flow limitation can be inspiratory, expiratory, or in both respiratory cycle phases. The collapsibility of the airway also influences upper airway patency (staying open).

Upper airway collapsibility can be determined by applying progressively negative pressure to the upper airway until the negative pressure reaches a critical closing pressure (Pcrit). Essentially, the sleeper is working so hard to pull air in that minor disruptions to sleep can happen numerous times throughout the night, leading to sleep that is not refreshing and causing daytime tiredness and fatigue.

A recent study found that about 3.1 percent of individuals (4.4 percent in women and 1.5 percent in men) have Upper Airway Resistance Syndrome In contrast, the prevalence of mild or more severe Obstructive Sleep Apnea was observed in 24 percent of men and 9 percent of women.[252] Recent international studies estimate that around one billion individuals worldwide are affected by OSA.

UARS is more common in pre and perimenopausal women than in men or postmenopausal women. In addition, women with UARS were found to have a higher reported need for sleep (approximately thirty minutes more) than men with UARS.

Patients with upper airway resistance syndrome often experience symptoms such as snoring, fatigue, daytime tiredness, morning headaches, depressive symptoms, and excessive daytime sleepiness. They do not have definitively witnessed apnea or gasping episodes. In addition, patients may complain of sleep disruptions and unexplained awakening from sleep, mainly after two to three hours of sleep. These frequent unexplained arousals are associated with increased respiratory effort and lead to sleep fragmentation, resulting in fatigue and excessive daytime sleepiness. Individuals with UARS and OSA have exhibited a low quality of life compared to the general population (five to six times worse). A current obstacle to diagnosis, or the "Gold Standard," is to have a sleep test using an esophageal manometry (the patient must swallow this tube and attempt to sleep with it in place).

Sleep Deprivation and Immunity:

In animal studies, a sleep-promoting factor found in the cerebrospinal fluid has been identified as adenosine. This discovery prompts me to pose a question to my patients: "What is the most commonly consumed medication globally?" It's neither an over-the-counter nor a prescription drug. Surprisingly, it's caffeine, which acts as a blocker of adenosine. Many people rely on caffeine throughout the day, often in the form of morning, mid-morning, afternoon, and sometimes even evening coffee.

Caffeine, like any medication, has a toxic dose, and one significant reason for this is its ability to block adenosine. Adenosine serves as the brain's metabolic waste product, akin to exhaust fuel.

Here's the mechanism: when the glial cells (often called the "glue" of the

---

252 Sankri-Tarbichi, A. G. "Obstructive sleep apnea-hypopnea syndrome: Etiology and diagnosis." *Avicenna Journal of Medicine*, vol. 2, no. 1, 2012, pp. 3-8. [PMC free article] [PubMed]

nervous system), which are not nerve cells in the central nervous system, are depleted of ATP (adenosine triphosphate, where adenosine is the "A"), they break down stored glycogen (the brain's glucose storage). This breakdown results in the formation of two ADP (adenosine diphosphate) molecules, which can then be utilized to generate an additional ATP molecule, leaving behind an excess adenosine molecule.[253]

Let me simplify that for you: Imagine the brain has worker cells called glial cells. These cells need a fuel called ATP, and when they run low, they can recycle two ADP molecules to create more ATP and a leftover molecule called adenosine. So, excess caffeine intake can strip the brain of necessary fuel, especially when glial cell ATP is already low from lack of sleep.

The process is that when ATP (adenosine triphosphate) is broken down into ADP (adenosine diphosphate) in the brain's glial cells, it releases energy. This energy can convert adenosine (a neurotransmitter) into ATP again,[254] providing energy for the cells. Caffeine intake can interfere with this process. Excessive or late-day consumption leads to depletion of essential energy reserves, especially when glial cell ATP is already low from lack of sleep, spiraling to even poorer sleep.

Adenosine is naturally synthesized in the body by merging adenine, a nitrogen-based compound, with ribose, a sugar. Apart from functioning as a neurotransmitter, adenosine falls under the category of chemicals called xanthines. Adenosine is ubiquitous in all cells, forming part of DNA and RNA molecules.[255]

Adenosine creates sleep pressure because it inhibits wakefulness in the arousal areas in the brain. It attaches to receptors there. If that is interfered with by a molecule like caffeine, which attaches preferentially to the same receptors that adenosine uses to increase sleep pressure, we stay awake. The longer a person is awake, the poorer the pressure to fall asleep builds. Typically, the average person will be awake sixteen to eighteen hours until enough sleep pressure is developed to cause a person to want to go to bed and sleep.

---

253 Zimmermann, H. "Extracellular Metabolism of ATP and Other Nucleotides." *NIH*, PMID: 11111825, DOI: 10.1007/s002100000309.

254 AK Neurochemie et al. "Extracellular Metabolism of ATP and Other Nucleotides." *Naunyn-Schmiedeberg's Archives of Pharmacology*, vol. 362, 2000, pp. 299–309. DOI: 10.1007/s0021000003092022.

255 Peters, Brandon, MD. "Adenosine and Sleep." *Verywell Health*, April 19,

If late afternoon habits or caffeine occur, they break the momentum of this sleep pressure, challenging going to sleep at the regular time slot, resulting in sleep onset insomnia.

One way of thinking about sleep pressure is to consider ATP the gasoline needed to run a car engine. The more the car runs, the more it burns gas, and the more tailpipe exhaust is made. Too much pipe exhaust and pollution will build up, causing dangerous air quality. Your brain will have a similar process occur as ATP is broken down to release energy needed for the cell's metabolism. The by-products of adenosine and ADP are essentially the pollution equivalent of cell metabolism. Once the brain is awake for sixteen to eighteen hours, the level of pollution in the cerebral spinal fluid from the adenosine forces the brain to sleep. In restorative sleep, the brain can clean up the cerebral spinal fluid and wash and drain this CSF to clean the brain and remove by-products of metabolism that cannot be recycled.

The glymphatic system is the wastewater management or sewer plant that drains CSF out of the brain during sleep. It is believed this CSF cleaning process only happens during sleep. Using the car analogy, your body driving the car throughout the day requires an oil change every night during sleep. Our bodies need dramatic maintenance and repair daily, which only happens during sleep. Not getting enough sleep means you don't get enough repair and maintenance of your car engine.

Adenosine is indeed a component of ATP, the primary energy-producing molecule in the mitochondria of our cells. Let's explore how consuming coffee, experiencing ATP depletion, and suffering from lack of sleep can profoundly impact the immune system, the formation of immunological memory, and various other healthy inflammatory functions.

The immune cascade triggered by infection initiates the activation of key white blood cells such as neutrophils, monocytes, and macrophages, which are the frontline soldiers of the immune system. These cells play a key role in producing inflammatory cytokines, which act as messenger proteins facilitating communication between cells.[256] These messenger proteins, like IL-beta, IL-6, and TNF-alpha, tell the liver to make C-reactive protein

---

[256] Krueger, James M. "The Role of Cytokines in Sleep Regulation." *Current Pharmaceutical Design*, vol. 14, no. 32, 2008, pp. 3408–3416. DOI: 10.2174/138161208786549281

(CRP). Doctors use high-sensitivity CRP (hs-CRP) as a marker to check for heart disease risk or general inflammation.

These cytokines are elevated the morning after as little as a night of four hours of sleep restriction.[257] Inflammatory mediators actually play a role in regulating sleep in the central nervous system (CNS). I'm optimistic that in the future, we may discover biohacks to help reduce inflammation caused by sleep deprivation. But for now, the most effective remedy is simply to avoid inflammation altogether by prioritizing good sleep habits.

During experiments where healthy volunteers were deprived of sleep, researchers observed an increase in blood pressure and other signs of heightened fight-or-flight nervous system activity. This increase in sympathetic output leads to the production of more blood clotting factors by stimulating the blood vessel endothelium—the lining of the arterial wall—which is typically very smooth in a healthy state. This change can elevate shear stresses due to higher blood pressure, consequently triggering inflammatory mediators.[258]

Other data support a connection between increased pain perception and sleep loss.[259] Inflammatory markers, such as prostaglandins and cytokines that increase inflammation, have been demonstrated to sensitize nociceptors, which are pain receptors. This sensitization contributes to the development of spontaneous pain and heightened sensitivity to pain, known as hyperalgesia.

Animal studies have observed decreased bone density in rats subjected to sleep deprivation. Dr. Everson's research on sleep highlighted that after ten days of sleep deprivation, rat blood stem cells were only half as effective. This decline in cell activity was associated with impaired migration ability of the bone stem cells.[260]

---

257 van Leeuwen, Wessel M. A., et al. "Sleep Restriction Increases the Risk of Developing Cardiovascular Diseases by Augmenting Proinflammatory Responses through IL-17 and CRP." *Online*, 2009 Feb 25. DOI: 10.1371/journal.pone.0004589 PMCID: PMC 2643002 PMID: 19240794

258 Meerlo, Peter, Sgoifo, Andrea, & Suchecki, Deborah. "Restricted and Disrupted Sleep: Effects on Autonomic Function, Neuroendocrine Stress Systems, and Stress Responsivity." *Sleep Medicine Reviews*, vol. 12, no. 3, 2008, pp. 197-210. DOI: 10.1016/j.smrv.2007.07.007

259 Schuh-Hofer, Sigrid, et al. "One Night of Total Sleep Deprivation Promotes a State of Generalized Hyperalgesia: A Surrogate Pain Model to Study the Relationship of Insomnia and Pain." *Pain*, vol. 154, no. 9, 2013, pp. 1613-1621. DOI: 10.1016/j.pain.2013.04.046 (Epub 2013 May 11)

260 Everson, C. A., Folley, A. E., & Toth, J. M. "Chronically Inadequate Sleep Results in Abnormal Bone Formation and Abnormal Bone Marrow in Rats." *Experimental Biology and Medicine (Maywood)*, vol. 237, no. 9, 2012, pp. 1101-1109. DOI: 10.1258/ebm.2012.012043 PMID: 22946089

Rodent models that were sleep-deprived died within two to four weeks.[261] The next group died within four to six weeks. The last group didn't die immediately but instead experienced a hyper-metabolic state, developed hypothermia, and were unable to control their temperature regulation. They then developed some ulcerations of the skin and of the GI tract, which ultimately resulted in an overwhelming infection resulting in death by sepsis.

Human trials have demonstrated reduced immunity in sleep-deprived subjects, as evidenced by vaccination experiments measuring antibody production in response to the flu vaccine. These subjects had one half the antibody response to the vaccine after volunteers were sleep-deprived for four hours a night for six days. This impairment persisted for an entire month.

Natural killer cells assail viruses and tumor cells.[262] Research has revealed that healthy volunteers who experienced four hours of sleep loss showed a significant 73 percent reduction in natural killer cells, crucial immune cells that help maintain our health.

From depleted brain fuel to heightened pain perception, reduced bone density, diminished natural killer cells, increased blood pressure, and heightened inflammation, it's clear that sleep deprivation profoundly impacts the immune system—even if individuals manage to remain awake and functional.

Sleep apnea results in sleep loss because it does not allow you to enter the restorative deep stage 3, and REM sleep, just like not scheduling enough sleep or insomnia, will do.

Sleep Deprivation and Glucose Metabolism

Current evidence suggests three pathways that connect sleep deprivation with an increased risk of diabetes and obesity:

1. Alterations in glucose metabolism.
2. Increased appetite.
3. Decreased energy expenditure.

PMCID: PMC3939802

261 Everson, C. A., Bergmann, B. M., & Rechtschaffen, A. "Sleep Deprivation in the Rat: III. Total Sleep Deprivation." *Sleep*, vol. 12, no. 1, 1989, pp. 13-21. DOI: 10.1093/sleep/12.1.13 PMID: 2928622

262 Hurtado-Alvarado, Gabriela, et al. "Sleep Loss as a Factor to Induce Cellular and Molecular Inflammatory Variations." *Journal of Immunology Research*, vol. 2013, Article ID 801341, 14 pages, 2013. DOI: 10.1155/2013/801341

The role of sleep in regulating glucose levels has been acknowledged for over a decade. Initial studies on sleep restriction involved short periods of total sleep deprivation. These studies discovered significant adverse changes in hormone levels and glucose utilization. However, when individuals were given the chance to recover with adequate sleep, these changes were rapidly reversed. Human physiology can tolerate one night of total sleep deprivation, provided there's an opportunity to catch up. However, more relevant experiments examine the effects of partial sleep deprivation over several days or longer periods.

The mechanisms influencing glucose metabolism following repeated partial sleep restriction are thought to be multifaceted. When insulin release drops suddenly, the sympathetic nervous system, particularly the part related to the pancreas, becomes more active. This is connected to the balance between the restful and active parts of our nervous system, and when sleep is limited, it shows up as changes in heart rate patterns in the form of reduced heart rate variability. We want more significant heart rate variability (a higher number).

Releasing hormones that counteract insulin, like Growth Hormone and cortisol, may play a role in the changes seen in glucose regulation when sleep is lost.[263] People tested at the height of sleep deprivation took 40 percent more time than usual to control blood glucose levels, and their ability to produce insulin dropped by around 30 percent.[264]

The disruption in the balance of catabolic (breaking down molecules in metabolism) and anabolic (stimulating protein synthesis, muscle growth, and insulin) hormones results in a dysregulation of the arcuate nucleus in the hypothalamus. This area contains opposing sets of neurons—one stimulating appetite and the other inhibiting it.

Epidemiological data suggest a connection between inadequate sleep (sleep deprivation) and disrupted eating habits, resulting in impulse-driven behaviors, such as irregular meals, frequent snacking, excessive food seasoning

---

263 Schmid, D. A., et al. (2006). Changes of sleep architecture, spectral composition of sleep EEG, the nocturnal secretion of cortisol, ACTH, GH, prolactin, melatonin, ghrelin, and leptin, and the DEX-CRH test in depressed patients during treatment with mirtazapine. *Neuropsychopharmacology*, 31(4), 832-844. doi: 10.1038/sj.npp.1300923.

264 Knutson, K. L., Spiegel, K., Penev, P., & Van Cauter, E. (2007). The metabolic consequences of sleep deprivation. *Sleep Medicine Reviews*, 11(3), 163-178. doi: 10.1016/j.smrv.2007.01.002.

(seeking sweeter or salty flavors), and reduced vegetable consumption.

Findings from the Wisconsin Sleep Cohort Study indicate that sleep loss may affect the accurate signaling of caloric needs by leptin and ghrelin.[265] This imbalance creates an internal perception of insufficient energy availability despite increased caloric intake. Dr. Carol Everson's research on rats subjected to sleep restriction for ten days revealed a persistent 20 percent increase in food intake, even with the opportunity for recovery sleep.[266]

The Nurse's Heart Health Study, which tracked 80,000 women, researchers noted a correlation between sleep duration and Body Mass Index (BMI). They found that nurses who reported sleeping seven to eight hours per night had the lowest average BMI. The bottom line is if we are not well rested, we seek out higher-calorie foods, feel hungrier, and take longer to reach fullness than when we get enough quality restorative sleep.

It's important to emphasize that continuous lack of sleep is a serious issue regarding blood sugar control, appetite, and fat loss.

While there's not a lot of research on how sleep loss affects female hormones, studies on male hormones provide solid evidence. For example, the National Heart, Lung, and Blood Institute funded a study where they deprived 24-year-old men of sleep. They found that their testosterone levels dropped by 10 to 15 percent when they didn't get enough sleep. This decrease seems to be connected to changes in LH (luteinizing hormone), which is made in the front part of the brain. So, if you're worried about your hormone levels, it might be worth adding some extra sleep to your routine and checking your testosterone levels after a month.[267]

Melatonin, often referred to as the circadian sleep hormone because of its role in regulating the twenty-four-hour sleep-wake cycle, holds significant influence over overall health. While research on the effects of exogenous melatonin supplementation exists, it may not replicate the same impact as simply increasing nightly sleep duration. The natural secretion of melatonin

---

265 Young, T., *et al.* (2009). Burden of sleep apnea: rationale, design, and major findings of the Wisconsin Sleep Cohort study. *WMJ*, 108(5), 246-249. PMID: 19743755; PMCID: PMC2858234.

266 Everson, C. A., Bergmann, B. M., & Rechtschaffen, A. (1989). Sleep deprivation in the rat: III. Total sleep deprivation. *Sleep*, 12(1), 13-21. doi: 10.1093/sleep/12.1.13. PMID: 2928622.

267 Greenfield, Ben. "The Terrifying Condition Of Sleep and Dying Earlier Without It." Ben Greenfield Fitness. Ben Greenfield Fitness, n.d. https://bengreenfieldfitness.com/article/sleep-articles/the-terrifying-condition-of-sleep-and-why-youll-die-earlier-if-you-dont-experience-it/ (accessed April 24, 2024).

sets off a series of biological processes. While many people know melatonin as the hormone that helps with sleep, its powerful antioxidant effects might not be as well-known. Surprisingly, melatonin is even better at fighting off harmful molecules than vitamins C, E, A, and carotenoids. And it's not just good for sleep—it also helps protect essential antioxidants in the brain, like glutathione. It is made in many body tissues and cells, not just the pineal gland in the brain.

Unfortunately, melatonin can't renew its antioxidant powers like other antioxidants. So, sleep is essential to restore this important antioxidant. Since sleep is crucial for our overall health, it makes sense that a key player in promoting sleep, like melatonin, also packs a punch as an antioxidant.[268]

Here's how it works: when melatonin is made, it acts like an antioxidant, helping to release glutathione. Why does this matter? Well, when we're low on antioxidants in general or missing one specific helper, glutathione steps in to clear out harmful molecules. But once this job is done, the amount of glutathione goes down, slowing down all the other important things it does in our body, like detoxifying, fixing DNA, recycling antioxidants, giving energy to our cells, and regulating our immune system.[269]

One of the effective ways to support the natural process of sleep, including the release of melatonin, is to steer clear of the light pollution that most of us encounter at night—avoiding bright light sources.

It has been widely reported that blue light is especially detrimental to sleep, but recent studies question that now and even question the effects of white light. Even Dr. Walker has changed his thinking on this topic. He condemned blue light for its impact on sleep in his book *Why We Sleep*, but in a recent interview with Dr. Peter Attia, he took a different position. He says that our engagement with our phones and pads activates our minds with information to the detriment of sleep.

Even though blue light can lower melatonin, it is not clear that it is the leading sleep disruptor. The best way to promote sleep physiology relating to melatonin secretion is likely by avoiding light pollution experienced by most people in the evening and avoiding bright light sources.

---

268 Ibid.

269 Monteiro, Karla Krislane Alves Costa, et al. "Antioxidant Actions of Melatonin: A Systematic Review of Animal Studies." *Antioxidants* 13, no. 4 (2024): 439. https://doi.org/10.3390/antiox13040439.

Using blue light at the right time of day can be beneficial. Bright light therapy, which involves exposure to full-spectrum bright light (10,000 lux) in the morning, is a popular method. It aims to enhance the morning circadian rhythm, especially for individuals with seasonal affective disorder (SAD), a form of depression linked to shorter days in regions with higher latitudes.

Melatonin, a hormone crucial for a healthy circadian rhythm, is produced in the pineal gland in the brain and excreted into the bloodstream to act as a hormone.[270, 271] After the age of forty, melatonin levels may significantly decrease. If considering melatonin supplementation, opt for a product with third-party testing to ensure quality, as the industry has faced issues with variable potency over the years. There has been recent speculation that melatonin can be synthesized, transported, and metabolized in mitochondria. Tryptophan can be converted into melatonin through four enzymatic steps in pineal, retinal, intestinal, and other tissues.[272]

However, even though these assumptions on the effects of light and device brain activation are being questioned now, these devices are with us. In some cases, they help people sleep. The jury is out, but keeping a device in the bedroom that is not in airplane mode is an invitation to disruption.[273] We also do not know how much the EMF radiation they produce disrupts sleep.

Sleep Duration, Genetics, and All-cause Mortality

Studies combining data from various populations, called meta-analyses, have examined how sleep duration relates to the risk of dying from any cause. They found that people who consistently sleep too little have a 10 to 12 percent higher risk of dying prematurely.[274]

---

270 Rahbarghazi, Afshin, *et al.* (2021). "Role of melatonin in the angiogenesis potential: highlights on cardiovascular disease." *Journal of Inflammation*, 18, article number 4.

271 Ibid.

272 Lei X, Xu Z, Huang L, Huang Y, Tu S, Xu L, Liu D. "The potential influence of melatonin on mitochondrial quality control: a review." *Front Pharmacol.* 2024 Jan 11;14:1332567. doi: 10.3389/fphar.2023.1332567. PMID: 38273825; PMCID: PMC10808166.

273 Bauducco, S., Pillion, M., Bartel, K., et al. (2024). "A bidirectional model of sleep and technology use: A theoretical review of How much, for whom, and which mechanisms." *Sleep Medicine Reviews, 76*, 101933.

274 Cappuccio, F. P., D'Elia, L., Strazzullo, P., & Miller, M. A. (2010). "Sleep duration and all-cause

But does everyone respond the same to sleep curtailment?

Recent twin studies have uncovered genetic variations that may protect some people from sleep deprivation. The mutations that occur to the p.Tyr362His BHLHE41 gene (this is just a name for a gene) appear to allow some to tolerate shorter sleep durations and maintain normal alertness and limited signs of inflammation.[275] This mutation is quite rare.

Unfortunately, the average person is currently trying to function like Thomas Edison, which won't end well for most genetically. I think Edison is probably one of those folks who may have had the p.Tyr362His BHLHE41 mutation (only an educated guess).

---

mortality: a systematic review and meta-analysis of prospective studies." *Sleep*, 33(5), 585-592. doi: 10.1093/sleep/33.5.585. PMID: 20469800; PMCID: PMC2864873.

275 Rosekind, M. R., *et al.* (2021). "Awake at the wheel: how auto technology innovations present ongoing sleep challenges and new safety opportunities." *Sleep*, 47(3), Editor's Choice. Oxford University Press.

CHAPTER 6

The Problem of Dental Profession Awareness

The Problem of Awareness

Even though sleep apnea has a widespread impact, many individuals remain undiagnosed, potentially leading to severe health complications, weight gain and inability to lose weight, upset microbiome balance in the gut, sugar cravings, including cardiovascular diseases, stroke, high blood pressure, erectile dysfunction in men, lower testosterone levels in men, lower sperm counts, loss of libido in women, kidney failure, osteoporosis, diabetes, cancer, mental illness, and various chronic illnesses.

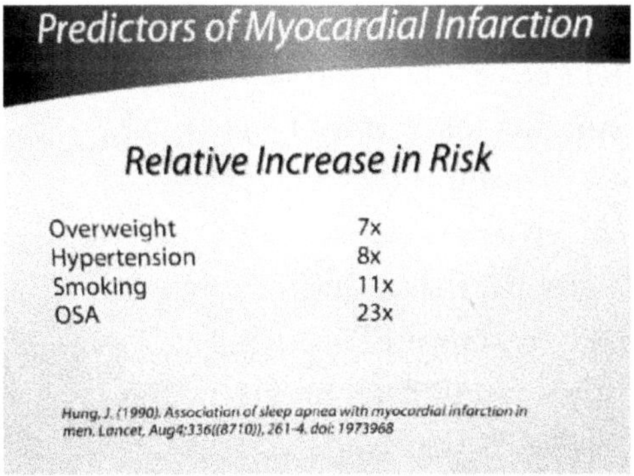

Predictors of Myocardial Infarction

Relative Increase in Risk

Overweight	7x
Hypertension	8x
Smoking	11x
OSA	23x

Hung, J. (1990). Association of sleep apnea with myocardial infarction in men. *Lancet*, Aug4;336((8710)), 261-4. doi: 1973968

Figure 40

You will note throughout this book, we will mention more medical conditions associated with obstructive sleep apnea in multiple places. There will be some we already mentioned, and then more that may not have been mentioned. The condition is quite extraordinarily impactful on all body systems. They are mentioned in various places and not just one long list because the impact of this human condition should become more alarming as you see the whole picture in this book.

Therefore, early identification with thorough diagnostic approaches and subsequent effective treatment options is crucial for effectively managing this condition. The following section will delve into various combined strategies currently employed to address sleep apnea while emphasizing overall health and facial aesthetics.

Combination Therapies

Until now, the utilization of combination strategies has received limited acknowledgment. For instance, a patient might find traditional CPAP treatment challenging due to the high air pressure required. However, combining CPAP with a conventional dental oral appliance therapy (OAT) that repositions the jaw and opens the airway might significantly reduce the CPAP air pressure to more tolerable levels. For certain individuals, using both devices concurrently might be the solution, whereas using either alone may not yield the necessary results. In addition to that, adding OMT may reduce or even eliminate reliance on the devices.

A recent meta-analysis of OMT alone for sleep apnea showed a reduction in AHI scores of 50 percent in adults and over 60 percent in children.[276]

At times, EPAP therapy (Expiratory Positive Airway Pressure) combined with OMT or even oral sleep appliances can achieve acceptable levels of airway sleep support. The BongoRx® is a well-known EPAP therapy (Figure 41). These EPAP nasal inserts have a one-way valve so that when you

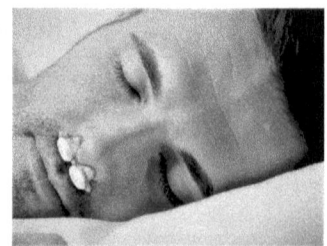

Figure 41: BongoRx®

---

[276] Camacho, Macario *et al.* (2015). "Myofunctional Therapy to Treat Obstructive Sleep Apnea: A Systematic Review and Meta-analysis." *Sleep*, 38(5), 669-6751(https://doi.org/10.5665/sleep.4652).

breathe in through the nose, there is no resistance, but when you breathe out through the nose, there is a slight resistance, and this inflates, and stents open their airway tissues somewhat like a CPAP would do at low-pressure settings. They do require a prescription to use them.

What are Sleep Studies?

Access to sleep testing or sleep studies is difficult for many, depending on where they live. They are expensive too. This is changing now with the astonishing advances in sleep technology, which allows for sleep studies that patients can order by mail. They are handy for many people's needs, including required sleep, health-regulated DOT drivers, ship captains, train engineers, and airline pilots. Some are disposable. They are so small that they can fit on one finger, and those wanting to limit their use face a near-impossible task.[277] You will see some of these sleep tests in the next section.

The initial sleep test and the most comprehensive sleep study is called a PSG or Polysomnography. This extensive sleep examination monitors various body functions and is commonly done in a dedicated sleep laboratory. Alternatively, home sleep tests (HST) or (HSAT) conducted in the comfort of an individual's bed also contribute significantly to finding those who suffer by assessing their apnea type and severity levels. A board-certified sleep physician reads the studies to determine whether these sleep disorders exist in each patient. It is mandated that the results of these tests be interpreted and diagnosed, and treatment plans are prescribed by either a medical doctor or a qualified sleep specialist nurse practitioner.

In the past, these testing services were only done in a hospital or medical sleep diagnostics in-lab center and have been highly regulated and restricted by insurance carriers and various medical and dental regulatory agencies. The restrictions have been justified on the issue of quality of care and who is qualified to order these tests in our various medical and dental professions.

As with many services and products that once were by prescription only or could only be performed in a medical lab or professional office and paid for by medical insurance, this test, along with many others, has been slowly evolving into a service that can be dramatically lowered in cost because of

---

277 Doctor Sleep Show, www.drsleepshow.com.

large volume, direct-to-consumer availability. Once these tests and products became available in direct-to-consumer and by mail order, insurance carriers and medical and dental boards began to try to restrict their distribution to physicians only, and some insurers will only pay for sleep apnea treatment if the sleep study was first prescribed by a face-to-face consultation with their family physician.

We do not want patients who order a sleep study to show up at a medical or dental office with the test data they got from a wearable device and direct those healthcare professionals to prescribe this or that type of therapy. This requires a discussion between the patient and healthcare professional and treatment must be authorized by the primary care physician or sleep physician.

In the past, a sleep study through face-to-face and written authorization by your primary care physician allowed you to get insurance benefits. However, this limits how many will be diagnosed, increasing the testing time and costs.

The restrictions on who can order a sleep study have also resulted in several states enacting rules to disallow dentists to dispense or order a sleep study for a patient. Most states have not enacted those restrictions. Many advocate that a dentist, who has been mandated to assess the symptoms and signs of a patient that might indicate they may be suffering from a sleep disorder and who also sees signs of sleep pathology in the mouth, should be able to order a sleep test. The sleep physician still interprets that test, issues the diagnosis, leads the team, and prescribes care.

Indeed, the American Dental Association recommends dentists screen all patients for sleep disorders. Dentists treat in the exact area where many signs of sleep apnea occur. Sleep apnea causes many dental diseases that we treat. Dentists order blood tests for systemic diseases that affect dental health. Dentists perform biopsies on cancerous lesions. I have ordered liver function tests, CBCs, urinalysis, MRIs, CT scans, antibiotic sensitivity tests, radiologist interpretations, arthrograms, TB tests, vitamin deficiencies tests, and more.

Even though I am retired from practice, I had the opportunity to provide many sleep studies to my patients. Iowa, like the majority of states, permits dentists to conduct sleep studies. Dentists are also authorized to perform other medical laboratory tests. Unfortunately, there is a perceived division between the medical and dental professions when classifying tests. No healthcare specialty should order tests that are not directly relevant to their field. Sleep apnea is closely connected to dental care. Therefore, tests ordered by dentists must be well understood by those who request them.

As a dentist, I do not use a radiologist to interpret my dental X-rays. I am better at interpreting teeth pathology than the radiologists are. Dentistry does have its own oral pathologists to help with other interpretations. On the other hand, if I take a large-volume radiograph of the head or CBCT scan, a general or dental radiologist is more qualified than I am to interpret that entire image. All tests should be used responsibly, including sleep tests, and, most importantly, ordering and interpreting must have the patient's best interest in mind.

Dentists do order sleep studies, tests for Sjogren's Syndrome (an autoimmune disease that dries the mouth), herpes simplex (cold sores), pemphigus (a skin disorder that can cause blisters in the mouth), bleeding time, lichen planus (an autoimmune disorder that causes lesions in the oral tissues), fungal tests, bacterial culture and identification tests, and many others. Alternatively, they may request that the patient's physician or specialists order and interpret these tests.[278]

The requirement that the patient must get authorization from their family doctor to get the sleep study adds a step that discourages patients from getting diagnosed and treated. Understandably, sleep disturbances can be caused or worsened by medical conditions the family doctor is most qualified to manage. At this time, there is a risk for the family doctor treating the comorbidities of sleep apnea and ignoring the epidemic of sleep disturbances causing them. The same risk is true for dentists and other healthcare professionals treating comorbidities instead of ruling out sleep disorders as a possible cause of the disease.

There are just too many people suffering to continue to promote this cumbersome, slow, costly, and rigid requirement to get authorization for a sleep study from the family physician. It is within the scope of dentistry to issue sleep studies when they determine they are warranted by conditions they see in the mouth.

---

278 Greenan, Shawn. "Lab Test Ordering Rights by State: The Ultimate Guide." *Rupa Health*, 29 Mar. 2023, (https://www.rupahealth.com/post/functional-lab-test-ordering-rights-by-state).

The Caution

I will paraphrase a post from the American Academy of Sleep Medicine (AASM) that was reported on LinkedIn. It is about the rapid expansion of home sleep studies and direct-to-customer smart watches and rings. The author of the article said this, and I will paraphrase:

> I've been anticipating this day for years.
>
> Samsung Electronics Co., Ltd. just announced that the sleep apnea feature on the Samsung Health Monitor app (accessible through their watch) has received De Novo authorization from the United States Food and Drug Administration (FDA).
>
> Samsung clarifies that this feature isn't meant to replace a diagnosis made by a qualified clinician and won't be initially accepted by insurance providers.
>
> But starting in the third quarter of this year, a patient, either paying out of pocket or with a high deductible, could walk into your office armed with FDA-approved data from their watch indicating severe OSA. They might decline to pay for a traditional home sleep test and request a CPAP prescription instead.
>
> What's the appropriate response?
>
> This Samsung device is just the beginning. Photoplethysmography (PPG) has already reduced the role of sleep clinicians in interpreting sleep testing results. Still, PPG has also made sleep breathing assessment more accessible for patients. This could further improve access but sideline sleep clinicians altogether. (PPG analyzes the optical blood volume variations of blood vessels, authors note.)
>
> The watch "detects signs of moderate to severe OSA," but what about false negatives?
>
> Could loud snorers with high BMI, excessive daytime sleepiness (EDS), cardiovascular disease (CVD), and type 2 diabetes mellitus (DMII) be walking around thinking they don't have OSA because of this watch? We need to address this before the third quarter arrives.
>
> And that's just one of the problems on the horizon. Currently, in the US, over 60 percent of home sleep studies are ordered by

non-sleep clinicians who often stop after a single inconclusive result. I don't see this trend slowing down. There simply aren't enough of us to handle all these patients anyway.

So, how do we protect patients without restricting access?

If we can't stop them, we can educate them.

As an academy, our best action may be to launch a campaign and develop educational content for providers outside our field (including information on HSAT technology), focusing on residency programs (and advanced practice provider programs).

To ensure it sticks, he said, we should push to increase the amount of OSA content on their board exams.[279]

(For your information, photo-plethysmography (PPG), mentioned above, is the type of technology used in the SleepImage Ring shown in this book.)

Dr. Zelk and I agree with much of what was said here by the AASM. More education of healthcare providers needs to be implemented. This should also occur with primary care medical providers, too.

Many dentists now know more about sleep disorders than the family physician from whom they are requesting authorization.

However, many allied health professionals and primary care providers may need more education to determine the significance or lack of significance of a single-night study or even multiple-night studies in ruling out obstructive sleep apnea. As the AASM statement says, over 60 percent of home sleep studies are ordered by non-sleep specialists. Some may conduct a study and fail to have it interpreted by a sleep specialist, believing it unnecessary after looking at the results. Dr. Zelk advocates all sleep studies be interpreted by a sleep specialist, regardless of whether the patient is deemed worthy of being referred for a prescription by a sleep specialist. No sleep test should be put in a record that is not, at least, interpreted by a sleep specialist.

The ADA has not taken a position (that we are aware of) on dentists dispensing or ordering sleep studies. The ADA did recommend dentists screen for sleep disorders in 2017 due to the high number of undiagnosed

---

[279] "Samsung Health Monitor App's Sleep Apnea Feature Receives FDA De Novo Authorization." *AASM Members Forum Post*. February 18, 2024. Available at: AASM Members Forum Post.

patients with sleep disorders. Dr. Zelk and I believe, this recommendation now makes it the standard of care in dentistry.

However, these restrictions against dentists ordering sleep studies in seven states do not prevent patients from ordering their sleep studies from a website offering those studies. It seems odd that a patient can order a study for themselves, but a dentist cannot order one for their patient in these few states. A dentist in a restricted state could have the patient go to one of these many websites and order their test.

As we said before, even though a patient can order their own sleep study, some insurance carriers will not cover the cost of the study or the cost of treatment because the study was not ordered by their MD, DO, NP or PA. In those cases, the patient can take the self-ordered test results to the family doctor and present it as the reason the patient needs a sleep study prescribed by the MD, DO, NP or PA. The sleep test is then retaken. This additional test adds to the diagnostic database as well.

The low cost of these tests makes them financially attractive, even with the extra tests they must take to navigate the gauntlet placed before them in the name of quality care. Even though the test costs more than it should because of these requirements, it is still less costly and faster than the traditional in-lab testing system. One must remember, however, that sometimes in-lab testing is the best choice, especially if the sleep disorder is something other than obstructive sleep apnea.

There are now sleep specialists who will evaluate a patient via telemedicine to issue a prescription for a sleep study so that the patient does not have to get authorization from their family doctor. Then, the patient can get that sleep study from their dentist, chiropractor, family doctor, or an online sleep study site and move on through the system.

Diagnostic Tools

As was previously mentioned, sophisticated diagnostic methods empower doctors to create personalized treatment plans for each patient. Polysomnography (PSG), the most detailed diagnostic instrument of sleep disorders, is like a comprehensive sleep detective computer monitor. It collects readings of various sleep-related indicators, monitoring brain activity, eye movements, heart rate, muscle patterns, airflow levels, blood oxygen saturation, and much more throughout a night's sleep. These insights unveil the frequency and duration of breathing pauses and help guide treatment choices for those with this condition. While polysomnography offers an in-depth understanding of sleep disturbances, the downside might be a clinic's cost and the unfamiliar sleep setting, potentially influencing test results. Despite its drawbacks, it remains a powerful tool for "sleep detectives"—the sleep experts.

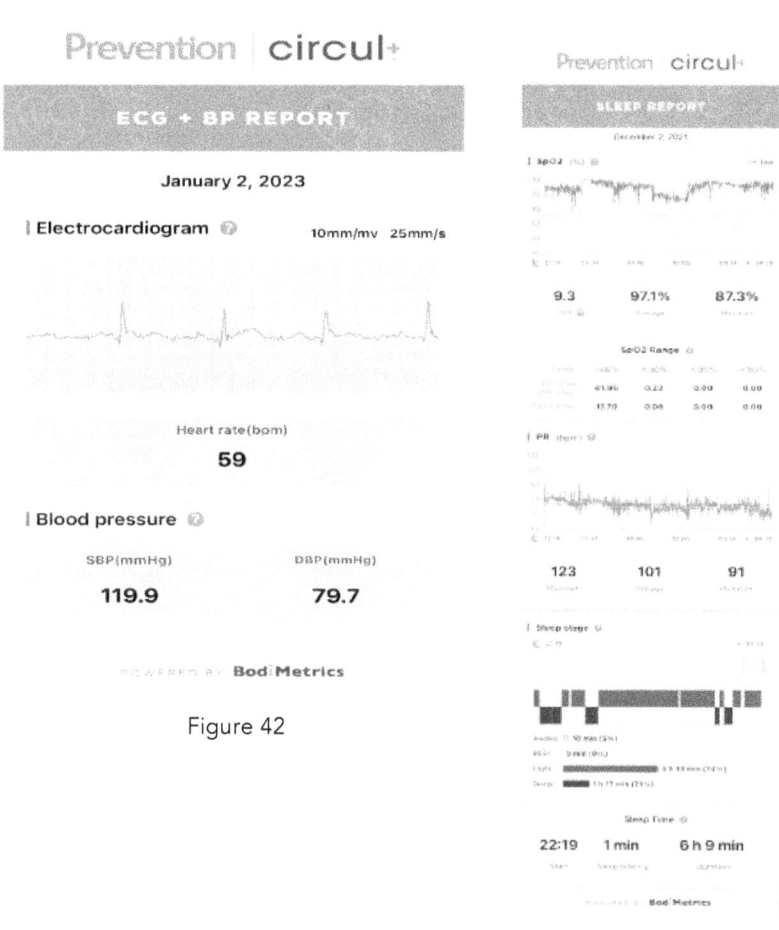

Figure 42

Figure 43

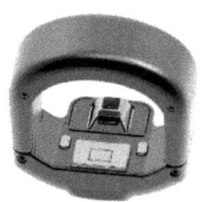

Figure 44: Circul+ ®

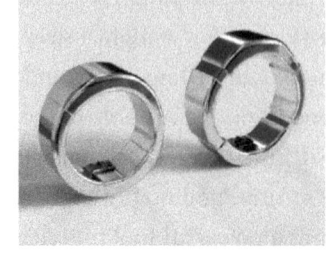

Figure 45: Circul IQ ®

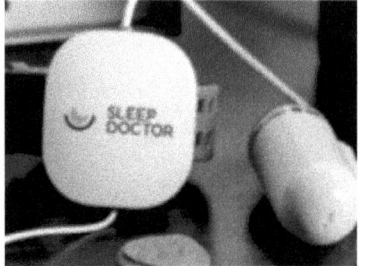

Figure 46: WatchPAT One®

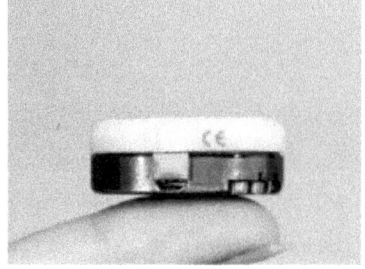

Figure 47: NightOwl®

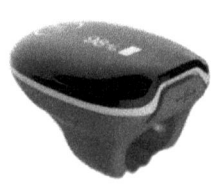

Figure 48: SleepImage®

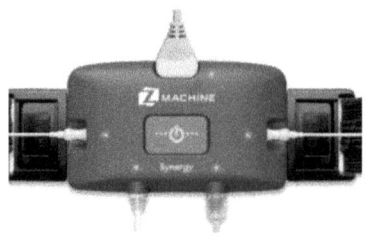

Figure 49: Z Machine®

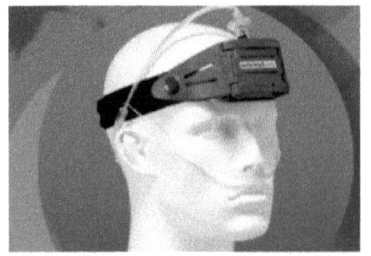

Figure 50: Ares®

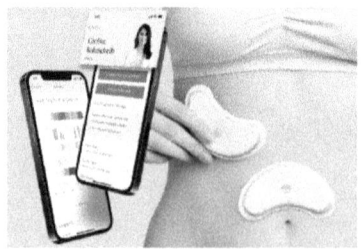

Figure 51: Wesper®

Today, many sleep clinics send patients home with a home sleep test device. They can also order them online.

Traditional polysomnography may be unacceptable due to financial or scheduling conflicts, while the home sleep apnea test offers an alternative. The HST or HSAT simplified diagnostic device can be conducted in a person's bedroom, measuring essential body functions such as airflow, oxygen levels, sleep interruption events, sleep latency or how long it takes you to fall asleep, sleep architecture (the sleep stages you go through during the night), and heart rate. They do not have leg monitors for limb movement disorders. Some do have ECG leads to measure brain waves.

Some HST devices approach the accuracy and measure close to the same number of physiologic parameters as the in-lab PSG. Although most HSTs or HSATs do not yield as much detail as a sleep clinic study, its convenience appeals to many seeking answers without the substantial expense or scheduling challenges.

As we have mentioned, new home HSTs have gotten so small and convenient that they can fit on one finger (Figures 47 and 48). This has made them quite popular. These devices can help diagnose obstructive sleep apnea, but most cannot be used to diagnose other types of sleep disorders. Most sleep apneas are obstructive apneas, and they, therefore, are helpful for most people. You will see a small sample of some home sleep studies here. The NightOwl®, The SleepImage Ring®, The Ares®, The Watchpat®, The Z Machine®, the Wesper®, and more are all home sleep studies that can be sent to a person by mail or dispensed at your medical or dental office.

Also shown in Figures 43, 44 and 45 are an FDA-registered pulse oximeters for any skin color called the Circul+® ring and Circul IQ® ring for monitoring oxygen levels at home and in clinics. This ring has overcome the racial bias in pulse oximeters for skin pigment color. It is accurate for all skin types. Although the Circul+® and Circul IQ® are not classified as home sleep studies in the U.S., they are in some other countries. Instead, they are high-sensitivity pulse oximeters.

It is superb for screening for sleep apnea and daily monitoring of oxygen levels, electrocardiogram, skin temperature, heart rate, blood pressure, sleep latency, oxygen desaturation index, sleep stages, sleep onset, and sleep time. It also measures the percentage of the time below 90 percent oxygen saturation, (heart rate variability for medical or dental clinic monitoring portals), and an oxygen saturation graph plotted all night and every one second.

We do not expect you to understand all these measuring tools. Still, it is provided so that you know this ring, and instruments like it are valuable for clinicians who want to "titrate" their treatment therapies to see where adjustments need to be made. This little device can also be used in some DOT driver sleep monitoring programs to help keep our roads safer. It can also be used to detect COVID-19 infections by measuring oxygen drops and does so much sooner than a temperature reading can do. "Titration" just means adjusting or fine-tuning an air pressure or jaw position settings to see which setting works best for a person to open the airways.

CHAPTER 7

The Dawning Awareness of the Dental Profession

A Dawning Awareness

In dental education, dentists receive comprehensive training spanning various specialties within the field. The National Commission on Recognition of Dental Specialties and Certifying Boards (NCRDSCB) recognizes twelve distinct dental specialties, which encompass:

- Dentist Anesthesiologist
- Periodontology (Diagnosis and Treatment of Gum Diseases)
- Prosthodontics (Involving Fixed and Removable Dentures)
- Endodontics (Root Canal Therapy)
- Pedodontics (Pediatric Dental Care)
- Oral and Maxillofacial Pathology
- Dental Public Health
- Oral Medicine
- Oral and Maxillofacial Radiology

- Oral and Maxillofacial Surgery
- Orofacial Pain
- Orthodontics and Dentofacial Orthopedics

General dentists have the opportunity to perform procedures in any of these specialty areas as long as they can demonstrate competence in these fields and maintain the same standard of care as a specialist. After dental school, many dentists further their expertise by becoming proficient in one or more specialty domains. Some pursue specialization after participating in general practice residencies, while others engage in continuing education programs. It's not uncommon for specialists to oversee these training programs, enabling general dentists to attain Fellowship or Diplomate credentials in specific areas of interest.

Upon graduating from dental school, I believed that the area of patient care in which had received the least training was orthodontics. Our education has equipped us for operative dentistry, periodontal care, and prosthodontics. We were well-versed in oral surgery, allowing us to perform tooth extractions and certain gingival surgeries.

The standard practice involved general dentists referring patients to specialists for procedures they didn't feel confident performing, which is a sound approach. We had the training to address any type of tooth requiring a root canal procedure. However, the extent to which dentists referred root canals and surgeries to specialists varied, with some opting to handle these procedures themselves while others preferred referring to specialized care.

On the other hand, orthodontic care, even minor orthodontics or tooth crowding in growing children, was not something I recall I felt confident treating. When I started my practice, I had some training to know when to refer to orthodontic specialists. To gain in-depth knowledge of orthodontic care, I and many of my general dentist colleagues had to take many courses. I even took courses from those offered by the American Orthodontic Association after graduation. I also took a two-year comprehensive straight wire program to learn the bracket philosophies and cephalometric analysis (referring to the dental and skeletal relationships of a human skull) used to diagnose and manage orthodontic cases effectively. Things are changing.

Both dentists and orthodontic specialists are paying more attention to airway and facial aesthetics.

Notably, general dentists are participating in orthodontic care. This does not mean that those general dentists address airway issues or understand the impact on tongue space and facial beauty. Still, it does show that they are moving forward to add the skills of orthodontic care to the general dental knowledge they gained at school.

A study was conducted by the University of Michigan that surveyed general dentists on the orthodontic services they provide. The study found that 76.3 percent of responding dentists offer orthodontic services to their patients, with only a few practitioners spending more than 50 percent of their time providing them. Most of these dentists refer more complex cases to orthodontists.[280]

The growing awareness of more airway-centered orthodontic care is now taught in postgraduate education by orthodontist specialists. Many of these general dentists and orthodontists have gained diplomatic status in the American Association of Dental Sleep Medicine, the strongest national organization in dentistry, educating and advocating for dental sleep medicine. They oversee the education of most dentists in this important partnership with the medical profession treating patients who suffer from these sleep oxygen suffocation conditions.

Since this is a medical condition being treated by dentists, this organization is also helping medical insurance carriers and government regulatory agencies navigate the definitions and rules regarding this care for dentists and their oversight by the State Boards of Examiners.

The downside is that dentists need to decide on their own that this airway education is worth their time and that they want to practice this style of dentistry when it should be a larger area of study in every dental curriculum, every orthodontic curriculum, and even in the dental hygiene curriculum before students graduate.

Dentistry has gone through at least four phases of airway health awareness.

---

280 Wolsky, Shari L., DDS, MS, and James A. McNamara, Jr., DDS, PhD. (1996). "Orthodontic services provided by general dentists." *American Journal of Orthodontics and Dentofacial Orthopedics*, 110(2), 211-2171(https://www.ajodo.org/article/S0889-5406%2896%2970111-7/ppt).

Dentistry used to be concerned with whole-body health, but it somehow lost its way due to the enormous amount of dental decay that started appearing in modern society. Once dental hygienists and fluoride came onto the scene, the focus on the enamel of the teeth wasn't as pressing. Cosmetic dentistry took giant leaps; the focus on the shrinking face was negligible. Instead, the crowded teeth were treated by tooth extraction and orthodontic alignment with little awareness of the airway. This lack of understanding was not only in orthodontic education but in all categories and specialties of dental education.

1. **Tunnel Vision.** Dentists looked at teeth, treated their diseases, and lined up the teeth to look straight and have what they call an ideal "class 1 bite," where the teeth fit into precise cusp-to-fossa relationships (this a correct pattern of the teeth bite relationship between upper and lower teeth). There was a limited vision of teeth and other oral tissues without consideration of airway health, even though they treated structures directly in a significant airway space. Teeth were aligned by trying to fit them into the jaw size rather than making jaw sizes larger to fit the teeth. We were taught to use Moyer's or Hixon and Oldfather's analysis[281] to determine when to do serial extractions. This is a procedure where, after measuring jaw space, baby teeth and permanent teeth are removed in sequential order and at a certain age in children to ensure teeth erupt into enough space not to be crowded.

   If the tongue space was infringed upon, the focus was whether or not a patient was biting their tongue, could speak properly, and ate normally, not airway patency.

2. The first glimpse of **awareness** for dentists that they could help with airways came from the realization that some of the splints we made for tooth grinding or bruxism helped with airways. The first oral appliances to create better jaw TMJ health that brought the jaw down and forward were introduced. Harold Gelb, DDS, was

---

281 Staley, R. N., and Kerber, P. E. (1980). "*A revision of the Hixon and Oldfather mixed-dentition prediction method.*" American Journal of Orthodontics, 78(3), 296-302. (https://doi.org/10.1016/0002-9416(80)90274-2).

among the first to advocate this new jaw position. The fact that this position was not a repeatable anatomic position resulted in furious debates. What I mean by repeatable jaw position is that dentists at that time were widely advocating pushing the jaw up and back and having the jaw open and close like a hinge. This movement is pretty repeatable for a dentist to build a person's bite. Still, it is not truly normal or comfortable because when human jaws open, the joint heads on each side of your face move forward and out of the sockets they are cradled in.

I attended one of his presentations early in Dr. Gelb's career at a national meeting in Chicago around 1976. I was stationed at the Great Lakes Naval Dental Center as a U.S. Navy dental officer. While at that meeting, I saw the dental audience's anger and accusations; it was eye-opening, but I believed Dr. Gelb was right. He and people like him helped patients get rid of jaw and headache pain and later gained awareness that their care improved the airway.

Dr. Gelb's son, Dr. Micheal Gelb, is now carrying on his father's legacy with equally significant jaw and airway advances. After Dr. Harold Gelb and others advanced these breakthroughs, dentists began working with physicians to help patients with jaw pain and headaches, mild to moderate sleep apnea, and those who do not tolerate CPAP wear.

3. The **expansion** of sleep apnea care in dentistry led to the establishment of the American Board of Dental Sleep Medicine, collaborating closely with the American Association of Sleep Medicine. Training and guidelines for achieving expert Diplomate status in dental sleep medicine primarily focused on oral sleep appliances and fundamental principles of sleep science. As we mentioned before, in 2017, the American Dental Association recommended that all dentists screen for sleep disorders in their practices. The recommendation urged screening and subsequent referral to an appropriate healthcare facility for testing and treatment.[282]

---

[282] American Dental Association. (2017). "Policy on Dentistry's Role in the Treatment of Sleep-Related Breathing Disorders." Accessed April 12, 2024, (https://www.ada.org/en/about-the-ada/

4. **Realization and Envisioning:** Recognition of the strong correlation between facial symmetry, facial form deficiency, and airway health, including sleep apnea, has become apparent. Traditional treatments for sleep apnea, such as oral appliances and CPAP, did not consistently yield successful outcomes. Some dentists who focused on enhancing the airway and promoting facial aesthetics observed additional benefits, with some patients experiencing a side benefit of improved sleep health for some patients.[283]

In the realm of clear aligner orthodontics, practitioners like Dr. Terry Coddington and Dr. Geoffrey Skinner, and many more, shifted their approach, opting to expand arches by uprighting teeth tipped into the tongue space with clear aligners such as Invisalign® and Candid Pro® rather than reducing tooth size to align them. This had a parallel improvement for many in airway volume.[284]

Another innovative approach by dentists like Dr. W. Moon, Dr. Kasey Li, Dr. Illya Lipkin, Dr. Kimberly Santiago, Dr. Marianna Evans, and others involve using mini dental implants to expand the bony palate, which is sometimes surgically assisted.[285] This often not only improves the oral airway but also can enhance nasal airway functionality because the roof of the mouth is also the floor of the nose.[286] By doing this, airways can be expanded beyond the limitations of orthodontics alone.

Dr. Kevin Boyd, DDS, MS, is a board-certified pediatric dentist with over twenty years of experience providing dental care to infants, children, adolescents, and young adults, including those with special needs.[287] He developed a medical theory called Darwinian

---

ada-positions-policies-and-statements/policy-on-dentistrys-role-in-the-treatment-of-sleep-related-breathing-disorders)

283 Miraglia, B. (n.d.). *Dr. Ben Miraglia - About Me*. Retrieved from https://www.benmiraglia.com/about

284 Coddington, T., & Skinner, G. (n.d.). *SmileWright Dentistry - Terry Coddington, DMD, MSD, GED & Geoffrey Skinner, DDS, GED*. Retrieved from l(https://www.smilewright.com/).

285 Moon, S. W. (2017). "The Use of Mini-Implants for Dental and Orthopedic Applications." Retrieved from https://jksom.org/journal/view.php?number=6921

286 *Your Health Magazine*. "Mouth Breathing and Dentistry." *Your Health Magazine*, n.d., https://yourhealthmagazine.net/article/dental-health/mouth-breathing-and-dentistry/ (accessed April 24, 2024).

287 Kids Dental World. "Meet Our Doctors | Antioch Pediatric Dentist | Brentwood Pediatric Dentist." *Kids Dental World*, https://www.kidsdentalworld.com/meet-our-doctors.html (accessed

Dentistry, based on studying prehistoric fossil remains of human ancestors. Dr. Boyd's theory aligns with his expertise as a dentist and offers much information about the past and future of children's healthcare. Dr. Boyd has been championing pediatric orthodontics, treating children with breathing and airway size discrepancies in the under-three-year-old crowd.[288]

Some orthodontists and general dentists have spoken to patients for many years, and even today, about fitting their teeth to the size of the jaws. With this philosophy, teeth are removed or shaped smaller to fit the jaw space. Today, many orthodontists and general dentists are shifting the philosophy of orthodontic care and newer science to airway-focused care. The language given to many patients is nearly the opposite of what it used to be. Today, many say we must fit our jaws to our teeth. This is a necessary mindset and treatment strategy change. When this approach is taken, teeth are less likely to be removed, and the jaw and tongue space is larger to fit crowded teeth.

The shifting away from the old alignment of teeth only focuses on a newer jaw and face approach by dentists and orthodontists educated in airway matters, which involves moving away from most tooth removal for orthodontic purposes. Instead, the focus is on helping to expand jaw and tooth arches to restore this lost genetic growth potential and re-accommodate the required airway space. The great side benefit of this approach is often enhanced facial symmetry and beauty.[289]

One of the champions in the orthodontic profession for beautiful faces and airway health is orthodontist Dr. William H. Hang, DDS, MSD, who has, on his website, said this about his Face Focused® philosophy of care. I will paraphrase his statements.

April 24, 2024).

288 Boyd, K. (2017). *Darwinian Dentistry*. Retrieved from https://www.findinggeniuspodcast.com/podcasts/darwinian-dentistry-kevin-boyd-dds-ms-pediatric-dentist-early-orthodontics-evolutionary-medicine-and-the-future-of-dentistry/

289 Harari, D., Redlich, M., & Miri, S. (2017). Impacted wisdom teeth—diagnostic imaging of a "silent" condition. *Oral Radiology*, 33(1), 18-23.

Dr. Hang has focused his career on advocating for a new approach to orthodontics that challenges traditional methods, particularly the practice of removing teeth, which often leads to pulling the front teeth backward to close the gaps. His treatment philosophy, "Face Focused®," aims to promote forward growth of the jaws, enhance facial symmetry, improve overall facial aesthetics, maintain an open airway, and achieve broad smiles extending to the corners of the mouth.

Regarding orthodontics, Dr. Hang's website says he does not believe one treatment can fit every patient. Over the years, experience has taught him that the easier way to treat is not always the best.

His website says he spreads awareness about the benefits of the Face Focused® philosophy to patients, parents, and professionals, and develops treatments based on these principles for patients of all ages, and teaches these methods to other dentists and orthodontists worldwide through seminars, workshops, and mini-residencies.[290]

Dr. Hang changed how he performed orthodontic care often without support from colleagues on non-extraction orthodontics, especially early in his transformation into the way he would practice his profession. When I watched one of his interviews online, he mentioned his growing realization and disillusionment over time about the methods he was taught to correct malocclusion, and he now believed it was wrong. He related some of the techniques he was taught in graduate school that he believed had poor supporting science to back up their treatment philosophies.

He also no longer believes general dentists should be barred from delivering orthodontic care as he once thought, as long as they become trained and can provide the standard of care as well as orthodontists.[291]

Dr. William Hang and Dr. Michael Gelb stated this in their publication for the magazine *Cranio*. I will paraphrase their statement. They said that they advocate optimizing the airway of every patient and avoiding any treatment that may compromise the airway, no matter how small, to be the standard of care in Airway Centric® Dentistry.[292] We agree with this statement. Dr. Hang

---

290 Hang, W. M. (n.d.). *Orthotropics*®. Retrieved from https://orthotropics.com/dr-bill-hang/.

291 Ibid.

292 Hang, W. M., & Gelb, M. (2017). "Airway Centric® TMJ philosophy/Airway Centric®

now recommends and teaches others about reversing extraction retraction orthodontics for those who might suffer from its consequences.[293]

Orthotropics is a term first coined by Dr. Michael Mew and his father, Dr. John Mew. Both Dr. Michael and his father are from England. They are British orthodontists who have been involved in developing the field of orthotropics, which is an approach to orthodontics that focuses on facial and jaw development to achieve a complete genetic expression of the craniofacial respiratory complex. And in doing so, optimal oral health and overall well-being are attained. Dr. John Mew, in particular, is known for his pioneering work in orthotropics and has contributed significantly to understanding facial growth and development. It also addresses biological, dietary, and cultural changes that have led to a rapid negative oral devolution shift towards smaller jaws and crooked, crowded teeth. These smaller jaws result in small nasal passages that predispose people to mouth breathing, which continues with a rapid reduction in proper facial development.

I want to highlight an important point. He said a reduction in jaw size is associated with smaller nasal passages. This connection arises partly because the palate, serving as the roof of the mouth, also acts as the floor for the nose. When the palate's width diminishes, the width of the nasal floor may similarly decrease, and the nose narrows, too. Additionally, the constriction of palate width can result in a high and vaulted roof of the mouth, pushing vertically into the nasal cavity. This elevation hinders the tongue from resting correctly on the roof of the mouth, leading to a low tongue posture and a propensity for open-mouth breathing.

Mewing

Since mewing has become a trendy subject on TikTok and other social media, a quick note about it is warranted. One of the concepts that John Mew was criticized for is a concept that suggests that proper tongue posture and correct oral posture can improve facial appearance and potentially correct specific dental and skeletal issues. According to the theory, maintaining the correct

---

orthodontics ushers in the post-retraction world of orthodontics." *CRANIO®, 35*(2), 68-78. doi: 10.1080/08869634.2016.1192315, Epub 2016 Jun 30.

293 Harari, D., Redlich, M., & Miri, S. (2017). "Reversing Retractive Orthodontics with Biobloc Orthotropics." *The Journal of Gnathologic Orthopedics and Facial Orthotropics*, 30(4).

tongue posture—pressing the entire tongue against the roof of the mouth, including the back—stimulates proper facial and jawbone development, leading to enhanced facial aesthetics and improved oral health. In theory, this agrees with orofacial myofunctional therapy in some respects.

The idea behind mewing is that when the tongue is positioned correctly, it exerts gentle pressure on the palate, potentially encouraging forward growth of the maxilla (upper jaw) and helping to create adequate space for the teeth. This, in turn, may result in improved facial symmetry, a more defined jawline, and potentially a straighter smile. It may improve muscle and nerve function.

Dr. John Mew was primarily concerned about facial appearance and did not emphasize these exercises to improve airways, as does orofacial myofunctional therapy. When considering the effectiveness of mewing, it's important to note that this topic sparks debate within the scientific community. While some anecdotal evidence supports that Mew's tongue posture can potentially influence facial development, robust scientific research cannot prove its efficacy.

I believe the mewing exercises are suitable for the face and jaw muscles. They might also help with other therapies to improve bony facial aesthetics. Muscles will work better if they get this exercise. As with any treatment, I also believe better-quality studies are needed.

Orthotropics

Some believe a heightened palatal vault can contribute to a deviated septum. This is because the upward movement of the palate leaves insufficient space for the septum's vertical growth, causing it to bow sideways.[294]

Orthotropics highlight the rarely discussed epidemic of poor jaw development leading to poor airway development that then results in poor breathing during sleep and when awake. The connections can and should be made more evident to the general public. These issues result in poor sleep and sleep deprivation. The opportunity exists to arm people with the information needed to help save their health and help prevent the problem of poor

---

294 Mayo Clinic. (n.d.). "Deviated septum - Symptoms & causes." Retrieved from https://www.mayoclinic.org/diseases-conditions/deviated-septum/symptoms-causes/syc-20351710

breathing in their developing children before it worsens. This issue should galvanize parents, general dentists, pediatricians, pediatric dentists, and orthodontists in significant ways.[295]

Small upper jaw size can also lead to the backward movement of the lower jaw due to its width restriction lagging behind the width restriction of the upper arch. To visualize, consider the dental arches somewhat V-shaped, with the front teeth closer together in arch width than the back teeth. If the upper arch narrows while the lower arch is slightly wider than the upper, the lower jaw must move backward to align the teeth when biting down. This adjustment is necessary to fit the narrower width space created by the upper arch by moving the lower jaw back so that the narrower width between the front teeth of the lower jaw can fit within the constricted upper width space. The lower teeth must move back enough to find an adequate width of the upper teeth to fit into. Consequently, this backward movement of the lower jaw restricts the airway space because the tongue moves backward with the jaw to a less optimal position.[296]

The controversy among professionals that these advocates for airway-centric care encounter persists. In 2022 Dr. Michael Mew was brought before a tribunal in London for his advocacy of these principles. Here is a summary from a news article at the time of his tribunal.

> Dr. Mike Mew, known for his 'mewing' techniques, which have garnered nearly two billion views on TikTok, is facing a misconduct hearing at the General Dental Council (GDC). They claimed his technique could be harmful to patients. They said he had been acting 'pejoratively' against the orthodontic profession. This tribunal resulted in Dr. Mew having his dental license revoked.[297]

---

295 Mew, J., & Mew, M. (n.d.). "Dr. Mike Mew & John Mew: Who Created Mewing and Orthotropics?" Retrieved from https://www.mewing.app/blog/dr-mike-mew-john-mew

296 Hang, W. M., & Gelb, M. (2017). "Airway Centric® TMJ philosophy/Airway Centric® orthodontics ushers in the post-retraction world of orthodontics." *CRANIO®*, *35*(2), 68-78. doi: 10.1080/08869634.2016.1192315.

297 PA Media. (2022, November 14). "Orthodontist advised treatment with risk of harm to children, tribunal told." *The Guardian*.

Dr. Zelk Presents Sleep Physiology and Then Screening Tools Used by Dentists

Soporific neurotransmitters refer to neurotransmitters or chemical messengers in the brain that induce sleep or drowsiness and have a calming or sleep-inducing effect. These neurotransmitters play a role in promoting sleep and relaxation. Examples of soporific neurotransmitters include:

- Serotonin, often linked with mood regulation, also plays a role in the sleep-wake cycle. It is a precursor to melatonin, a hormone essential for regulating sleep.
- GABA, (Gamma-Aminobutyric Acid), an inhibitory neurotransmitter, helps calm the brain by reducing neural excitability, thus promoting relaxation and sleep.
- Melatonin, primarily a hormone, also functions as a neurotransmitter. It plays a critical role in regulating the circadian rhythm and inducing sleepiness.
- Adenosine, Adenosine levels increase during wakefulness and decrease during sleep. It has a calming effect on the brain and is involved in homeostatic sleep regulation.

These neurotransmitters work together to modulate the sleep-wake cycle and contribute to the overall regulation of sleep. Soporific neurotransmitters are involved in signaling the transition from wakefulness to sleep, helping to induce and maintain a state of rest.

Serotonin, which is known for affecting our moods, also plays a part in controlling when we're awake or asleep. It's kind of like a starter for melatonin, which is super important for making sure we sleep well.

GABA (Gamma-Aminobutyric Acid) is a neurotransmitter that calms the brain. It tells the brain to calm down and prepare for sleep by making things less exciting.

Melatonin, even though it's mainly a hormone, also works as a neurotransmitter. It's in charge of keeping our body's internal clock in check and making us feel sleepy when it's time to hit the hay.

A regular sleep schedule allowing for approximately 16 hours of wakefulness will maintain a normal homeostatic sleep drive. The longer a person is awake, the more adenosine builds up in the cerebral spinal fluid (CSF). This drives the person to feel sleepy. A common habit of drinking caffeine blocks adenosine receptors and fools the brain into thinking it is more alert despite these high levels of adenosine in the CSF. The average sleeper will use this strategy to increase the sleep-promoting neurotransmitter adenosine in the cerebrospinal fluid to allow for natural sleep onset. This will reduce the need to add amino acid precursors for GABA neurotransmitters or melatonin supplements.

It's a good idea to dim down bright lights to below 80 lux after 6 p.m. to help your body prepare for sleep. But it can be tricky because most indoor lights are much brighter than that, usually over 100 lux. Many electronic devices also emit bright light, which can interfere with melatonin production, making it even harder to wind down for bedtime. Adding blue wavelength-blocking glasses may improve natural melatonin production. Putting lights on a dimmer in the kitchen, bedroom, and family room can make a big difference, too.

Avoid electromagnetic frequencies disrupting slow wave sleep (SWS) generation and Rapid Eye Movement (REM) sleep. Try not to leave relaxation until the very end of your day. Incorporate some calming activities into the hour before bedtime, like reducing the amount of light around you. You might also consider using a sleep induction mat with acupressure points (it's my personal favorite), trying heart rate variability training, or using brainwave entrainment techniques. These can help you unwind and get into a more relaxed state before hitting the hay,[298] deep, slow breathing (box breathing), tapping (EFT), and don't go to bed until sleepy. The period between the time your head rests on the pillow in bed and the time you fall asleep is called sleep latency. The recommended sleep latency is about five to twenty minutes.

Brainwave entrainment works with neuroplasticity (the neurons in the brain adapting and changing through growth and reorganization) using specific frequency sound waves and binaural beats. The science on this is

---

[298] Huang, T. L., & Charyton, C. (2008). "A Comprehensive Review of the Psychological Effects of Brainwave Entrainment." *Alternative Therapies in Health and Medicine*, 14(5), 38-50.

not well developed. Binaural beats happen when you hear two tones with different frequencies—one in each ear. Your brain then creates a third tone that seems to "swing" back and forth between the two tones. These beats can be detected within the frequency range of approximately 1–30 Hz, aligning with the primary human EEG frequency bands. The brainwave entrainment theory suggests that external stimulation at a specific frequency can synchronize the brain's electrocortical activity to that frequency, forming the foundation for investigating the impact of binaural beat stimulation on cognitive and emotional states.[299] Braintap® at braintap.com is a source for more information on brainwave therapies and is headed by Patric Porter, PhD.

One of the worst things to do for someone with insomnia is going to bed early and then lying awake for hours. Doing this repeatedly can train your brain to associate the bed with being awake. Over time, the brain can create pathways that reflect our sleep habits, so years of neglecting our sleep needs may wire us to become poor sleepers as we get older. This is especially problematic for people aged fifty or older, as sleep tends to become less solid and less deep with age, adding to the challenges of an aging brain.

The evidence emphasizing the importance of getting enough sleep is becoming increasingly clear. For those aiming to enhance performance or maintain optimal health, paying attention to sleep is essential. Most individuals require at least seven to eight hours of actual sleep each night, not just time spent in bed.

As evident from the increasing concerns about inflammation, immune system issues, weight gain, high blood pressure, and hormonal imbalances, many people are striving to manage these health challenges. However, these issues could potentially be prevented by harnessing the power of our natural healing resource: sleep.

---

[299] Ingendoh, R. M., Posny, E. S., & Heine, A. (2023). "Binaural beats to entrain the brain? A systematic review of the effects of binaural beat stimulation on brain oscillatory activity, and the implications for psychological research and intervention." *PLoS ONE*, 18(5), Article e0286023. doi: 10.1371/journal.pone.0286023.

Ways to achieve goals for optimal sleep

1. The easiest way to gauge if you're getting enough sleep is by monitoring your alertness during the day.

2. If you find yourself relying on an alarm clock to wake up in the morning, nodding off during the afternoon or meetings, or dozing off in front of the TV in the evening, it's a sign that you're not getting sufficient rest.

3. Another way to assess your sleep quality is by measuring your morning heart rate variability (HRV), which reflects the variations in your heart rate from beat to beat. Practice good breathing exercises such as box breathing (a type of yogic deep breathing that can lower stress and activate the parasympathetic nervous system. A high HRV rating is good and is parasympathetic. HRV readings are available on some health rings. Calm the mind,[300] or do so via the Heart Math app.[301]

4. Blood testing showing elevated CRP (CRP is a blood inflammation protein) may represent sleep duration shortening as well. If you have elevated CRP, consider possible periodontal (gum disease) inflammation and infection as one potential source. The bacteria, yeasts, and viruses that cause gum disease can be reduced by clinically validated mouthwash named OraCare™ Health Rinse®.[302]

5. This measure would likely need to be assessed after a whole week of recovery sleep, noting the long duration that CRP persists in the bloodstream. A new test measuring the reduced concentrations of nitric oxide present in an exhalation of breath may help with screening for undiagnosed OSA in the future. This test needs more validation testing.

6. Measuring oxygen levels in the blood with wearables like the Circul+® or Circul IQ® Rings and monitoring HRV with Oura Ring® are other strategies.

---

300 Young, M. (2024, January 10). "Grounding Techniques to Reduce Anxiety." *Cleveland Clinic Health Essentials Podcast*. Retrieved from https://my.clevelandclinic.org/staff/18244-melissa-young.

301 HeartMath. (n.d.). *HeartMath App*. Retrieved from https://www.heartmath.com/app/

302 OraCare. (n.d.). "OraCare - The Professional Alternative to Chlorhexidine." Retrieved from https://www.oracareproducts.com/

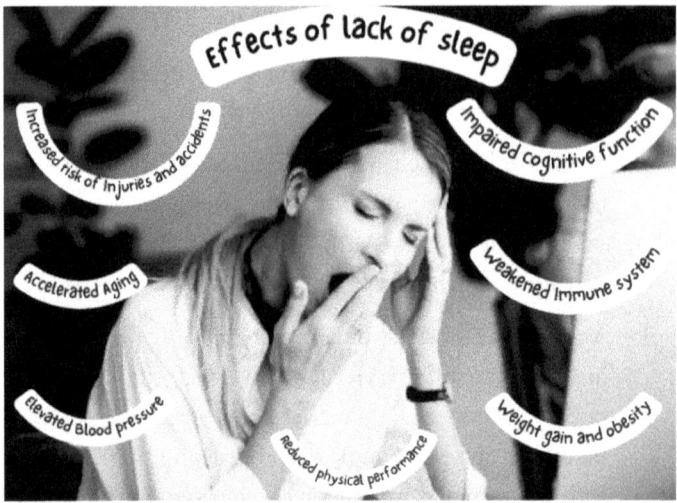

Figure 52: An AI-generated graphic image by Pearl Maisiri, Harare, Zimbabwe, using Canva® Placed on a Pixabay® free Photo.

7. If you or a bed partner snore—tame the snoring and improve your breathing as a snorer and improve your bed partner's sleep with less exposure to "second-hand snoring noise."

8. Emerging therapies like essential amino acid supplementation, creatine supplementation, CBD preparations, low inflammatory personalized eating (for your susceptibility to trigger inflammation), peptide treatments, and liposomal formulations of antioxidants are new options for the well-informed clinician.

9. My preferred modality for maintaining muscle mass is exercise and strength training. Consider an infrared sauna three to four times a week for twenty minutes and a cold plunge daily.

10. Eating within your circadian rhythm and limiting meals to one to two meals daily with time-restricted eating, also known as intermittent fasting.

11. Add digestive enzymes daily to improve the delivery of nutrition and rob the bad actors (opportunistic microbes) of nutrients.

12. Focus on nasal breathing and avoid mouth breathing with myofunctional therapy, addressing nasal restriction (allergies or

anatomical anomalies), Buteyko breathing (a learned technique of breathing out through the nose to slow air intake), and other methods.

13. Continuous glucose monitoring to identify suspect foods that may contribute to unknown glucose fluctuations after a meal. This will also help look for cortisol-related glucose fluctuations related to "OSA - Sleep Suffocation."

14. Avoid invisible environmental pollution, EMF microwave pollution, high indoor particulate levels, mold spores, and exposure to volatile organic compounds (VOCs) and related chemicals in everyday cleaning products (especially now with the constant disinfection post-COVID-19). HEPA filtration in the home and bipolar cold plasma air cleaning.

15. Clean water (ultrafiltration) and possibly add hydrogen, ozonated, structured, or deuterium-depleted water to your water choices and avoid sodas.

16. Obtain a consultation with a naturopathic physician or functional medicine clinician to better assess the health of your digestion, metabolism, diet, and exercise. These evaluations often include advanced biomarkers assessing for any level of systemic inflammation. Lifestyle changes related to these evaluations can often reduce weight, improve physical conditioning, and improve daytime alertness and feeling of restful sleep.

Managing Sleep Apnea—Practical Tips

SCREENING TOOLS

First, you might ask how you know you have sleep apnea or that you might have it. How do you know you need a sleep test? There are screening tests you can take, and they all have strengths and weaknesses. I will include two of the most common ones for you so that you can do a self-assessment. Here is a list of some of the types of screening tests:

- **Epworth Sleepiness Scale (ESS):** Assessing daytime sleepiness involves measuring the likelihood of falling asleep in various situations.
- **Pittsburgh Sleep Quality Index (PSQI):** Assesses overall sleep quality and disturbances over one month.
- **STOP-Bang Questionnaire:** A screening for obstructive sleep apnea by evaluating snoring, tiredness, observed apneas, high blood pressure, BMI, age, neck circumference, and gender.
- **Berlin Questionnaire:** Identifies individuals at risk for sleep apnea based on categories such as snoring, daytime sleepiness, and hypertension.
- **Insomnia Severity Index (ISI):** Assesses the nature, severity, and impact of insomnia.
- **STOP questionnaire:** A simple screening tool for identifying individuals at risk of having moderate to severe OSA.
- **Athens Insomnia Scale (AIS):** Assesses the severity of insomnia and its impact on daily functioning.
- **Rapid Eye Movement (REM) Sleep Behavior Disorder Screening Questionnaire:**[303] Helps identify individuals at risk for REM sleep behavior disorder.
- **Berlin Questionnaire for Chronic Obstructive Pulmonary Disease (COPD):** Identifies individuals with COPD who are at risk for sleep apnea—children's **Sleep Habits Questionnaire** (CSHQ): Assesses sleep habits and disturbances in children.
- **Earl O. Bergersen, DDS, MS: Children sleep screening questionnaire.**

The choice of a specific questionnaire may depend on the suspected sleep disorder, or the population being assessed. These questionnaires should be used with clinical assessments and other diagnostic tools. These questionnaires do not tell you that you have a sleep disorder but instead help your healthcare provider know when to issue a sleep test overnight study to help find out if you have a disorder.

---

303 Mckinney Pulmonologist et al. "Watermark Medical ARES Questionnaire." Mckinney Pulmonologist, https://www.mpsleepcenter.com/watermark-medical-ares-questionnaire/ (accessed April 24, 2024).

One of the most popular assessments is called The Epworth Sleepiness Scale. This self-assessment should be answered when you are not caffeinated and not using alcohol. I suggest you answer these questions on a separate piece of paper.

Epworth Sleepiness scale:[304] You would rate how likely you are to doze off or fall asleep in[305] various situations compared to just feeling tired. This assessment should reflect your typical behavior or habits, even if you haven't experienced these situations recently or have not done these things recently. Try to work out how they would have affected you. Answer the questions using the following scale. 0 = would never doze, 1 = slight chance of dozing, 2 = moderate chance of dozing, 3 = high chance of dozing.

(Scores 0-7, low risk; scores 8-10, moderate risk; score 11 or more, higher risk.)

____0 ____1 ____2 ____3   Sitting and reading

____0 ____1 ____2 ____3   Watching TV

Total Epworth Total Score   _____

____0 ____1 ____2 ____3   Sitting and talking to someone

____0 ____1 ____2 ____33   Sitting quietly after lunch without alcohol

____0 ____1 ____2 ____3   Sitting inactive in a public place (theater, meeting, etc.)

____0 ____1 ____2 ____3   As a passenger in a car for an hour without a break

____0 ____1 ____2 ____3   Lying down to rest in the afternoon when circumstances permit [306]

____0 ____1 ____2 ____3   In a car, while stopped for a few minutes in traffic

---

304 Mckinney Pulmonologist et al. "Watermark Medical ARES Questionnaire." Mckinney Pulmonologist, https://www.mpsleepcenter.com/watermark-medical-ares-questionnaire/ (accessed April 24, 2024).

305 iCare Platform. "SLEEP CHECK EN." https://my-icare.com/divi_overlay/sleep-check-en/ (Accessed April 24, 2024).

306 Ibid.

This is another popular assessment. The STOP-BANG

STOP-BANG Sleep Apnea Questionnaire [307]

STOP

Do you **SNORE** loudly (louder than talking or loud enough to be heard through closed doors)?   Yes____ No____

Do you often feel **TIRED**, fatigued, or sleepy during Daytime?   Yes____ No____

Has anyone **OBSERVED** you stop breathing during your sleep?   Yes ____No____

Do you have or are you being treated for high blood **PRESSURE**?   Yes____No____

BANG

BMI more than 35 kg/m2? (7.1547 pounds/foot²)   Yes____ No____

AGE over 50 years old?   Yes____ No____

NECK circumference > 16 inches (40cm)?   Yes____ No____

GENDER: Male?   Yes____ No____

TOTAL SCORE _____

High risk of OSA: Yes 5 - 8

Intermediate risk of OSA: Yes 3 - 4

Low risk of OSA: Yes 0 - 2

---

307 Rigdon, O. A. "An examination of the association between traumatic brain injury and sleep disruptions among athletes in contact and non-contact sports." 2017. https://core.ac.uk/download/222992688.pdf (Accessed April 24, 2024).

Earl O. Bergersen, DDS, MS: Children sleep screening questionnaire.
This is a modification of Bergerson's questionnaire to simplify its inclusion in the book.[308]

Does Your Child:

1. ____ Snore
2. ____ Experience labored, hard, difficult, loud breathing at night
3. ____ Have interrupted snoring/breathing where they stop four or more seconds
4. ____ Experience stoppage of breathing more than two times per hour
5. ____ Exhibit hyperactivity
6. ____ Mouth breathes during the day
7. ____ Mouth breathes while sleeping
8. ____ Experience frequent headaches in the morning
9. ____ Display allergic symptoms, the appearance of dark circles under the eyes, adenoid facies with a drooping face
10. ____ Experience excessive sweating while sleeping
11. ____ Talk while sleeping or sleepwalk
12. ____ Exhibit poor ability in school
13. ____ Fall asleep watching TV
14. ____ Wake up at night or experience nightmares or night terrors
15. ____ Experience restless sleep, move all over the bed
16. ____ Grind teeth
17. ____ Experience frequent throat infections/ear infections
18. ____ Have a hard time listening and frequently interrupt
19. ____ Ever wet the bed
20. ____ Exhibit a bluish color at night or during the day
21. ____ Experience speech problems

---

308 Bergersen, Earl O., DDS, MS. "Sleep Disordered Breathing Questionnaire for Children." *First published in 2019*. Available at: Sleep Disordered Breathing Questionnaire for Children, accessed from https://www.thehealthystart.com/earl-bergersen-dds-msd-abo.

22. ___ Have sleepy, irritable, and aggressive behavior above normal
23. ___ Fidgets with hands and will not sit quietly
24. ___ Has ADHD
25. ___ Sad or depressed

Each of the above assessments is helpful but can miss some needing testing. For example, some people are not sleepy with obstructive sleep apnea and are "keyed up." The questions have equal value when, in my opinion, dozing off to sleep while stopped at a red light on the Epworth Assessment is an automatic score of 11, necessitating a recommendation of a sleep study.

The STOP-BANG is weighted toward age and gender when we know that women begin to catch up to the men in incidents of sleep apnea after menopause, and the protective effects of estrogen and progesterone wane.[309] It does contain a fundamental question, though: "Has anyone told you that you stop breathing while sleeping?" This is a highly indicative sign of sleep apnea.

None of these screening tests have any questions about grinding of teeth, except for Bergersen, which is a correlating sign, nor do they have any questions on teeth crowding, broken teeth, tongue scalloping, or how low the soft palate drapes down toward your tongue. For this reason, I and other dentists have also developed versions of screening forms for dental offices. There are patient-filled-out screening forms and clinical exam screening forms. A healthcare provider may use more than one screening form. Most patients with undiagnosed OSA don't recognize a reduction in daytime alertness. This means the Epworth Sleepiness Scale may miss the majority of OSA patients if they are too heavily relied upon for screening for OSA.

Sleep Hygiene

Sleep hygiene refers to practices or adjustments made outside of the bed to enhance sleep quality. For individuals with conditions like sleep apnea or insomnia, implementing sleep hygiene strategies can sometimes improve

---

309 Peters, B. (2020, January 06). "Menopause and the Higher Risk of Sleep Apnea in Women." *Verywell Health*.

sleep quality and overall health, particularly if the condition is mild. Cognitive behavioral therapy is a well-established therapy for insomnia. There are sleep coaches trained in this therapy and sleep hygiene that can help via telemedicine. Those who have asthma must use their medications as prescribed. All prescribed medications must be used as directed by your doctor.

Establishing a consistent bedtime routine creates an ideal environment conducive to restorative sleep (red light, cool room, made bed). Not eating two hours before sleeping and avoiding electronic devices are all important steps toward achieving better results from treatment plans.

Additionally, relaxation techniques such as deep breathing, Buteyko slowed breathing exercises, and meditation can help alleviate stressors that may contribute negatively to poor sleep patterns. Regular follow-up with qualified professionals remains crucial in monitoring progress made over time by adjusting treatment strategies where necessary.

Sleep apnea is a condition that poses significant health risks when left undiagnosed and untreated. Early detection and timely intervention are crucial because of its alarmingly high prevalence and potential consequences on cardiovascular health and overall well-being. The current number of estimated undiagnosed OSA patients is too high and greater than 80 percent. This fact has been unfortunately true for decades. Little progress has been made in treatment options relying on the current gold solution, CPAP. This is partly due to OSA's poor branding. Most patients have only heard of CPAP from their doctor and would rather delay treatment due to the "unsexy" idea of wearing a CPAP.

Sleep-disordered breathing OSA can brew slowly for decades before it has gotten bad enough to cause the OSA patient to notice it is negatively impacting their daytime function and metabolic health. Suppose patients had an awareness of less invasive treatments and better attractiveness. In that case, more people may start looking into the issue earlier and prevent some of the damage that can arise from years of untreated "sleep suffocation."

Diagnostic methods were cumbersome before relying on spending an expensive night at a strange sleep laboratory. Fortunately, there are many more accessible options for testing a patient for OSA at home. The diagnostic methods, treatment options, and practical steps discussed in this chapter provide doctors and patients with valuable tools to help them effectively manage sleep apnea or ask better questions of their physicians, dentists, and chiropractors. By raising awareness and implementing proper screening protocols, physicians, dentists, chiropractors, and allied healthcare providers should play a crucial role in addressing the impact of undiagnosed sleep apnea and enhancing patient quality of life.[310]

When sleep disorders began to be explored, understood, and treated more systematically, dentistry's role in tackling airway issues and their solutions gained prominence in the later decades. This includes sleep treatment and testing. Again, before this, the prevailing method for addressing sleep-disordered breathing, specifically obstructive sleep apnea, involved using a positive pressure airway machine and later variations known as CPAP, BiPAP, or AutoPAP, all of them blowing air into the airway.[311] In the US, CPAP, or its cousins, is the dominant treatment of obstructive sleep apnea, but in Europe, dental oral sleep appliances outpace the use of CPAP. They are sometimes called an OAT (oral appliance therapy) oral sleep appliance, or MAD, which is short for mandibular advancement appliance. There are other acronyms, too.

The introduction of dental care into airway treatment brought with it the innovation of oral sleep appliances. Currently, there are more than one hundred variations of these appliances, and for many patients, they offer the most effective means of addressing airway issues associated with nighttime breathing.[312] They are better tolerated, and more people use them than CPAP devices.

Nevertheless, it's important to recognize that no single treatment is universally effective. Even the CPAP, which is considered the gold standard for obstructive sleep apnea treatment, is not consistently worn by patients. In fact, it is unused by approximately 50 percent of patients, and of those who do use it, many fall short of the recommended nightly usage. The recommended night usage standard is a dismal four hours of use. This four-hour nightly use goalpost is a poor standard of success, and we are not alone in

---

310 Johns Hopkins Medicine. (n.d.). *Sleep Apnea*. Retrieved from https://www.hopkinsmedicine.org/health/conditions-and-diseases/sleep-apnea

311 Dieltjens, M., & Vanderveken, O. M. (2019). "Oral Appliances in Obstructive Sleep Apnea." *Healthcare*, 7(4), 141. doi: 10.3390/healthcare7040141.

312 SomniFix. (n.d.). "The Foolproof Way to Increase Your CPAP Compliance Score." Retrieved from https://somnifix.com/blogs/snews/cpap-compliance

that view. Here are some sources on its use and success rates. According to a study conducted between 2011 and 2015, the adherence rate for CPAP therapy varies widely.[313] Another source reports that the national adherence rates for CPAP therapy are anywhere from 30 to 60 percent within the first year of treatment.[314] It is widely known that adherence statistics are even worse after the first year of wear.

Along with the growing influence of dentists in sleep disturbance awareness, an area of contention that already existed within the dental profession was also reopened. We will deal with orthodontic care again.

We have spent some time on the basics of airway and sleep apnea, but we will get to the more exciting stuff soon.

Dawning awareness of the airway is taking place in general dental and orthodontic care, especially regarding the issue of premolar extraction orthodontics.

Recent research has shed light on a potential consequence of this approach—a potential worsening of the airway opening and a less aesthetic appearance.

Traditional Premolar Extraction Orthodontics

See the figures below. The model on the right shows how much area exists on the roof of the mouth after tooth removal and closing of those tooth spaces.

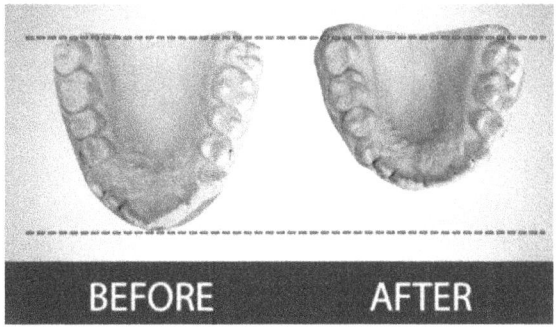

Figure 53: Courtesy of Dr. Geoffery Skinner.

---

313 Wells, Audrey. "Improving CPAP Adherence and Compliance for the Long-Term Health of the Patient." *Everything CPAP*, June 29, 2021, everythingcpap.com.

314 Park, Steven. "CPAP Success for Sleep Apnea: What You Must Know." *Everything CPAP*, June 29, 2021, Retrieved from https://doctorstevenpark.com/cpap-success-for-sleep-apnea-what-you-must-know.

In the photos shown here, you can see a dramatic reduction in the size of the roof of the mouth once two teeth were removed to create space for alignment. One reason for this is that the arch of the mouth is roughly like an open-ended circle. In a circle, if you reduce the size of the circumference (for simplicity's sake, let's assume by 50 percent), the area within that circle is reduced by 75 percent. In other words, a slight reduction in the circumference of the dental arch accomplished by removing two teeth creates a much more disproportionate loss of interior space for the accommodation of the tongue.

This loss of space for the tongue then creates a loss of airway space posterior to the tongue in the throat area. This is where the Bernoulli principle begins to influence this cascade of consequences.

Bernoulli's principle, named after Swiss physicist Daniel Bernoulli, helps us understand how fluid pressure, speed, and elevation are connected. Think of it like this: when a fluid speeds up, its resting pressure decreases, or its potential energy decreases.

In simpler terms, if a fluid moves faster, it either uses up some of its potential energy (energy from its position) or gets extra internal energy, which creates pressure.[315]

This principle is crucial for physicists studying fluid dynamics. The key takeaway? Faster-flowing fluids have lower pressure on the surfaces they touch. Remembering this helps explain many phenomena of an airplane wing lifting the plane. The upper part of the wing is rounder than the bottom, so air must go faster over it to catch back up to its underwing half. This faster air pressure on top of the wing causes it to have less pressure on top of the wing than the flat lower surface, which has higher pressure and pushes it up.

So, if your airway is narrowed by the tongue forced into it, air must go faster through that space. This creates a lower pressure on the sides of your throat airway, and they collapse inward, choking off the air and making noise. This is why your soft palate is fluttering, too. This is why you snore. This is why snoring is nothing to ignore. It is telling you that you do not have enough airway space.

---

315 Lee Johnson, Bernoulli's Principle: Definition, Equation, Examples, *Science.com*, December 28, 2020, https://sciencing.com/bernoullis-principle-definition-equation-examples-13723388.html

You can get an idea of the size reduction of the roof of the mouth in traditional orthodontic premolar extractions and headgear retraction of the front teeth.[316] This has been a common approach to relieve dental crowding. While this method effectively might achieve aesthetically aligned teeth, it often reduces the overall volume of the width and length dimensions of the oral cavity. The extractions often result in less room for the tongue and a smaller smile, leading to a narrower maxilla and potentially compromising the airway and a less beautiful result. If this type of care is implemented early in life, it can redirect growth, and some have attributed severe headaches and TMJ or jaw joint damage to the practice.[317]

Orthodontists have pointed to studies showing no worsening of sleep apnea or jaw joint damage from this type of care. The debate on premolar removal has been ongoing for many years. It is not just a debate between general dentists and orthodontists but one within the orthodontic profession and general dentists' profession. Dentists and orthodontists are colleagues in the field of dentistry. Both are respected and highly valued. Both branches of dentistry are working together to improve the quality of dental care. Consensus is growing.

For example, orthodontists, for many years, have used reverse-pull headgear to move the upper jaw forward away from the airways. This can also open up airways even if there is a need for tooth removal to line up teeth. This is done on children, not adults.[318] This treatment can also dramatically improve the beauty of faces for those who need it.

This debate is entering a new phase now that the FDA has recognized and cleared Vivos®' DNA, mRNA, and mmRNA jaw devices. This means it is now medically recognized that a type of airway expander made by dentists can increase airway volume and lessen sleep apnea events. Let's expand the understanding of just what that FDA clearance is.

---

316 Koh, H., & Lew, K. K. K. (2007). "A randomized clinical trial of two orthodontic headgear strap systems." *American Journal of Orthodontics and Dentofacial Orthopedics*, 131(4), 470.e1-470.e5.

317 Michelotti, A., Farella, M., Martina, R., & Pellegrino, G. (2002). "The relationship between headache and symptoms of temporomandibular disorder in the general population." *Journal of Orofacial Orthopedics / Fortschritte der Kieferorthopädie*, 63(1), 21-28.

318 Hill, Alyssa. "Orthodontic Headgear: Types & When Treatment is Necessary." *New Mouth*, November 8, 2023.

Vivos® FDA 510(k) Clearances

While researching the Vivos® airway therapies, I was fortunate enough to remember a lecture I listened to by Dave Singh, DMD, PhD, DDSc. Dave Singh, Todd Huntsman, Braden Bennett, Justin Harris, and Cathryn Bonar are the names listed as inventors on patent No. 11,723,790 B2 for the DNA®, mRNA®, and mmRNA® appliances.[319] The lecture was in Arizona at the American Sleep and Breathing Academy. I then contacted Vivos® for more information.

Kirk Huntsman, co-founder and CEO of Vivos®, was kind enough to grant me a phone interview about Vivos® and the FDA 501(k) clearances they received. He explained that there are two clearances. First, he said three appliances were cleared to treat severe OSA on November 28, 2023. They are the DNA appliance®, the mRNA appliance®, and the mmRNA appliance®,

Huntsman said they are changing the names of these appliances because they can be confusing and imply meanings they do not have. They now refer to them as the CARE® appliance system, which stands for Complete Airway Repositioning and Expansion.

In the first FDA clearance (granted Dec. 2022), Vivos® demonstrated functional airway improvement with the DNA appliance. More importantly, they demonstrated that sleep apnea (or AHI) scores were significantly reduced, and 26 percent of those cases showed complete resolution of sleep apnea! No therapy I know of has shown actual cures for sleep apnea other than this system. To be clear, the FDA did not approve of any language regarding a cure for sleep apnea. This December 2022 clearance was for treating mild to moderate obstructive sleep apnea with the DNA appliance.

In July 2022, researchers from Mount Sinai and Stanford University published a groundbreaking study in the Journal of Sleep Medicine showing that one out of four OSA patients (26 percent) treated using CARE oral appliances had seen their post-treatment AHI scores *drop below five with no device in the mouth*—technically within a normal score range most commonly used to measure obstructive sleep apnea. Vivos® was encouraged to apply for even more clearance for severe sleep apnea patients.

---

319 Singh, Dave. "Dr. Dave Singh Talks About the DNA Appliance." *Oral Systemic Link*, May 4, 2017. Accessed May 22, 2024. https://oralsystemiclink.net/health-care-providers/profile/dr-dave-singh-discusses-the-dna-appliance.

With this result, Vivos® applied for clearance of all three appliances for severe sleep apnea and received that in November 2023. It is the only line of dental appliances to have that clearance. In other words, Vivos® is cleared to treat mild, moderate, and severe obstructive sleep apnea. This is a monumental event. This means that nearly anyone with obstructive sleep apnea can benefit from Vivos®' oral sleep appliances.

In severe sleep apnea, CPAP was once the only therapy available, and the high air pressures made those who suffer often unable to wear the CPAP devices. With Vivos® some will be able to get the relief they need with Vivos® alone, or some may use Vivos® in combination with CPAP to lower their air pressure and make them tolerable to wear. Vivos® technology has been used to treat more than 45,000 people worldwide safely and successfully since 2010.

When I asked Mr. Huntsman what was improving the sleep apnea scores, he said they were not entirely sure, although they had some good theories. With the DNA appliance, for example, there is no forward advancement of the lower jaw, and the tongue, as most dental sleep appliances work. It might be that muscles and nerves work better. He assumes the expansion of airway space is part of the answer, but they have not proven it to the satisfaction of the FDA.

Typically, the palate is widened and increased in the anterior/posterior direction, and the nose airway is increased, too. They typically achieve a two to three-times size increase in the volume measures of the airway. The FDA is less interested in knowing how it works and far more interested in the product's safety, efficacy, and repeatability across a broad spectrum of adult population demographics.[320]

Here is my paraphrase of a statement by Julie Gannon on a Vivos® blog.

> According to a study published in the *Journal of Sleep Medicine* in 2022, one in four patients using Vivos® products experienced a complete resolution of their obstructive sleep apnea (OSA) symptoms. Vivos® asserts that its products mark the first instance where a significant resolution of OSA has been conclusively demonstrated within a limited treatment period, in contrast to the ongoing intervention needed for CPAP therapy or surgical neurostimulation implants.[321]

---

320 Huntsman, R. Kirk, Vivos® Therapeutics, Inc.
321 Gannon, Julie. "Vivos Therapeutics Receives First Ever FDA 510 (K) Clearance for Oral Device

When you have results like this that are cleared to treat obstructive sleep apnea and it comes with airway expansion on nearly every treated case, with improved facial beauty, there is no excuse to treat orthodontically on any patient without also trying to improve airway volume. The idea that premolar extraction has not been proven to worsen sleep apnea is not defensible as a routine procedure to correct crowded teeth. It is not optimal care, in my opinion.

Because of this, the discussions are now shifting. The differences of opinion and conflicting science are taking a new focus. I say this because if you can perform orthodontic care with the guiding principle of increasing airway space and improving misaligned teeth, that is becoming the standard of care. In our opinion, the argument that teeth removal may not cause or worsen airway health or sleep apnea is now a weak one or less relevant. Even though Vivos® is not an orthodontic appliance, with this FDA clearance showing we can improve airways by combining their use with orthodontics, the focus should now be to combine airway care and orthodontics.

Stay tuned because some beautiful cases are shown in this book. Dentistry has now intersected with medical care in instances like these, and this unique role cannot be fulfilled by any other health profession.

Treatment of Severe Obstructive Sleep Apnea." *Vivos Blog News*, November 29, 2023.

CHAPTER 8

The Transition from Traditional to New Approaches

Treatment options include but are not limited to traditional methods, Traditional Dental Sleep Appliances, and The New Airway Bone and Muscle Development Integrated Approaches.

Traditional Treatment Plans

The current state of obstructive sleep apnea care is massive underdiagnosis of no less than 80 percent of those with OSA currently affected. Again, this may be partly related to bad branding for OSA. Many patients, at this point, are familiar with OSA but choose to do nothing because all they think they will have offered to them is a CPAP machine. Some would lose their livelihood if they had an OSA diagnosis. Many people would prefer to delay treatment due to the "hassle factor." Patients who are aware of the new treatment options are much more willing to undergo diagnostic testing and treatment. Effective traditional management of sleep apnea typically involves the use of CPAP, AUTOPAP, or BiPAP therapy, regardless of the severity of the condition. This is almost exclusively the case in the United States, whereas Europe's statistics differ. See Figure 54.

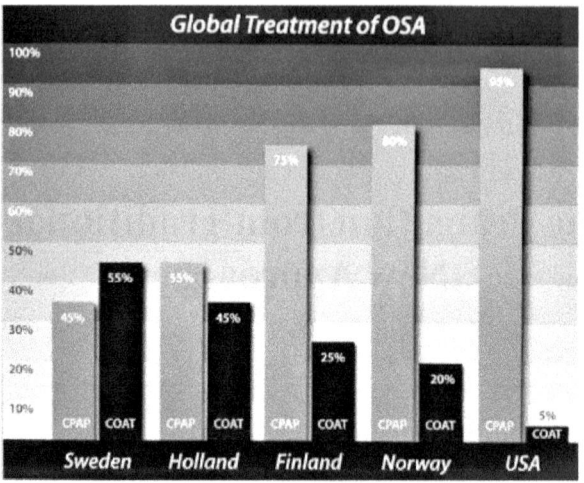

Figure 54: Source, Somnomed®

Continuous Positive Airway Pressure (CPAP) therapy stands out as a widely used medical intervention for treating sleep apnea, as we said, particularly in the United States. This method employs a mask worn over the nose, mouth, or both during sleep, delivering a continuous pressurized airflow to open the airway artificially. By exerting a steady air stream, CPAP helps support the tissues from collapsing into the airway, similar to inflating a balloon.

While CPAP effectively eliminates breathing interruptions, enhances sleep quality, and decreases daytime fatigue, some individuals struggle with exhaling against the air pressure or face challenges due to air leaks, especially if the air pressure has to be set too high to hold the airway open.

Think about driving, and the passenger puts their head outside the window. This is a liberating experience and comfortable at ten to twenty mph. But driving at sixty mph feels very different and uncomfortable and can make it feel like the air blowing in your face is unmanageable and jarring. CPAP is not magic; it is basically a vacuum cleaner exhaust blowing into the lungs, stenting your throat open throughout the night. A gentle pressure is well-tolerated, while a high pressure is uncomfortable and can disrupt the CPAP user's sleep. The higher the pressure, the more challenging it is to keep your CPAP mask in place. This can result in losing the mask seal and blowing air into and under the eyelids, where the mask makes annoying noises at night, waking the sleeper. Some unlucky people actually have air pushed into their stomachs, called aerophagia.

A tighter mask fit can also cause sores on the face and, like orthodontic treatments, can alter the underlying bones of the face. According to a study conducted in Japan, there have been significant changes in the facial structure of people who have used CPAP machines for two to three years. The study observed a reduction in the prominence of the upper and lower jaws, demonstrating that constant pressure on the jaws can cause dental changes.[322]

Another study found that after using CPAP, cephalometric variables (these are X-ray measurements of the bones in the head) demonstrated a significant remodeling of the maxilla or upper jaw, an increase in upper and lower jaw size discrepancy, a setback of the supramentale (it is a bony point or B point in the depression of the middle of the lower jaw just under the teeth and above the chin) and chin positions, a retroclination (sloped back into the mouth or rabbit-like) of upper jaw front teeth, and a decrease of convexity of the face.[323]

These effects from CPAP are especially concerning when they have to be worn by children. Their faces are easily deformed. According to a *Chest* article, there is a condition called "Smashed Face Syndrome" that can occur in some child patients who use CPAP for a long time.

Dr. Zelk is leading an initiative to trial the use of iNAP® for some of these children. It uses negative suction pressure instead of positive pressure to open airways. The mouth interface of the iNAP® looks a lot like a pacifier and will not smash the face. This is not an approved procedure and needs extensive study to determine if it will work for these children before it becomes available.

Another issue is where the mask seal is compressed excessively tight on the face, the dreaded morning CPAP mask imprints are a common complaint of the users. These imprints on the face may not become unrecognizable for up to three and four hours after waking.

It is not uncommon to see those who advocate this traditional CPAP approach issue a prescription for CPAP for almost all cases, mild, moderate,

---

322 Iida, J., et al. (2016). "Long-term use of continuous positive airway pressure therapy and changes in the facial profile of patients with obstructive sleep apnea." *The Angle Orthodontist*, 86(5), 788–795.

323 Sutherland, K., et al. (2014). "Craniofacial phenotyping in Chinese and Caucasian patients with sleep apnea: Influence of ethnicity and sex." *The Laryngoscope, 124*(5), 1268–1275. DOI: 10.5664/jcsm.7212

and severe. To be fair, CPAP therapy may indeed be the optimal solution for individuals with severe sleep apnea, central sleep apnea, or a combination of both obstructive and central sleep apnea.

In central or mixed sleep apnea, the brain is not signaling the person to breathe; therefore, just opening the airway with an oral sleep appliance, iNAP®, widening the jaws, or shrinking the tongue will not work. This is also why purchasing sleep devices from the internet or over-the-counter sleep therapies is dangerous. Treating a condition without a diagnosis is reckless and may worsen the condition if a person has central sleep apnea. Fortunately, these non-obstructive sleep apnea conditions are not as common as the obstructive form of sleep apnea; therefore, non-CPAP therapies can be used if appropriately applied.

A mix of strategies can also be included in traditional care embracing, lifestyle adjustments, weight loss, medical interventions, drugs, and rarely surgical procedures, and adapted according to the severity and root causes. There are various solutions ranging from free or inexpensive to surgical solutions that can be permanent. Lifestyle changes, including shedding excess weight, regular physical activity, getting eight hours of sleep for adults and ten to twelve hours for children, going to bed and waking at the same time each day, having a cool sleeping area, turning off cell phones and even routers, avoiding alcohol, smoking, sedatives, illicit drug use, and adjusting sleep positions for better breathing, play a pivotal role in alleviating symptom severity. Healthcare professionals worldwide highly recommend integrating these practices into daily routines.

Surgeries include sometimes extreme measures like tracheostomies (creating an opening in the trachea or windpipe from outside the neck), surgically moving one or both jaws forward, called MMA, deviated septum correction, sometimes turbinate (turbinates are tiny structures inside the nose that cleanse, heat, and humidify air) reduction, removing tissues in the throat and soft palate, and now recently an implanted electrical stimulator with the registered trademark name of INSPIRE®, which is an electrode placed under the jaw to stimulate the nerve to stick the tongue out while sleeping.

These traditional strategies are based on what are called phenotypes and endotypes. Please take a moment to understand what Joseph has written here. Joe will also explain INSPIRE® a bit later.

Individualized Care Based on Phenotype for Obstructive Sleep Apnea,

Current approaches to managing obstructive sleep apnea (OSA), often follow a standardized model, where diagnosis and treatment, usually starting with continuous positive airway pressure (CPAP), are applied universally. If CPAP proves challenging, alternative interventions like oral appliances may be considered a secondary option. However, this generic strategy overlooks the diverse nature of OSA, which can stem from various risk factors, such as different causes and clinical features.

We also must understand that not all obstructive sleep apnea is related to this modern dolichocephalic head (a relatively long head) and facial structure that much of the book has been focused on. If a person has a wide and well-formed dental arch, wide palate, open nasal passages, and good facial bone structure and yet has obstructive sleep apnea, the approach to treatment with widening arch therapies and opening the nasal areas may not be as helpful. This likely is due to the different phenotypes of people we encounter.

This section of phenotypes and endotypes is primarily genetically influenced instead of epigenetically influenced factors for sleep disorders. Yet it is important to mention certain aspects about them.

Recent analytical studies aim to unravel this diversity by identifying distinct OSA phenotypes or patient subtypes with unique characteristics. This nuanced approach holds the potential for more personalized and effective treatments tailored to individual needs.

Phenotypes include such types as ethnic differences, where Whites appear to be more susceptible to the shrinking face of modern lifestyle influences, Blacks have more musculature of the tongue, and there is a somewhat more posterior placement of the zygomatic bone in Asians that can change a person's susceptibility to apnea events. Other differences like gender and age have some bearing. Knowing them helps health professionals plan and implement better treatment.

As with many diseases, some racial differences do have an influence. Here are some conclusions paraphrased from the Cleveland Clinic on this subject.

The Sleep Heart Health Study revealed a slightly elevated prevalence of moderate to severe obstructive sleep apnea among Black individuals (20 percent) and American Indians (23 percent) compared to Whites (17 percent). Another study indicated OSA prevalence rates of 30 percent among Whites, 32 percent among Blacks, 38 percent among Hispanics, and 39 percent among Chinese individuals. Moreover, a higher incidence of OSA was observed in young Black individuals (≤ 25 years) compared to Whites, although no disparities based on race were found in older patients. These discrepancies across racial groups may stem from differences in craniofacial anatomy.[324]

The same article discusses sex differences.

Men are at a higher risk of developing obstructive sleep apnea (OSA) compared to women, although postmenopausal women face a similar risk once they reach menopause. Research indicates that postmenopausal women who undergo hormone replacement therapy tend to have lower rates of OSA, indicating that hormonal changes after menopause contribute to an increased risk of OSA. Furthermore, women typically experience more OSA episodes during rapid eye movement (REM) sleep and fewer when sleeping in a supine position. In contrast, most men predominantly experience OSA when sleeping on their backs. Additionally, the severity of OSA tends to be less pronounced in women with similar body mass index (BMI) compared to men. Symptoms of OSA also vary between genders, with men more frequently reporting snoring and witnessed apneas, whereas women often complain of insomnia and excessive daytime sleepiness. These differences in symptoms may result in delayed diagnoses and higher mortality rates among women compared to men.[325]

---

324 Rundo, J. V. (2019). "Obstructive sleep apnea basics." *Cleveland Clinic Journal of Medicine, 86*(9 suppl 1), 2–9. DOI: 10.3949/ccjm.86.s1.02

325 Ibid.

An endotype is a specific version or type of health issue. It focuses on the inner workings, biological factors, and molecular details that drive the development and progress of a condition. This is different from the more general term "phenotype," which looks at the visible symptoms or characteristics of a condition.

One recent line of investigation has delved into the various understandings of how the body's normal functions are altered due to illness or injury and the risk factors contributing to OSA, seeking to refine our understanding of why OSA develops. This research has spotlighted three key endotypes or categories:

> **Arousal Threshold:** Examining how easily an individual wakes up in response to external stimuli, such as noise or pain, sheds light on one contributing factor to OSA. Some people are easily awakened, while others are not.
>
> **Craniofacial Morphology:** Addressing the "shrinking face conundrum," particularly the impact of smaller jaws and airways in contemporary populations, which this book often discusses. This offers insights into another endotype related to OSA.
>
> **Chemoreflex Sensitivity:** refers to the responsiveness of the chemoreceptors, (these are areas where carbon dioxide levels are monitored by how much it makes the blood acidic).

The chemoreflex sensitivity receptors we're talking about are chemoreceptors located in the carotid and aortic regions. They're sensitive to alterations in blood composition, such as shifts in oxygen and carbon dioxide levels. These receptors are vital for controlling respiratory function. When chemoreceptors detect alterations in blood gasses, they send signals to the brainstem, prompting adjustments in breathing rate and depth to maintain the body's internal balance.[326] They can even cause the nose tissues to let in more or less air.

---

326 "Hypoxia and Hypercarbia." USMLE Forums, https://www.usmle-forums.com/threads/hypoxia-and-hypercarbia.2626/#post-9190 (Accessed April 24, 2024).

In obstructive sleep apnea (OSA), chemoreflex sensitivity becomes relevant because imbalances in respiratory function, such as chronic mouth breathing or hyperventilation, can impact the chemoreceptor response. For example, habitual mouth breathing, associated with OSA, may alter the chemoreflex in the blood, potentially contributing to respiratory disturbances during sleep. Mouth breathing generally results in less carbon dioxide in the blood, which would result in an increase in pH or more alkaline blood. Researchers and clinicians often examine chemoreflex sensitivity to understand its role in respiratory disorders and explore interventions to optimize respiratory function.[327]

High-performance Weightlifting Athletics

This likely will not be considered an endotype by experts. It is self-imposed, so it is not technically an endotype or phenotype; however, it is related to the African ethnic phenotype group because they have about 10 to 11 percent more muscle on average than other ethnic groups.[328] This is also why the BMI is not necessarily applicable to African individuals.

It is interesting to note that muscle-enhancing weightlifting competitors often have thicker necks due to highly enhanced muscles. It is common to see them using CPAPs as an essential weight and competition aid. This is because they have narrower airways due to this constriction of the muscles in the airways. The same thing happens when you become overweight. Excess fat in the neck and tongue will constrict airways.

While these endotypes appear promising in capturing the diversity of causes and expression of OSA, further clinical validation is necessary to confirm their relevance and application in refining OSA management strategies.[329]

---

327 Forbes, J., & Menezes, R. G. (2023). Anatomy, Head and Neck: Carotid Bodies. *StatPearls [Internet]. Treasure Island (FL): StatPearls Publishing.* Available from: StatPearls - Carotid Bodies

328 Silva, A. M., et al. (2010). "Ethnicity-related skeletal muscle differences across the lifespan." *American Journal of Human Biology, 22*(1), 76–82. DOI: 10.1002/ajhb.20956.

329 Zinchuk, A., Gentry, M., Concato, J., & Yaggi, K. (2017). "Phenotypes in obstructive sleep apnea: A definition, examples, and evolution of approaches." *Sleep Medicine Reviews, 35,* 113–123. DOI: 10.1016/j.smrv.2016.10.002.

Let's Now Discuss the New Team Approach to Airway Health and Beauty.

We will first address orofacial myofunctional therapy, then oral dental appliance therapy. Chiropractic is an overlooked profession that is well-positioned to find and collaborate with this epidemic of sleep and airway neglect. We will then cover combination therapies, including EPAP therapy, Nightlase® therapy, orthodontic care, allergies, Myo Munchee®, ToothPillow® and Myobrace® for child facial development. We will also cover nasal dilators, nasal hygiene, chiropractic care, diet and weight control, sleep hygiene, traditional surgical approaches, iNAP® eXciteOSA®, Vivos®, positional therapy, INSPIRE® and Invisasleep® with HPAP. Ultimately, we will cover aligners (the most well-known is Invisalign®), airway therapy specialized for airway and beauty, Nightlase®, MARPE, SARPE, DOME, EASE, MSE, and MMA. These terms will be explained.

Even though some of these have been mentioned, you will be excited to see what they can do for real people. Those practitioners presenting these cases and the amazing patients who have given permission to see their photos and hear their stories are real heroes.

Traditional Treatment with Dental Sleep Appliances

As mentioned, traditional care eventually included a slow acceptance of dental oral sleep appliances. When dentistry began helping in sleep airway care, dental sleep appliances became the standard of care for many dentists.[330] They essentially did not provide any other care related to sleep health.

However, the entry of dentists into the area created a bit of a dilemma because dentists were considered separate from medicine. The insurance industry and those tackling this dilemma decided to label the oral sleep appliance a DME, which stands for durable medical equipment. The appliance was treated the same as a CPAP and classified as DME.

But they went further. Not only did they classify the oral sleep appliance as a DME, but they also designated the dentist as a DME provider rather

---

330 Kushida, C. A., et al. (2006). "Practice parameters for the treatment of snoring and obstructive sleep apnea with oral appliances: An update for 2005." *Sleep, 29*(2), 240–243. DOI: 10.1093/sleep/29.2.240.

than a treating medical provider. This designation is unfortunate and will have to change because dentists now perform many procedures with lasers, surgeries, and orthodontics that will not fit into a DME provider category.

What is an Oral Sleep Appliance?

Dr. Zelk will summarize this section since he has placed over 15,000 of these and is familiar with the advantages and nuances of each appliance.

The oral appliance, dental appliance, mandibular advancement device, or splint are all synonymous with one device. OAT stands for oral appliance therapy. Confusing, yes, but let's just use the abbreviation of MAD for this discussion.

This treatment option has been around for decades but has only had the attention it deserves in the last several years. The OAT or MAD (mandibular advancement device) is a compact, low-impact device that supports the airway to treat snoring and OSA. The technology has continued to improve the size, fit, and options of MAD. It is portable, so it has been popular for travel use.

When surveyed, the majority of OSA patients were given the option to undergo treatment for OSA with either the CPAP or the MAD, and the majority of patients chose the MAD. Unfortunately, most patients are not given that option in the U.S.

A custom-fitted mandibular advancement device offers several benefits for managing snoring and obstructive sleep apnea. A recent study showed that MADs are not inferior to CPAP in controlling sleep apnea-related blood pressure.[331] Let's explore these benefits of oral sleep appliances:

Reducing Snoring

MADs effectively reduce snoring by temporarily holding the jaw and tongue forward. This action helps prevent throat constriction, allowing for better airflow during sleep.[332] If you're fed up with getting punched in the ribs to

---

331 Cox, C. E. (2024, April 6). "Oral Device Noninferior to CPAP for Reducing BP in Sleep Apnea: CRESCENT." *tctmd.com*.

332 Steph Coelho, CPT. reviewed by Raj Dasgupta, MD, (2020, July 13). "Mandibular advancement device: What to know." *Medical News Today*. Accessed at https://www.medicalnewstoday.com/articles/mandibular-advancement-device

roll over and stop snoring, it's a compelling reason to investigate solutions for your snoring issue. It's similar to the head tilt or jaw thrust maneuver used in CPR, which involves maintaining an open airway to enable passive breathing.

In this analogy, CPAP plays a role similar to rescue breaths in CPR, functioning like a balloon-blowing machine. This is one reason why many patients struggle to tolerate CPAP; its pressure creates a sensation opposite to natural respiration, where instead of sucking in, air is blown in.

Minimal Side Effects: Unlike other treatments, MADs have minimal side effects. They are easy to use and generally well-tolerated by users. [333]

Cost-Effective: Custom MADs' prices are decreasing, with more dentists learning how to fit these devices. Compared to continuous positive airway pressure machines, MADs are more cost-effective. These savings can add up since most MADs have no replacement parts to buy, like CPAP therapy, over the long term. It is also covered under most medical insurance plans, as is CPAP.

The MAD can come in many configurations to help treat more people with different treatment needs. They can be used with CPAPs, too.

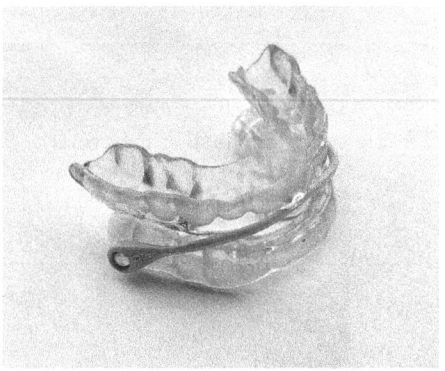

Figure 55: Avant®
The Avant® is a strap mechanism connecting the upper and lower jaw splints. The strap's direction goes from the posterior part of the lower splint to the center of the upper splint.

---

333 Ibid.

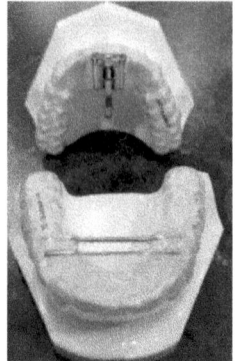

Figure 56: TAP®
The TAP® device has a center hook attaching the upper and the lower trays.

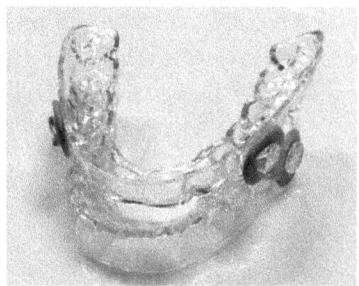

Figure 57: EMA®
The EMA® has flexible straps connecting the upper and the lower trays.

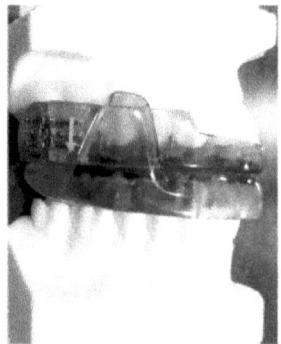

Figure 58: Clear Dream®
The dorsal wing devices have a bilateral ramp-style mechanism.

These are some of the most commonly used devices. There are many configurations and designs to choose from.

Remember that while side effects like some initial overproduction of saliva or increased tooth sensitivity are common and generally mild, they typically resolve on their own after a few days. Consult a dental professional if you experience persistent discomfort or issues of severe side effects.[334] For most people, the devices, if managed diligently, should not change the dental bite. The treating dentist should avoid being too aggressive, pushing the lower jaw forward at night. A jaw moving too far forward can result in a high occurrence of pain and dental changes.

Every patient responds differently to OAT or MADs. A patient with loud snoring, UARS, and mild or moderate OSA are just as likely to have a good treatment response as they would using the CPAP. In the Severe OSA patient, the MAD can optimally treat around 50 percent of these patients. There is typically some improvement in oxygenation, snoring, and subjective feeling of being rested. If a patient with severe OSA cannot tolerate or is not willing to use a CPAP, the MAD is a better option than doing nothing. This patient will likely need to look at combining different types of treatment to get a more synergistic improvement in the overall treatment of their OSA.

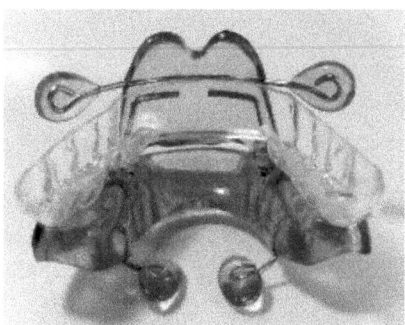

Figure 59: A combination of oral, tongue, and nasal appliance called Oasys®

---

[334] "Temporomandibular Joint Syndrome." tmjtreat.com, https://tmjtreat.com/temporomandibular-joint-syndrome/ (Accessed April 24, 2024).

For those unable to tolerate CPAP or experiencing limited effectiveness, alternative treatments present viable options. However, you do not have to use these options solely because you failed with CPAP. For many, they not only can be your first choice but can also be a better choice. As we just mentioned, these may include oral appliances, which realign the jaw to maintain open airways. In addition to that, surgical procedures involving tissue removal,[335] non-surgical laser treatments for tongue size reduction, firming the soft palate with non-surgical lasers,[336] reshaping the jawline, tongue nerve stimulation devices resembling pacemakers, orofacial myofunctional therapy, nasal dilators, nasal rinses, EPAP devices, chiropractic care, growth stimulating chewing devices for children's jaw development (MyoMunchee®, Tooth Pillow®, Myobrace®), orthodontic care, clear aligner care, or specialized negative pressure airway opening devices during sleep (iNAP®).

Orofacial myofunctional therapists began to treat with nasal breathing exercises and mouth exercises to improve the strength of airway muscles, which can also improve breathing capacity both during sleep and during wake times. Daily nasal and oral hygiene began to receive more attention. It can improve the health of the membranes of the nasal and oral airways as well as help prevent the increase in the size of the tonsils and adenoids, improving the likelihood that a sleeping person will keep their mouth closed.

New CPAP Alternative for the Treatment of OSA and Snoring

Positional Therapy: As discussed with phenotypes, women seem to have fewer apneas while sleeping on their backs while men have less sleeping on their side. This shows how phenotypes play a role in how we treat patients.

Raising the head of the bed with a wedge or using a body pillow to stay off the back when sleeping seems to be useful for all phenotypes.

---

335 Mayo Clinic. "Sleep Surgery Clinic - Overview." Otolaryngology (ENT)/Head and Neck Surgery. Mayo Clinic. Accessed at https://www.mayoclinic.org/departments-centers/sleep-surgery-clinic/overview/ovc-20469499.

336 Picavet, V. A., Dellian, M., Gehrking, E., Sauter, A., & Hasselbacher, K. (2023). "Treatment of snoring using a non-invasive Er:YAG laser with SMOOTH mode (NightLase®): A randomized controlled trial." *European Archives of Oto-Rhino-Laryngology*, 280(1), 307–312. DOI: 10.1007/s00405-022-07539-9.

The Latest Traditional Approaches

INSPIRE® and StimAireE™ – Dr. Zelk

INSPIRE® is an FDA-cleared implantable upper airway stimulation (UAS) device for obstructive sleep apnea. The device works inside the body, stimulating key airway muscles and allowing the airway to stay open during sleep.

The INSPIRE® Upper Airway Stimulation (UAS) system is approved to treat moderate to severe obstructive sleep apnea.[337] The device is an implantable nerve stimulator. It is approved for use in some people who have not had success with continuous positive airway pressure machines. Some insurance carriers are not allowing benefits for this treatment until the patient has demonstrated failure in the use of oral sleep appliances for their sleep apnea.

INSPIRE®, a compact device that bears resemblance to a pacemaker, is implanted into the chest wall in a same-day, outpatient surgery. To fit the device, one small incision is made under the chin, and another is made below the collarbone. The device includes a small machine that creates an electrical pulse to stimulate a nerve in your tongue. This causes the tongue to move forward at night as you breathe. This keeps your airway open if the tongue is causing the obstruction. A handheld remote control turns the device on and off. The INSPIRE® battery lasts about eleven years. INSPIRE® therapy is recommended for a specific group of patients diagnosed with moderate to severe obstructive sleep apnea who find it challenging to tolerate continuous positive airway pressure therapy.

As with any surgical procedure, there are both potential risks and benefits associated with INSPIRE® therapy. Risks may include, but are not limited to, discomfort, nausea, temporary tongue weakness, and the possibility of infection. Prior to treatment, a drug-induced sleep endoscopy (camera scope exam in the airway) will need to be performed by the ENT physician to assess the airway because not all airways are

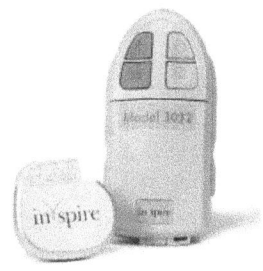

Figure 60

---

337 "Neurostimulator Long-Term Patient Management Is Easier." *Sleep Review*, https://sleeppreviewmag.com/sleep-treatments/therapy-devices/neurostimulators/digital-solutions-neurostimulator-long-term-patient-management/ (accessed April 24, 2024).

appropriate for INSPIRE®. It is an implanted battery under the skin with a wire to the base of the tongue that sometimes can be visible in certain types of patients.

StimAire™

StimAire™ is a non-surgical hypoglossal nerve stimulator that could become much less expensive and has immediate results with less post-treatment complications.[338] I will paraphrase part of the press release. This is not yet available to patients.

> TUCSON, Ariz., Oct. 11, 2023 /PRNewswire/ — Innovative neuromodulation firm StimAire™ has successfully completed its initial clinical trial in Australia. This pioneering study, involving the first human subjects, evaluated a small injectable device designed to treat obstructive sleep apnea (OSA). The trial focused on the safety of the injection procedure, the functionality of the patented device, and the overall feasibility of the treatment method. Additionally, the study included overnight sleep tests on an OSA patient, both with and without the StimAire™ device, which modulated the hypoglossal nerve during sleep.
>
> The trial reported no adverse events and minimal pain or discomfort from the injections. Efficacy results showed that the patient experienced the expected reduction in obstructive events. The patient slept two and a half times longer with the device and achieved thirty minutes of REM sleep, compared to none without the device.

Nasal Stent Devices

Nastent™ is a device that effectively treats snoring and sleep apnea syndrome. Nastent™ is a nasal stent that fits through the nose, and the tip reaches the soft palate.

---

338 UAVenture Capital Fund, LLC. "UAVenture Capital Portfolio Company StimAire Completes First-In-Human Study of Injectable Stimulator for Obstructive Sleep Apnea (OSA)." News release, October 11, 2023. *PR Newswire*. Accessed June 4, 2024. https://www.prnewswire.com/news-releases/uaventure-capital-portfolio-company-stimaire-completes-first-in-human-study-of-injectable-stimulator-for-obstructive-sleep-apnea-osa-301953742.html.

It is made from a flexible silicone tube and designed with a natural curve. Each Nastent™ box contains seven devices of your chosen size for one week of use.

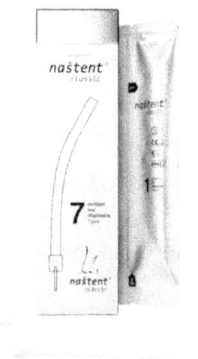

Figure 61

The Alaxo™ Nasal Airway Stents mechanically splint open the nasal airway, indicated to treat snoring. The stents are self-inserted by the user and can be worn for up to eighteen hours at a time.

The smooth stent braid is made from memory metal nitinol. It has a ball-shaped widening positioned at the nasal valve (nose opening area) and a longer cylindrical section that splints the turbinates open. Some patients have snoring worsened by nasal alar collapse (outer wall of the nasal opening), nasal valve collapse (there is an inner and outer nasal valve), or turbinate hyperplasia (swelling).

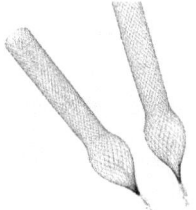

Figure 62

eXciteOSA®

Neuromuscular electrical stimulation (NMES) applied to the tongue is a novel approach to treating mild obstructive sleep apnea and snoring. With FDA clearance, eXciteOSA® offers a patient-friendly daytime therapy that targets the upper airway muscles and tongue to prevent airway collapse during sleep. Just a twenty-minute session during the day can lead to improvements in nighttime sleep apnea severity. This therapy enhances tongue muscle endurance, reduces mild obstructive sleep apnea, and enhances overall sleep quality. Notably, it addresses both daytime and nighttime breathing concerns.[339]

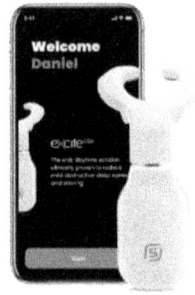

Figure 63: eXciteOSA®

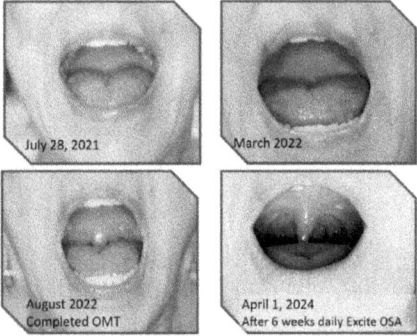

Figure 64: This case study photo series courtesy of Shirley Gutkowski, Primalair

iNAP®

CPAP uses positive air pressure to open up the airway (balloon-like); iNAP®, which is the opposite, uses a light suction in the mouth to move the tongue forward and open up the airway. The best way to think about the treatment is that it is similar to the suction felt in the mouth while we are swallowing. The tongue and soft palate are pulled forward out of the back of the throat with the intraoral negative pressure (suction). It is recommended for all severities of obstructive sleep apnea. It is FDA-cleared for all severities of obstructive sleep apnea.

---

339 "How It Works." eXciteOSA®, https://exciteosa.com/how-it-works/ (accessed April 24, 2024).

The benefits of iNAP® over a CPAP device are no mask or headgear, it is battery-powered, it is quiet, compact, and portable. For the best response with iNAP®, the patient should have improved nasal breathing and hygiene. The user must be able to breathe well through the nose during sleep, and it is not useful for central sleep apnea, which is sleep apnea where the brain does not signal your muscles to take a breath.

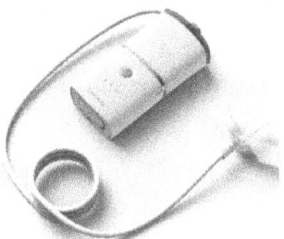

Figure 65: iNAP®

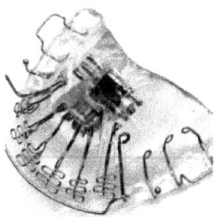

Figure 66: Vivos® DNA

MARPE

Miniscrew-assisted rapid palatal expansion (MARPE) offers a non-surgical and non-extraction method for widening the upper jaw or maxilla. A narrow maxilla is often linked with issues like nasal congestion, crowded teeth, and impaired facial development, which are characteristic features of obstructive sleep apnea.

Traditional treatments for a narrow maxilla typically involve conventional maxillary expanders, but these are mostly suitable for children since the mid-palatal suture, which holds the maxillary bone together, typically fuses by around twelve to fifteen years of age. MARPE extends this treatment option by utilizing mini-screws or mini-implants to directly connect the expander to the palatal bone, allowing for expansion even in older individuals.[340]

Sometimes, the appliance is attached to the bone only and sometimes to both bone and teeth. MARPE can be effective for young adults whose sutures have already fused. It can be adapted for older adults too, with specialized procedures to reopen the fused suture of the maxilla. In older adults, piezotome instruments or lasers may be used to weaken the suture prior to expansion. Often, this procedure also widens the nasal and oral airways.[341]

MARPE has gained popularity due to its ability to achieve significant maxillary expansion in a shorter period. It is often used in cases where there is a need for significant skeletal expansion, particularly in adult patients with transverse maxillary deficiencies (narrow upper jaw). However, MARPE is a complex procedure that requires careful planning and expertise from a well-trained general dentist, orthodontist, or other dental specialist who has gained this knowledge.

Each person's experience with the procedure varies, particularly in how it affects speech. Some may notice slight changes in facial appearance, such as increased width and accentuated cheekbones.

Postoperative discomfort typically lasts two to three days, though usually mild. While MARPE often improves nasal breathing, these benefits may not always be permanent and could regress due to external factors like allergens or air pollution.

Complications can arise, including inflammation or infection that may require additional or replacement of mini-screws or even early removal and replacement of the device, incurring additional costs. Tissue overgrowth on the screws and palatal tissues may necessitate surgical intervention, while lost screws or broken TADs (temporary anchorage device) might require replacement or removal.

---

340 Lipkin, I. (n.d.). *Westwood Orthodontics*, Accessed from Westwood Orthodontics (gotbraces.com)

341 Kapetanović, A., et al. (2023). "Efficacy of Miniscrew-Assisted Rapid Palatal Expansion (MARPE) in late adolescents and adults: A systematic review and meta-analysis." *European Journal of Orthodontics*, 43(3), 313–323. DOI: 10.1093/ejo/cjab005.

In rare cases, faulty appliances or maxillary expansion can lead to skeletal discrepancies or facial imbalances, which may require surgical correction. Some individuals may require additional procedures if the upper jaw expands unevenly.

It's important to note that MARPE treatment has been in use for around ten years, and while uncommon, unforeseen complications may still occur and it may not improve sleep apnea and airway health for everyone. Nothing works for every person, including mouth widening, ENT surgeries for deviated septum, or soft palate removal.

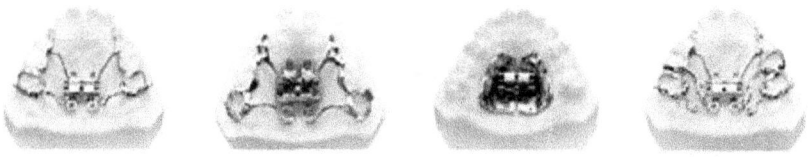

Figure 67

SKETATAL EXPANSION – The Future of Optimizing Nasal Breathing and Sleep – Kimberly Santiago, DDS

Understanding How to Optimize Your Airway: It All Starts with the Nose!

Let's talk about something really important for your health: your nose! Believe it or not, the key to having a functional airway begins with how well your nose works.

The Importance of Nasal Anatomy

In the past, our ancestors had noses that were perfectly designed for breathing through them. But over time, as our lifestyle changed, our noses stopped developing to function as well as they used to. Imagine the shape of the nasal opening (called the nasal aperture)—in modern humans, it looks like an almond, but ideally, it should look more like a pear for optimal breathing.

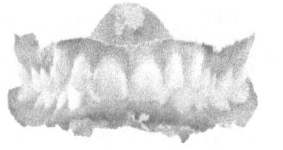 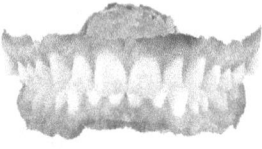

Figures 68 and 69: These are before and after MARPE Scans of Patient C

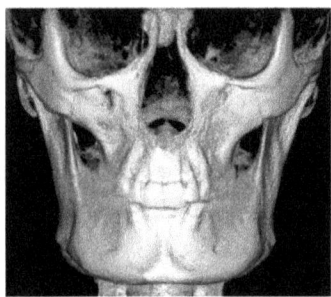 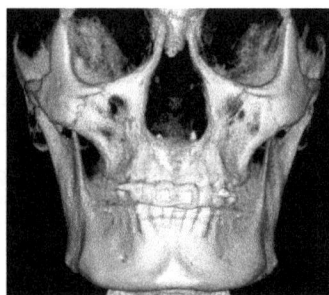

These figures 70 and 71: These figures are of the same patient C. Notice the widened nasal opening and jaw structures. These results use a minimally invasive MARPE solution that is often better than surgery.

How Nasal Function Affects Breathing

Your nose plays a crucial role in how air moves through your airways. If your nose isn't functioning properly, it can cause turbulence and resistance when you breathe. This can lead to airway collapse, which means you might stop breathing because of obstructions caused by narrow anatomy and inflamed nasal tissues.

Why Focus on the Nose and Not Just Airway Volume?

It's not just about the size of your airway; it's about how well your nose functions. If your nose works efficiently and has the right resistance, your airway can stay open and allow you to breathe easily.

Expanding the Nasal Passages

One way to improve your nasal function is by expanding the internal nasal passages. While traditional nasal surgeries focus on reducing or removing parts of the nasal tissue, there's a newer approach that involves expanding the nasal and upper jaw bones. This method has only recently become more well-known.

MARPE has not worked for everyone, and here is an article comparing it to control and to another expansion done in children called RPE or rapid palatal expansion.[342] In this article, pharyngeal airway was significantly better in MARPE, but not all measurements were significantly improved long-term. I believe that there are a number of variables that may not have been considered during their study. The age of the patients is a factor. How long were expanders left in for passive retention? Were the expander screws locked in a way to prevent unwinding during retention?

I keep retention for RPE for six months and for MARPE for ten to twelve months to prevent bone remodel relapse. I also always have these patients in concurrent myofunctional therapy during the treatment for lip competence and tongue tone. I doubt that was present in this study. This study is important reading, nevertheless, because it cautions us on overly optimistic expectations from this type of care.

UNDERSTANDING SKELETAL EXPANSION

The upper jaw is made of two bones joined at the midline by a seam called a suture. It was once believed that this suture fuses early in adulthood, but recent research and clinical practice have shown that it can be gently teased apart using a skeletal expander. This process, known as skeletal expansion, can be done by a dentist or orthodontist using various dental appliances. MARPE is a variation of MSE (Maxillary Sagittal Expansion) (widening) and has been shown to improve airway volume in a number of studies.[343]

---

342 Mehta, S., Wang, D., Kuo, C.-L., Mu, J., Lagravere Vich, M., Allareddy, V., Tadinada, A., & Yadav, S. (2021). Long-term effects of mini-screw–assisted rapid palatal expansion on airway: A three-dimensional cone-beam computed tomography study. *Angle Orthodontist*, 91(2), 195–205. doi: 10.2319/062520-586.1

343 Dominguez-Mompell, R., et al. "Breathing Changes Following Mini-Implant-Supported Maxillary Skeletal Expander Treatment in Late Adolescent or Adult Patients: Assessment of Objective

How Skeletal Expansion Works

Skeletal expansion literally widens the upper jaw by separating the two halves at the seam. This makes the entire upper jawbone wider, which directly widens the base of the nose, improving airflow. It also creates more room for your tongue inside your mouth, which is beneficial for breathing.

Dental vs. Skeletal Expansion

While dental expansion focuses on widening the bone that holds the teeth, it doesn't provide the same long-term stability or improvements to nasal function as skeletal expansion. Skeletal expansion offers true, long-lasting benefits by widening the upper jaw and enhancing nasal passages.

The MARPE Appliance

One of the most effective methods for skeletal expansion is the MARPE appliance. This custom-designed device combines 3D CT scans and digital impressions to precisely fit your anatomy. It's cemented to your teeth and attached to the bone with mini anchors, applying constant, gentle force to open the suture slowly.

Benefits of Skeletal Expansion

Skeletal expanders do more than just widen the upper jaw. They also optimize the bones connected to it. There is weak evidence of improved vision. It can lead to higher cheekbones, and even better facial aesthetics. Additionally, they can move the upper jaw forward, further enhancing the airway and correcting underbites if necessary.

The Process and Timeline

The entire process is minimally invasive. You start noticing breathing improvements in about 3-4 weeks, sometimes even sooner. The benefits continue to grow as the expander is slowly adjusted. The expansion is

---

and Subjective Functional Breathing Changes." *Journal of Orofacial Orthopedics*, Epub ahead of print (2024). doi: 10.1007/s00056-024-00521-6.

followed by carefully planned orthodontics to minimize the loss of growth that was just developed. Not all MARPE providers offer the same success; it is important to vet their education and technique.

Here are some of the things to consider when evaluation of a patient's treatment is contemplated. Is the practitioner expanding to correct a crossbite? What I mean is, are they uprightling the lower molars in order to match the upper expansion to the lower?

Are they treating anthropologic norms or norms where the first molars are between 38-42mm? The width of the cortical plate (the outside covering of a bone) at the joining of the roots of the first molars of the upper arch relative to the lower should be at least 5mm wider. I know this is technical, but I want readers to understand that this care must be done by knowledgeable dentists.

As mentioned before, how long should a practitioner retain the MARPE appliance after the active expansion is completed? Is there an evaluation using a CT scan to confirm that the bone has fully remineralized, ensuring stability and consistent short-term and long-term effects?

Furthermore, if the nose is not re-trained or orofacial myofunctional therapy (OMT) is not utilized, the results may be limited. An untreated tongue-tie could also compromise the volume, as the patient would be unable to elevate the mid and posterior blade of the tongue. If NightLase^{TM} therapy is not applied, the soft palate may occupy excessive space, preventing it from returning to healthy dimensions and function.

We are attempting to overcome a host of modern facial and airway damage. It can be a challenge for some patients.

Initially developed at UCLA over a decade ago, MARPE appliances have succeeded in older teens, adults, and even those in their late 60s.

SLEEP APNEA (BOOK AUTHORS NOTE)

Improved airway volume achieved by MARPE does not directly mean sleep apnea is improved, but a study by Brunetto D. et al., 2022 showed improvements in snoring and sleep apnea metrics. A number of contributors in this book show significant improvements in daytime airway and in sleep apnea with expansion of mouth and nasal airways as you will see. They also improved facial beauty.

Moving Forward

While some patients might still need jaw surgery, many can benefit from skeletal expansion using the MARPE appliance. This innovative approach has opened up new possibilities for improving airway function, breathing, sleep, and overall health.

SARPE, MSE, DOME, EASE

A number of palatal expanders related to MARPE are listed below and all of them work for some people but not all. A number of practitioners use these techniques to widen oral and nasal airways and correct dental misaligned teeth. They are selected by the outcome they want to achieve and by the skill levels each practitioner has developed using a particular technique. SARPE means surgically assisted rapid palatal expansion that often uses a tooth bone expander and bone expander.

MSE and MSE II mean maxillary skeletal expansion. It is a non-surgical expander using a combination of tooth and mini-implant-secured palatal expander appliances. It was developed by Dr. Won Moon.

DOME means distraction osteogenesis for maxillary expansion, which involves a bone-releasing surgery. It is a two-step process that involves the use of mini-implants to secure the expander to the palate. It was developed at Stanford. The DOME procedure expands the palate but does not necessarily expand the nasal airway.

EASE means endoscopic assisted surgical expansion. It uses TAD or mini-implant-secured expanders and opens nasal and oral airway space. The approach is through the nose with a piezo instrument with minimal bone scoring to release the palatal suture. Developed by Dr. Kasey Li.[344] All of these expander treatments also require orthodontic care in addition to the expansion to close spaces between the teeth created by the expansion and to align the bite.

---

344 Li, Kasey, Tomonori Iwasaki, Stacey Quo, Eileen B. Leary, Connor Li, and Christian Guilleminault. "**Nasomaxillary Expansion by Endoscopically-Assisted Surgical Expansion (EASE): An Airway-Centric Approach**" *Journal of Experimental Zoology* 345, no. 2 (n.d.): 234-245.

Chiropractic Care as a New Collaborative Profession

Four years ago I began to seek the services of chiropractors to screen for and find patients who suffered from obstructive sleep apnea. In that quest, I found Dr. Shane Smith, DC of Chico, California who had a keen interest in the subject and saw the immediate application of what he was focused on regarding the health of his patients. He also recognized the huge impact his profession could make on the health of our country and the world. He saw that his profession could be another source of help in finding the 70 million people who are undiagnosed in the United States.

He then became one of the first in that profession to complete the basic sleep medicine education and training Dr. Zelk, and I created for the documentation of training for dentists, nurses, and chiropractors. The courses are recorded online for those PACE-approved continuing education achievements and requirements. Dr. Shane is now a faculty member of Sleep Balance Academy and heads the chiropractic division.

Later, we also got to meet Dr. Karen Hannah, DC of Morton, IL. She explained the challenges of being a medical examiner for the Department of Transportation and its regulations on sleep apnea management for commercial drivers.

Here are those reports. First, Dr. Shane Smith will cover his journey in sleep medicine, and then Dr. Hannah will illuminate the DOT challenges.

SHANE SMITH, DC

> When I was first introduced to sleep dentistry, I had no idea airway dentistry existed. We began exploring the applications in all health areas, including the central nervous system. As an upper cervical chiropractor, I specialize in restoring the function of the central nervous system.
>
> When I told Dr. Downs about my goals in chiropractic nervous system function, he mentioned that the airway was critical to this function. When someone has an apnea event, their airway is blocked for various reasons. The body goes into a state of suffocation, stimulating and triggering a sympathetic response inside the central nervous system.

They also often have a forward neck posture.

My job as an upper cervical chiropractor is to first, and foremost, measure the responsiveness of the nervous system to determine its state. If a patient is in a constant or chronic state of sympathetic tone, then we call that sympathetic dysafferentation. Essentially, it means that the nervous system is constantly in a fight-or-flight state.

In this fight-or-flight state, the body no longer has the capacity or ability to recognize its surroundings as safe. It has a lowered ability to drop into a parasympathetic state or rest and digest. It's solely operating all bodily functions in a state of fight-or-flight or sympathetic neurological activity. When I adjust a patient's upper cervical spine, first, we measure to see if the patient is in that fight-or-flight state using digital infrared thermal imaging.

The imaging takes a reading of heat from each side of the body at like points, bilateral and symmetrical points, and measures the tip and the temperature of each blood vessel from each side. The software then plots out a graph on one side versus the other, so left versus right. Most importantly, the middle graph shows us a delta, or, in other words, the difference between the two sides. We know through countless studies that blood vessels at like places, at like points, are consistently and persistently asymmetric.

That is a sympathetically dysafferentation state. When a patient exhibits this response on our measuring device, we take three-dimensional and motion X-rays of their upper cervical spine to determine if the neurological response is due to a misaligned and fixated upper cervical spine.[345]

When this is, in fact, the case, a corrective adjustment is made based on the three-dimensional X-ray findings. In other words, X-rays will tell us in which direction the misalignment is and which joint is fixated. When a joint becomes fixated, there's

---

[345] Fitz-Ritson, D. (n.d.). "Cervicogenic Sympathetic Syndromes." In *ClinicalTree*. Retrieved from https://musculoskeletalkey.com/cervicogenic-sympathetic-syndromes/, May 19, 2024.

no motion in the direction you want, creating an abnormal compensating movement pattern for the patient. To address this, we reverse engineer the area that isn't moving properly and free it up to restore proper movement. This may involve making adjustments tailored to the patient's X-rays. It may only be a millimeter of movement. Once the adjustment is delivered, the patient rests in a zero-gravity chair to decrease external stimuli for at least twenty minutes.

They're laid in a nice, cool, dark room and allowed to rest in a neutral position—again, a zero-gravity experience. After the rest, the patient is returned to the exam room, where they are thermographically measured again. In an ideal setting, the delta differential between the thermal output of the left and the right blood vessels is now less than zero to three degrees.

Once this is obtained, we now know the patient is, at least at that moment, in a parasympathetic state and, ideally, is allowed to switch back and forth between the parasympathetic and the sympathetic states. In other words, the brain should then, in an adjusted state, be able to determine what is safe and, therefore, be able to run in a parasympathetic state versus a constant stressful or dangerous sympathetic state.

When a person's nervous system can effectively and accurately assess the surrounding environment and make the correct choice as far as which way to operate the body, then the patient has a successful outcome regarding the upper cervical care being received. The next stage of care is to try to get the patient to stay in that adaptive state for as long as possible so that the nervous system can operate at 100 percent capacity, 100 percent of the time. They have a hard time doing that if they are suffocating at night in their sleep.

After speaking with Dr. Downs about another stimulus creating a sympathetic effect, which in this case would be apnea or suffocation, it occurred to me that measuring these apnea events and episodes in our patients would be very worthwhile. That is when I was introduced to measuring devices.

We utilize the Circul+® ring to measure various parameters including hypoxic events, apneic events, heart rate variability, pulse rate, finger temperature, sleep cycles, and SpO2 (this is an oxygen concentration measurement in the blood). This device provides valuable data to assess patients' sleep quality and detect apnea events before they begin upper cervical care. We gather information on these events' frequency, severity, and duration, enabling us to better understand each patient's sleep patterns and overall health status.

Then, we administer prescribable care just like we always have. But now we have one more metric to measure again, how the patient sleeps. The thought is that if we can achieve a parasympathetic state for the patient while they're sleeping, the patient ought to have a better sleep cycle, and our care will last longer.

We were able to show that that was the case. However, there were still other variables and factors causing the patient to have an apnea episode or hypoxic events. These episodes could have been caused by various factors such as the patient's weight, lack of tone in the tongue and throat muscles, inability to breathe through the nose, malformation or inflammation, adenoids in the nose, and issues in the mouth from allergies and infections.

We started implementing strategies within my chiropractic practice to address nasal congestion and airway obstruction issues. These strategies include using nasal dilators, hypochlorous acid, nasal sprays, xylitol-based sprays, and other methods to improve nasal airflow and increase oxygen intake. The primary goal is to promote effective and efficient nasal breathing, which stimulates a parasympathetic response in the brain. By facilitating better nasal airflow and triggering a parasympathetic response, we aim to enhance our patient's sleep quality.

As more air is transmitted across the membrane of the nose, we also see evidence that a person will secrete and produce more nitric oxide. Nitric oxide is a chemical our bodies make that increases blood perfusion. It dilates blood vessels, essentially allowing more blood and oxygen to go to the deeper recesses of the body without any negative impact on heart rate or blood pressure.

Nitric oxide, a chemical we produce, is very effective. Interestingly, it's also the active ingredient in medications like Viagra and Cialis, known for their ability to dilate blood vessels. We studied our patients more closely and implemented a sleep apnea screening questionnaire.

We asked new and existing patients to complete the questionnaire, assessing their overall sleep quality and various aspects of their well-being. Questions covered topics such as how they felt throughout the day, how quickly they fell asleep, and whether they felt rested after sleeping. Additionally, we utilized data from the Circul+® ring to obtain objective, quantitative, and repeatable measures of their physiological well-being.

We coupled the questionnaire responses with thermographic readings, a standard practice in upper cervical chiropractic. Additionally, we followed our established protocol while integrating data from the Circul+® ring and questionnaires to gather more information about our patients' sleep patterns.

The goal was to minimize apnea or hypoxic events during sleep, aiming to prolong the patient's adaptive or parasympathetic response during rest. This approach sought to promote a longer period of parasympathetic dominance, particularly during sleep, when it is most beneficial.

Thus far, we've observed various factors influencing these outcomes. The severity of apnea events, the extent of tissue laxity, individual weight, and other variables play significant roles. However, now that we can identify and quantify these factors, we're equipped to treat patients effectively. We can facilitate appropriate interventions by leveraging sleep study data and collaborating with sleep specialists to interpret the results. This enables us to assist patients in breathing better at night, enhancing oxygen intake through the nasal passages and ultimately improving overall patient outcomes.

Again, the main focus of my profession, as an upper cervical doctor, is helping a patient restore normal neurological function. This involves allowing the patient's brain to automatically assess a situation, external or internal, through the autonomic nervous system and allowing the body to operate in an appropriate sympathetic or parasympathetic state.

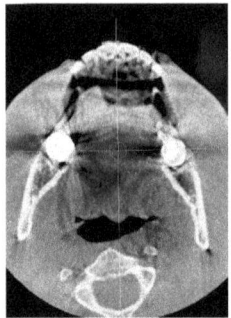 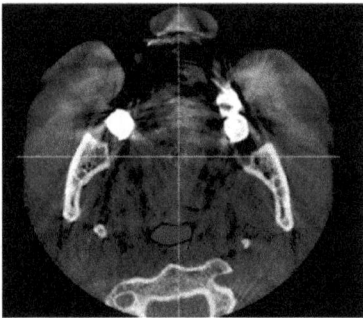

Figures 72 and 73: Courtesy of Dr. Geoffrey Skinner, DDS showing neck vertebrae misalignments and airway distortions on a CBCT scan. The airway on the left is the black area. On the right it is the gray surrounded by a black border area. The spine is the bone just under those areas and is rotated left

Most importantly, the body must adapt rapidly and accurately to any situation. In other words, if the body recognizes a threat, it must trigger a fight-or-flight response to protect itself. However, once the threat is eliminated or is deemed no longer a threat, the body should, under normal circumstances, be able to switch back into its default mode, a parasympathetic state, and be allowed to operate in a more resting and digesting capacity. This is one example that I use with my patients.

The patient can be likened to a car engine. When they're driving at freeway speeds, which are more stressful, more demand is placed on the engine, causing its RPMs to increase. For example, if someone travels eighty miles per hour on the freeway, their RPM might be 3,000. The vehicle can handle upwards of 5,000 RPMs before reaching the red line.

When the engine operates at maximum capacity, it will sustain damage unless something changes quickly. Once the stress is removed, a healthy engine can return to a lower RPM. For example, if they exit the freeway and come to a stoplight on a side street, the RPM gauge drops to 500.

The human body should operate at around 500 to 700 RPMs most of the time. When stress is applied, the body goes up to 3,000. When it's in a very stressful state, the body can redline and operate at 5,000 and even 6,000 RPMs for a short period of time. It's similar to an engine.

When the body operates at those high RPMs for too long, damage will begin to be sustained. So, I tell patients who are stuck in this fight-or-flight mode that their idle speed is, say, 3000 RPMs at every stoplight. They only have about 2000 RPMs worth of external stressors that they can tolerate before they hit the redline.

My goal as their doctor is to adjust and keep them adjusted so that their internal engine can drop down to 500 RPMs. Then, they can tolerate 4,500 more RPMs before they hit the redline at 5,000.

Adding the idea of measuring and monitoring sleep and hypoxic events to our patient care has increased positive patient outcomes. Delivering just upper cervical treatment to a patient with sleep apnea has improved their overall sleep scores. It's not the sole cure by any means, but it is effective in helping someone with sleep apnea improve.

Now that we've incorporated these additional modalities and measurements into our treatment process and are collaborating with sleep professionals, we are fully equipped to assist our patients, and I am incredibly enthusiastic about the opportunity to do so.

Certainly, we work with experts in dentistry and medicine to achieve the desired goal. Below is my daughter, who has Down Syndrome (Figures 74 and 75). Children with this genetic disorder have enlarged tongues and often narrow arches. As you can see from the before and after images, I referred her to an orthodontist for widening of her dental arches to give her more space for her tongue. It also improved her smile.

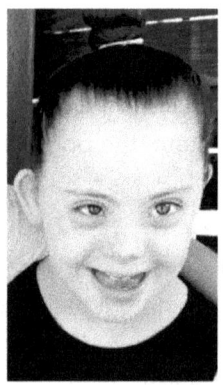 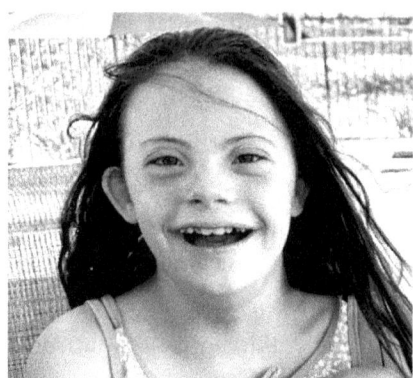

Figure 74   Figure 75

KAREN HANNAH, DC

Dr. Hannah begins with a discussion about CPAP compliance and its standard definition of compliance for DOT.

The implications of this standard are sad. CPAP compliance is better defined as four hours of effective use on 70 percent of nights. If a patient uses the device for only three hours and fifty-nine minutes one night, that night is typically not considered compliant. This is the standard DOT medical examiners have for our truck drivers on our roads, as explained to me by Dr. Karen Hannah, DC, a DOT medical examiner. I think this is frightening, as do many of my colleagues. Here is the situation in her own words.

> This DOT standard is even more frightening because truck drivers often avoid sleep tests and will lie on screening questionnaires for fear of losing their jobs because they don't want to bother with a CPAP machine.

If a driver is diagnosed with diabetes, they are given a period of time to bring it under control and comply with the DOT standards by their next physical (which could be either six months to a year). The standard for controlling diabetes is vague, but if the driver presents with an A1C below ten, they are qualified to drive.

The same can be said for sleep apnea, but the hoops to jump through for compliance and the time it takes a driver to schedule a sleep test, get the results, set up, and receive the CPAP machine can sometimes take weeks to months to set up. This is quite concerning regarding the safety of the drivers and others on the road with them, as well as putting the driver in a determination pending status for driving.

If an existing diagnosis of obstructive sleep apnea has already been given to the driver, they are found to be not compliant with their CPAP usage; they are only given a thirty-day medical card. They must return for a new physical while demonstrating CPAP usage compliance over those thirty days. They must then do the same process for sixty, ninety, and one-year intervals. If at any point they are found to be non-compliant, they are automatically disqualified and must wait until they can show CPAP compliance within the most recent thirty-day interval.

This could take so long that the driver is penalized with no work, especially if their CPAP machine has an error, the chip can't be read, or the data doesn't upload properly. It is especially true for traditional testing.

In some parts of the country, they cannot get a sleep test for many weeks. Then, the treatment period adds to the dilemma, especially if they want something other than a CPAP. Dental devices are not easily fitted with automatic monitoring for compliance, Many CPAPs are also not easily automatically monitored for compliance at this time.

Dr. Hannah is pioneering new monitoring methods to help truck drivers comply, even using treatment devices other than CPAP. This compliance monitoring may include the use of the Circul + ring.

By definition, many truck drivers are sedentary and, consequently, overweight. Sleep apnea is a much more significant issue than our truck drivers tell us.

CHAPTER 9

The Transition in Orthodontic Care

The Connection Between Dental and Airway Health

The relationship between dental and airway health is intricate. Changes in dental arch dimensions can influence the positioning of the tongue, palate, and soft tissues within the oral cavity, all of which play a very important role in maintaining an open airway.[346] A narrower maxilla (upper jaw) can result in a more crowded oral space and nasal airway, reducing tongue space and potentially leading to airway obstruction during sleep.

Individuals exhibiting more normal Class I bite but with crooked teeth (teeth positioned with no overbite or underbite) and those with Class II crooked teeth (teeth positioned so that there is an overbite) and who also have an abnormally tall or short face tend to possess upper throat airways that are noticeably narrower compared to individuals with Class I and Class II malocclusions and typical normal growth patterns.[347]

---

[346] Trenouth, M. J. "The Relation Between Dental Arch Measurements and the Anatomy of the Human Palate." *American Journal of Orthodontics*, vol. 83, no. 4, 1983, pp. 299-303.

[347] Alves, M., *et al*. "Upper and Lower Pharyngeal Airways in Subjects with Class I and Class II Malocclusions and Different Growth Patterns." *American Journal of Orthodontics and Dentofacial Orthopedics*, 148(6), 969-977.

The Impact on Airway Dimensions

Studies have shown that premolar extraction orthodontics can lead to a decrease in airway dimensions, particularly in the upper airway. A narrower maxilla can contribute to a constricted upper airway space and loss of soft tissue facial support. See the facial images of Miss America before and after tooth extraction orthodontics by scanning the QR Code below. The QR code will lead you to a photo of Miss America in the Beautiful Faces Resource folder.

Premolar extraction potentially increases the risk of airway-related issues such as snoring and obstructive sleep apnea[348] and a compromised smile. Not long ago, a dentist who treated orthodontically without premolar extraction for quite crowded teeth cases could be brought before the Board of Examiners and sanctioned for that. Orthodontic treatment without premolar extraction was not considered standard of care unless the crowding was considered minor. However, with advancements in orthodontic techniques and technology, non-extraction orthodontic treatment has become more common.

Figure 76: This is the QR code link to the Beautiful Faces Resource folder. Here is the website link as well. https://www.beautifulfacesbook.com

Note: Although she is smiling wider in the photo to the right, there is a tendency toward larger dark spaces at the corners of the mouth. It appears she has had premolars removed.

---

348 Orabi, Noha, *et al.* "Pharyngeal Airway Dimensional Changes After Orthodontic Treatment with Premolar Extractions: A Systematic Review with Meta-Analysis." *American Journal of Orthodontics & Dentofacial Orthopedics*, August 31, 2021, DOI: 10.

Many orthodontists now prefer non-extraction treatment plans for patients with moderate crowding, Class II malocclusions (overbite and overjet), and severe crowding cases.[349] It is important to note that each patient's case is unique and requires individualized treatment planning. Not all orthodontic cases can be done without tooth extraction. This is the crux of Dr. Mew's argument: Why do they want to know if dental crowding exists? Why are the maxillae too small for all the teeth? Often, the orthodontic treatment model marches on without answers. Many say genetics is the cause, but there are few, if any, skulls in any archive or museum on the planet that show dental crowding before the Industrial Revolution in the late 1800s.

There is a skull showing dental crowding in a specimen from over 100,000 thousand years ago.[350] The citation for this is a human specimen in Israel, in the Anthropological Collection at Tel Aviv University. Even though this paper clearly shows misaligned teeth, the jaws are broad and generally well-developed, in my view.

I also believe that one conclusion from this study is an overreach. That statement is that there is no evidence supporting the idea that early anatomically modern humans had a better alignment between teeth and jaw size.[351] This conclusion is difficult to justify with a study of one prehistoric skull. The malocclusions on prehistoric jaws appear less common than today, and the jaws are almost always larger and broader. This finding is supported by a study from Dublin by an international team of scientists. Here is a summary of that article.

Researchers uncovered intriguing findings by analyzing the lower jaws and teeth crown dimensions of 292 archaeological skeletons from the Levant.

They found that hunter-gatherers exhibited minimal malocclusion and dental crowding, with these conditions becoming prevalent among the earliest farmers approximately 12,000 years ago in Southwest Asia, as reported in a study published in the journal *PLOS ONE* on February 4, 2015.

---

349 Altamash, Sara, *et al*. "Non-extraction Orthodontic Treatment for Severe Dental Crowding Using Miniscrew-Assisted Rapid Maxillary Expansion." *Journal of Surgical Case Reports*, Volume 2022, Issue 11, November 2022, rjac509, (https://doi.org/10.1093/jscr/rjac509).

350 Sarig, R., *et al.* "Malocclusion in Early Anatomically Modern Humans: A Reflection on the Etiology of Modern Dental Misalignment." *PLoS One*, 8(11), e80771. doi: 10.1371/journal.pone.0080771. PMID: 24278319; PMCID: PMC3835570.

351 Ibid.

An international team of scientists observed notable differences in jawbone structures among European hunter-gatherers, Near Eastern/Anatolian semi-sedentary hunter-gatherers, transitional farmers, and European farmers from 28,000 to 6,000 years ago in Anatolia and Europe.

Professor Ron Pinhasi from the School of Archaeology and Earth Institute at University College Dublin, who spearheaded the study, highlights that the lower jaws of the earliest farmers in the Levant didn't simply reduce in size compared to those of hunter-gatherers. Instead, they underwent a series of shape changes linked to the transition to agriculture.[352]

The research reveals that hunter-gatherer populations displayed a remarkable alignment between their lower jaws and teeth, indicating a nearly perfect harmony. However, this harmony diminished in the lower jaws and teeth of the earliest farmers.

For hunter-gatherers, the analysis demonstrated a correlation between inter-individual jawbone and dental distances, suggesting a near-perfect equilibrium between the two. Conversely, semi-sedentary hunter-gatherers and farming groups showed no such correlation, indicating disruption in the harmony between teeth and jawbone with the adoption of agricultural practices and sedentism in the region.[353]

These studies are brought to your attention to focus on the idea that treating modern-day small jaw size misaligned teeth by fitting the teeth to the size of the small jaw instead of attempting to fix both the malocclusion and the jaw size is a philosophy losing ground to the approaches being highlighted in this book.

Compounding the lack of airway space already too small in modern humans by removing teeth to align them and making that space even smaller is logically and practically losing favor. It also often does not create beautiful faces.

---

352 Ibid.
353 Ibid.

The Emergence of Orthodontic Alternatives

In response to the concerns associated with premolar extraction orthodontics, alternative approaches have gained recognition. Orthodontic techniques, such as non-extraction and arch expansion, aim to create dental alignment while preserving or even enhancing airway dimensions.[354] The term expansion includes both widening and, for some, increasing the length of the jaw. In some cases, reverse pull headgear pulls the maxillary jaw forward away from the posterior airway, potentially increasing its size. By addressing both dental and airway concerns simultaneously, these techniques offer a more holistic approach to orthodontics.

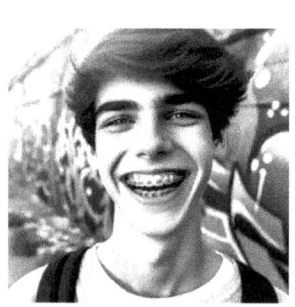

Figure 77: Traditional orthodontic care most often involves fixed brackets and bands. Dall E 3® Bing® and Copilot® image.

The potential for premolar extraction orthodontics to compromise airway dimensions and impair the attainment of beautiful faces highlights the importance of considering dental alignment and airway health in orthodontic treatment planning. As the field of orthodontics continues to evolve, practitioners increasingly recognize the need to prioritize the aesthetics of a smile and the broader health implications of their treatment decisions.

In the upcoming sections of this book, we will further explore these alternative orthodontic approaches and their potential to promote facial aesthetics while safeguarding airway health. You will see the progress airway-centered dentists, orthodontists, and other healthcare providers have achieved. Smiles shown by these practitioners are no longer collapsed, and the resolution of negative space issues in those broad smiles will be explained.[355]

One of the driving forces of change in orthodontic care is that many general dentists also provide that care.

---

354 Bennani, F., Semlali, A., Zoaoui, M., & Tazi, M. "The Effect of Rapid Maxillary Expansion on Nasal Breathing and Some Anatomic and Functional Aspects of the Nasal Cavity." *The Pan African Medical Journal*, 29, 130.

355 Cozza, P., Marino, A., & Mucedero, M. "Analysis of the Changes in the Pharyngeal Airway Space and in the Position of the Mandible Produced by Activator Treatment." *The Angle Orthodontist*, 75(2), 215-223.

The Participation of General Dentists in Orthodontic and Airway Care

General dentists were allowed to provide Invisalign® treatment as early as 2002. Invisalign®, a brand of clear aligners used for orthodontic treatment, initially began with orthodontists as the primary providers. However, in 2002, Align Technology, the company behind Invisalign®, started offering certification and training programs to general dentists, allowing them to become certified Invisalign® providers.

The decision to expand Invisalign® certification to general dentists was driven by several factors, including recognizing that aligning teeth is not limited solely to orthodontic specialists. General dentists have extensive training in oral health and are well-positioned to provide orthodontic treatments like Invisalign®, as well as traditional brackets and wire orthodontics. This expansion allowed more patients to access Invisalign® treatment from their general and family dental care providers, making it more convenient and widely available.

As a result, many general dentists have since become certified Invisalign® providers, and Invisalign® has become a standard option for both orthodontists and general dentists to offer their patients a more discreet and comfortable alternative to traditional braces. Including general dentists in the provision of Invisalign® has expanded patient access to orthodontic care and increased the popularity of this treatment option.

Align Technology®, the company that manufactures Invisalign®, faced legal challenges related to its distribution and certification practices for Invisalign® treatment when it first began offering its services. One notable legal case in the early 2000s resulted from a lawsuit filed by the American Association of Orthodontists (AAO). As a result of this legal action and similar challenges, Align Technology settled with the AAO and agreed to make Invisalign® available to general dentists as well. This settlement, reached in 2006, allowed general dentists to become certified Invisalign® providers and offer the treatment to their patients.

Many transparent aligner companies have since entered the marketplace and are helping treat these conditions with new knowledge of how to use them. However, the attempts to fit teeth to the size of the jaws rather than make the jaws fit the teeth was and is still emphasized by many providers.

The result is that teeth removal is being done to make space for tooth alignment and IPR (interproximal reduction) or shaving between the teeth to make them smaller to fit the space.

This is not always wrong to do. There is a limit to how large you can make a person's jaws so that you can avoid shaping teeth smaller or removing teeth to align them. Some teeth are also abnormally large in some instances. Yet, this is not the philosophy many now believe should be emphasized in planning treatment. Planning, if at all possible, to preserve teeth and tooth structure is the goal we believe should be the starting attitude in the airway, dental alignment, and aesthetic care.

CHAPTER 10

Emerging Science and Healthcare

As you know, this book explores a new direction in healthcare, driven by a visionary team of dentists and a growing awareness within the medical community. It addresses the issues in modern society: structural airway insufficiency, deformed faces, and the pervasive problem of sleep disorders. Remarkably, it's only within the last seventy years that the medical community began recognizing the existence of an epidemic of sleep disorders, thanks to the pioneering work of psychologists in the field of sleep science.

This relatively short time frame saw the emergence of a new field within medicine and their takeover of the science of sleep disorders from the field of psychology, where sleep disorders are explored, understood, and treated more systematically, resulting in a whole new specialty in sleep medicine.

Dentistry's role in tackling airway issues and their solutions has only gained prominence in the last three decades. Before this, the prevailing method for addressing sleep-disordered breathing, specifically obstructive sleep apnea, involved using a positive pressure airway machine called CPAP, BiPAP, or AutoPAP.

Introducing dental care into obstructive sleep apnea treatment brought the innovation of oral sleep appliances. For many patients, they offer the most effective means of addressing airway issues associated with nighttime breathing. Nevertheless, it's essential to recognize that no single treatment is universally effective.

Dentistry is uniquely positioned because our expertise lies directly in the path of a significant airway, the mouth. However, we also have a shared interest in the nasal and sinus airway because teeth are connected to the maxillary sinuses, and the soft palate has both oral and nasal functions. We share this interface with the ENT physicians. When an orofacial myofunctional therapist (OMT) or speech and language pathologist (SLP) treats patients for swallowing, speech, or airway issues, they also work on the palate muscles. When a Nightlase® non-surgical procedure is performed by a dentist, dental hygienist, or nurse with a laser, the tongue and palate are treated.

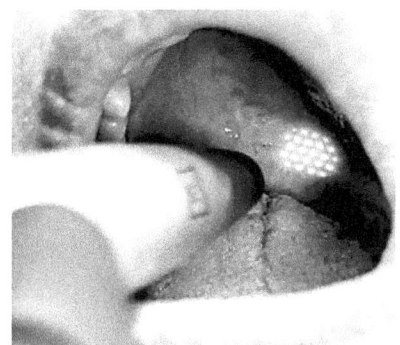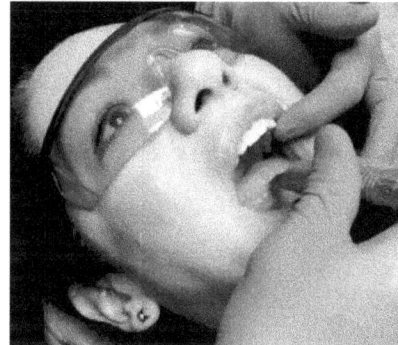

Figures 78 and 79: Nightlase® of the palate.
Photo courtesy of Dr. Nitish Kamboj, Left.- Richard Downs' photo Right.

When a dentist expands the roof of the mouth, he or she also often expands the nose floor. The nasal passages are also developed in many instances with these airway expansions, and when surgeries are performed, we can influence how the nasal passages work. We also see the upper jaw teeth projecting into the maxillary sinuses, and infections in teeth can infect the nasal sinuses. When we place dental implants, we often must also graft bone into the sinuses to create more anchorage for these implants. Oral and maxillofacial dental surgeons also frequently treat many of the same diseases as ENT physicians. No health professional can do more to transform the airway and facial contours (especially non-surgically) than dentistry can. It is no wonder that dentistry is making considerable strides in this critical area of health care.

Tongue Lab – Tongue Right Positioner (TRP®)

As we navigate the landscape of sleep-disordered breathing, exploring emerging sciences and healthcare that complement existing therapies is helpful. One example is Tongue Lab therapy, which complements oromyofunctional therapy. While this new approach will be available in the United States and awaits FDA clearance, it holds promise in addressing muscle-related issues with greater efficiency and effectiveness.

This oral device focuses on targeting muscles involved in sleep-disordered breathing. By addressing muscle function with reduced effort, we anticipate that this treatment modality will seamlessly integrate into the practices of oromyofunctional therapists and speech-language pathologists.

We anticipate using this device for snoring even before regulatory approval, and we remain optimistic about the potential of this new therapy to enhance the care of sleep-disordered breathing and improve patient outcomes. Stay tuned for updates on its availability and effectiveness as we continue to advance in the field of sleep medicine.

Moreover, we see this new therapy as a complement to the eXciteOsa tongue toning device, which has already received FDA clearance for treating OSA. Our belief in the synergistic potential of these two therapies is reinforced by our introduction to this company through Olivier Lauzeral, the head of Somnics Corporation, which owns the FDA-cleared iNAP® therapy. This therapy can potentially enhance combination therapies, offering a multifaceted approach to addressing sleep-disordered breathing and improving patient outcomes.

I am grateful for the introduction of this next section from Björn Ulrich Winter and Jean-Michel Mauclaire.

The Tongue-Right-Positioner – (TRP®) Device for Sleep Apnea Treatment

Dr. Björn Ulrich Winter, specialist in Craniofacial Orthopedics and Dental Sleep Medicine, Oslo, Norway, www.airway.no

Jean-Michel Mauclaire, Founder and Owner of Tongue Lab, Paris, France, www.tonguelab.com

Obstructive sleep apnea (OSA), a prevalent sleep disorder characterized by recurrent pauses in breathing during sleep, poses significant challenges to individuals seeking restorative rest and optimal health. In response to this pervasive issue, function-related causative alternative therapies are expanding. Improving OSA management may be challenging because changing neuromuscular functions requires lengthy work.

A new functional solution has emerged. The Tongue Right Positioner (TRP®).

Understanding the relationship between mouth breathing, tongue function, and sleep disturbances requires not just addressing a jaw position, forced air, or surgery to open the airway. We believe those therapies have a place, but often, the function of the airway muscles is not addressed and left in a poor functioning state. Like oromyofunctional therapy, (TRP®) reestablishes muscle tone and proper muscle function so that airway tissue collapse is lessened.

Mouth breathing, often linked to tongue positioning and airway constriction, can significantly disrupt sleep quality. When individuals breathe through their mouths, it can lead to a downward and backward tongue position, narrowing the airway and increasing the risk of conditions like snoring and OSA. Addressing these factors through techniques like myofunctional therapy, nasal breathing exercises, and utilizing devices like the TRP® is essential for improving sleep quality and overall health.

The TRP® Advantage – Mechanisms of Action:

TRP® operates on natural neuromuscular stimulation, targeting tongue position and oropharyngeal muscle activity to optimize airway patency (keeping the airway open) and mitigate mouth breathing and OSA events. Through precise sensorimotor feedback, TRP® facilitates the toning and coordination of oral-pharyngeal musculature, thereby reducing the upper airway collapsibility and enhancing breathing efficiency throughout the sleep cycle. Furthermore, its design enables the tongue to learn its new (or lost) functions and positions effortlessly during sleep, when the brain reprograms itself. Treatments with TRP® may thus have lasting outcomes.

Ergonomic Design and Comfort:

A hallmark of TRP® lies in its ergonomic design and patient-centric approach to therapy. Unlike traditional interventions such as continuous positive airway pressure (CPAP) therapy or mandibular advancement devices (MADs), TRP® offers a discreet, non-invasive solution that prioritizes patient comfort and compliance. Its compact form factor and customized fit have no iatrogenic effects (side effects), thus ensuring optimal comfort and ease of use. This fosters adherence to therapy, facilitating sustained therapeutic benefits.

Personalized Care and Comprehensive Support:

A multidisciplinary team of healthcare professionals collaborates closely with patients from initial evaluation to ongoing management. This holistic approach encompasses education, behavioral modification strategies, and lifestyle interventions to optimize treatment outcomes and promote long-term sleep wellness.

Unveiling Research Insights - Clinical Efficacy of TRP®:

A rising body of clinical research underscores the efficacy of TRP® in mitigating OSA severity and improving sleep quality. Rigorous observational and controlled studies have consistently demonstrated significant improvement in airway size,[356] nasal patency,[357] tongue strength,[358] and reductions in the apnea-hypopnea index (AHI) among TRP® users,[359] indicative of reduced respiratory events during sleep.

Furthermore, enhancements in nocturnal oxygenation parameters (increased oxygen in the blood while asleep), reduction in arousal frequency

---

356 Mauclaire, et al. "Physiological correction of lingual dysfunction with the 'Tongue Right ..." *International Orthodontics*, vol. 13, no. 3, 2015, pp. 370-389. DOI: 10.1016/j.ortho.2015.06.007.

357 Mauclaire, et al. "Importance of the lingual reeducation by the tongue right positioner on the upper airway's permeability in young orthodontic patients, *Sleep Medicine*, vol. 40, 2017, e288. DOI: 10.1016/j.sleep.2017.11.846.

358 Yanagida, et al. "Effects of tongue right positioner use on tongue pressure: a pilot study, *Scientific Reports* volume 13, Article number: 3289 (2023) . DOI: 10.1186/s40101-023-00323-6.

359 Wulleman, et al. "Facteurs favorisant le traitement rééducatif des troubles respiratoires du sommeil par Tongue Right Positionner, " *Médecine du Sommeil*, vol. 17, no. 1, 2020, pp. 51. DOI: 10.1016/j.msom.2019.12.049.

(reduced sleep micro-awakenings), and improved subjective sleep quality has consistently been documented during and after TRP® intervention.[360] These findings underscore TRP®'s therapeutic advantages and practical value in managing OSA and cardiovascular comorbidities,[361] particularly in mild to moderate OSA.

Additionally, TRP® can be seen as a beneficial adjunct to CPAP or iNAP® therapies for severe OSA cases.

Beyond objective measures of sleep-disordered breathing, TRP® has been shown to exert favorable effects on patient-reported outcomes and quality-of-life metrics. Reduced snoring intensity, reduced number of sleep bruxism (teeth grinding) events, and improvements in mood, exercise, and cognitive function have been documented or reported among individuals undergoing TRP® therapy.

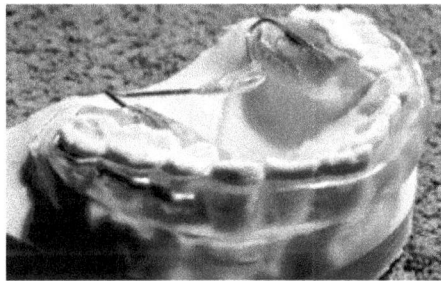
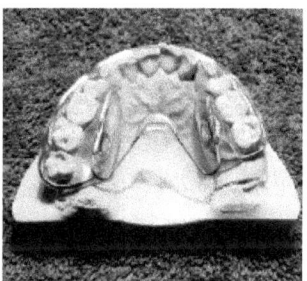

Figures 80 and 81: TRP® Oral Appliances.

Alohaligners™

Dr. Terry Coddington,[362] is a co-founder of the Air Institute and an active lecturer for clear aligner therapy. He is a master of Invisalign® therapy and a top provider of this treatment. He has contributed immeasurably to the success of creating beautiful faces with his care. The patients shown here represent some amazing transformations. Before we start, here are a few words from Dr. Coddington.

---

360 Winter, et al. "Oropharyngeal stimulation with the Tongue-Right-Positioner (TRP) device on OSA patients." *Sleep Medicine*, vol. 100, 2022, S1eS307. Doi: 10.1016/j.sleep.2022.05.707.

361 Belattar, et al. "Impact of Obstructive Sleep Apnea treatment with the Tongue Right Positioner on Arterial Hypertension: a case study," 45th annual meeting of Japanese Society of Sleep Research 2022

362 Coddington, Terry, DDS, Aloha Dental Group, Kahului, HI.

My treatment process always begins with establishing a comprehensive, healthy occlusion for all of my patients. If orthodontic treatment is warranted, I utilize clear aligner therapy with the Invisalign system.

In my orthodontic treatments, I always strive to expand the arches and develop ideal arch forms. My aim is to achieve ideal occlusion with anterior and canine guidance, as well as proper overbite and overjet.

While I am not seeking a reported cure for my OSA patients treated with Invisalign, I am looking for positive changes relative to airway improvements. In my evidence-based experiences with OSA-Invisalign patients, I have witnessed general improvements. Most report a decrease in snoring and a more restful sleep pattern. As we continue to conduct studies to confirm data showing OSA improvements related to orthodontic expansion, we remain hopeful that this will soon be an accepted treatment pathway for doctors moving forward.

He has now created Alohaligners™ to allow the use of clear aligners on children. Invisalign® and other clear aligner companies have only been available for those with adult teeth. Now, with his aligners and system a new and exciting tool has been added to child face development and airway enhancement.

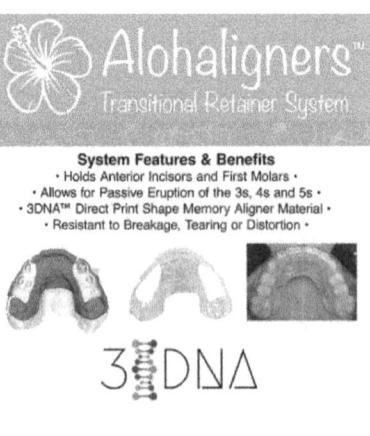

Figure 82

Oralase™ and Babylase™ by Lindsey R. Zeboski, DDS

In this section, Dr. Lindsey Zeboski, DDS[363] presents emergent care for infants and children. Dr. Zeboski is a key opinion leader in the Academy of Clear Aligners and has lectured for the Air Institute on childcare, using airway expansion as a foundation of care. This information is another example of an important treatment for infants and small children. It is the use of non-cutting lasers to help infants and children.

> Some of the best adjunctive procedures I have found and integrated into my airway-focused dental practice are Oralase™ and Babylase™. Oralase™ was created by Darick Nordstrom, DDS, and later on, Babylase™ was developed for infants and babies up to age two. Babylase™ was developed in conjunction with Oralase™ by Angie Tenholder, DDS.
>
> Oralase™/Babylase™ utilizes a specific sequence of laser energy to the mouth, head, and neck areas. Treatments use non-ionizing radiation laser exposure in a specific sequence to alleviate muscle and fascia restrictions while enhancing neurological function. This process engages the body's natural reflexive systems and stimulates C tactile fibers, cranial nerves, and both the limbic and autonomic nervous systems following a standardized technique, which is customized for each patient. Providers must assess the patient's specific needs to determine the appropriate dosage and sequence for the treatment.
>
> Dr. Nordstom developed this sequence using the Fotona Lightwalker® and Fotona X-Pulse® lasers, only. To be clear— this cannot be done with just any laser or in any sequence to receive positive and optimal patient benefits. Like so many other procedures in dentistry— proper training is required.
>
> Providing Oralase™ and Babylase™ as part of my overall treatment plan for my patients with breathing and sleeping issues has optimized how they respond and feel. One of the patient populations that experiences the most profound effects

---

363 Zeboski, L. R., The White House Comprehensive Dentistry, North Platte, NE.

is babies that have trouble nursing and/or sleeping. As a mother of two daughters who did not sleep well, I know how taxing this can be for a family. When my daughters were babies, I was unaware that Babylase™ existed, but I would have loved to have seen what it could have done for them. However, I can help other mothers and babies get on track with this procedure.

One of the things I like the most about Oralase™/Babylase™ is that it allows fascial tongue tie release in a non-surgical way. Tongue tie is not the only treatment it is used for. When babies experience difficulties with nursing, it can sometimes be attributed to tethered oral tissue (TOT), such as a lip or tongue tie. Additionally, their neurological regulation might be affected, as the stress or 'trauma' from the birthing process can disrupt their nervous systems. This disruption can interfere with their ability to latch and nurse effectively.

In babies, their tissue is so pliable that by using Babylase™ and stretching, we can see and feel the release of the tight fibers restricting their improper breathing and swallowing patterns. Yes, there are times when a surgical release is still required and necessary—but if this is something we can avoid, it's better for everyone involved. I always recommend Babylase™/ Oralase™ before surgical releases because it helps improve the final outcome. Even if we still have to release it surgically—it is less invasive because only the very resistant fibers are left to cut. I also see faster and better healing when Oralse™ is done pre- and post-surgical release.

The other key component of Oralase™/Babylase™ is that it provides a neurological reboot or what Dr. Tenholder calls a "CTRL+ALT+DELETE" of the cranial nerves. When our bodies experience trauma—whether it be physical (simply the birthing process), mental, or emotional—our brains and nerves work differently (and not optimally). This all impacts how we swallow, eat, breathe and FEEL. By decreasing the sympathetic output and balancing the parasympathetic system, our bodies can find a more normal and optimal way of functioning. This includes breathing, swallowing, sleeping, and improvement in mood and disposition.

Activating the vagal nerve during OraLase™ provides additional benefits by inducing a profound sense of calm and wellness, which enhances and amplifies the patient's healing capacity due to the procedure. Oralase™ [364] is a type of photobiomodulation (PBM).[365]

I have helped many mothers and babies get to a place where moms can nurse, which is critical for proper jaw growth and development. To prevent more airway issues in our society, everyone must look closer at how we can help our youngest patients.

After Babylase™, parents will notice an improvement in the baby's sleep and temperament (reduced colic). It is easier for the baby to nurse, and less painful for the mother. It should also be noted that mothers are advised to continue working with a lactation consultant during this process to optimize improvement. I have also found that if the mother is treated with Oralase™ while the baby is treated with Babylase™, it also helps them "sync up" and "bond."

Dr. Leboski also uses airway expansion for her patients. Here is a case for Teghan by permission using a combination of fixed expansion and Healthy Start® System appliances.
We address childcare more thoroughly in Chapter 11.

Visionaries in Emerging Science

This awareness of what dentistry can do for facial beauty and airway health is rapidly expanding. Dental sleep medicine courses that were once only teaching oral sleep appliance therapies are rapidly adapting to combination

---

364 MedX Health Corp. "MedX Receives FDA Clearance for Oralase™, an Advanced Laser Treatment for Pain." *BioSpace*. Last modified October 6, 2008. Accessed May 29, 2024. https://www.laserfocusworld.com/home/article/14192939/fda-clears-medxs-oralase-laser-pain-treatment-device

365 Moro, Cecile, et al. "The Effect of Photobiomodulation on the Brain During Wakefulness and Sleep." *Frontiers in Neuroscience*, Section Neuroenergetics and Brain Health 16 (27 July, 2022). https://doi.org/10.3389/fnins.2022.942536.

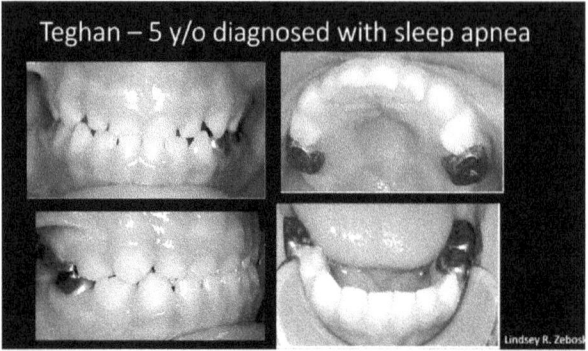

Figure 83

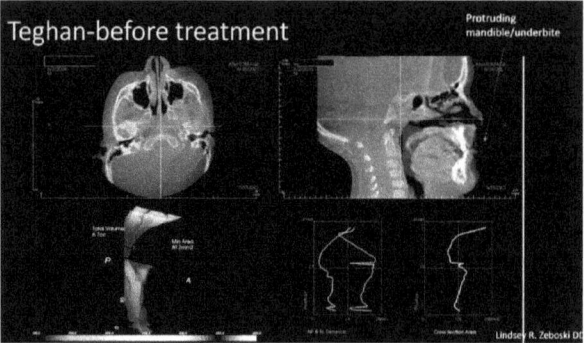

Figure 84

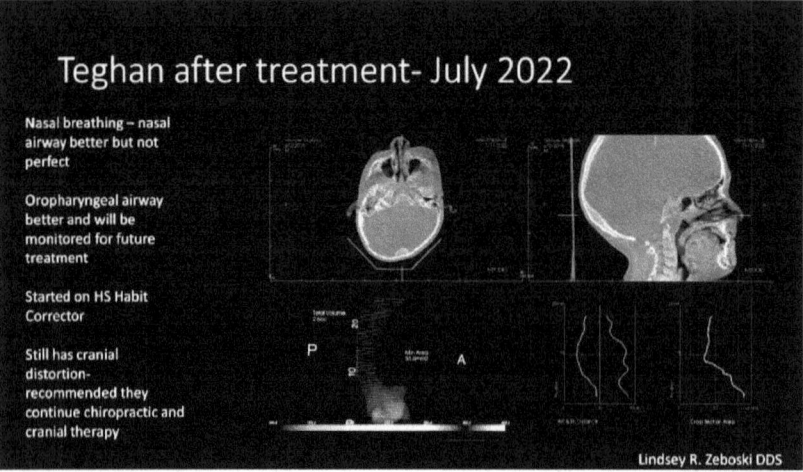

Figure 85: The initials "HS" stand for Healthy Start® appliances.

Emerging Science and Healthcare | 253

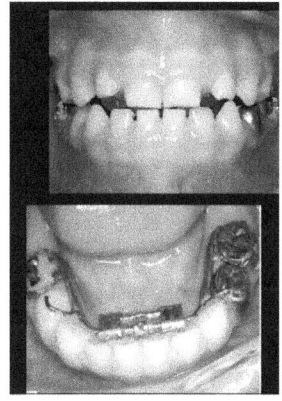

Figure 86

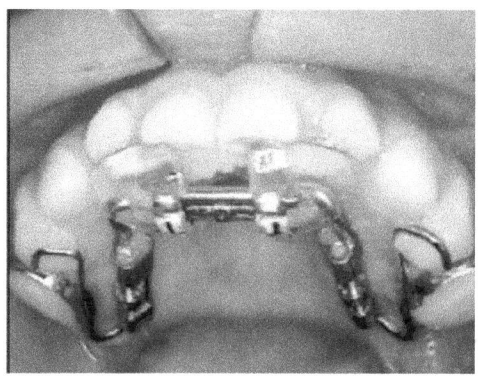

Figure 87

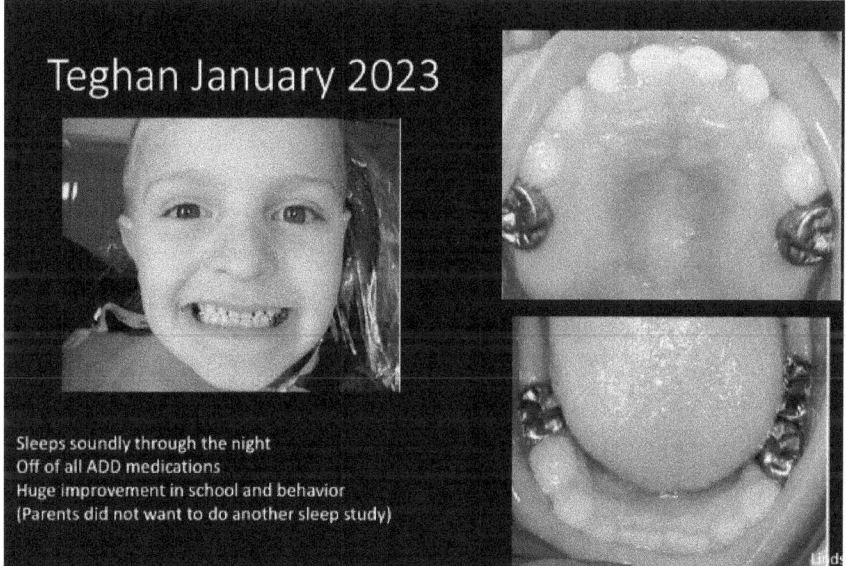

Figure 88

I have a 5 yr old son named Teghan that has been working with Dr. Lindsey for 8 months and I have seen such a huge change in him, even in the very first week of having all his expansion metal in his mouth. It all started with a referral from our speech therapist, Teghan was having issues with speech, hearing, major mouth breathing, sleeping, snoring and behavioral issues. He had been having these issues since he was 2 and we just needed to figure something out. We went to a sleep specialist who then told us that Teghan had mild sleep apnea. With that we also went with the referral from our speech therapist and sleep specialist and went to the orthodontist side to see what she could do. Within the first week of having his expansion metal in he was sleeping through the night, behavioral issues went down, and his mouth breathing even went down majorly.

We have seen so much change in Teghan since we started that I am truly happy with where we are. He breathes out of his nose like 95% of the time, he lets us tighten his appliances like a champ 100% of the time, and he sleeps through the night with very little snoring depending on a head cold or allergies, so now mom can sleep through the night. Also on another note I truly love the atmosphere in this office and so does Teghan. He is not as scared as he used to be going to the dentist, they know him by name and he loves the extra attention. I am truly grateful for the staff and Dr. Lindsey and the outcome we have had and will have when we are finished with his appliances.

-Tiffany & Teghan

Figure 89: Mother's observations of Teghan's treatment progress.

therapies that, in some instances, are placing the recommendations of oral sleep appliances as a last resort to care rather than the foundation of care dentists perform.

This has led to pioneering work by such leaders as Dr. Geoffrey Skinner of Portland, Oregon, the co-founder of the Portland Protocol. Dr. Joseph Zelk, medical director for Dr. Skinner, who co-authored this book, is a medical sleep specialist who understands combination therapy's role. Dr Marc Abramson, who recently retired from the private practice focused on jaw joint pain and disease, has remained on the faculty of Stanford University in their mindfulness studies. Dr. Terry Coddington lectures on Invisalign and Alohaligners^{TM}.

Dr. Felix Liao is a children's facial growth expert in orthodontic airway-centric care. Dr. Kevin Goles and Dr. Kamran Fattah are leaders in Vivos® airway expansion. Dr. Ben Miraglia is an expert in childhood airway development. Dr. Ilya Lipkin is an orthodontist with expert knowledge of many orthodontic issues, including MARPE use for the airway.

This field is expanding so quickly that I cannot list all the leaders in the dental, orthodontic, and medical fields pioneering this movement. I mention these few. Some have developed the Air Institute, and others have developed other institutes to advance this field of knowledge. As we mentioned before, we will call them the "A" (Air) Team, and you will see examples of their cases in this book and sections of text they have expertly written. They are champions of transformative dental and medical care in airway health and beautiful faces.

CHAPTER 11

Children and Sleep Suffocation

Children are unique in this area of airway medicine. They are still growing. They are more adaptable. Shirley Gutkowski, RDH, BDH, has published many articles and is an orofacial myofunctional therapy (OMT) expert. Orofacial myofunctional therapists work with adults and children to retrain muscles in the tongue and throat to function correctly. Using telehealth technology, OMT uses techniques to retrain the snoring complex, nose, mouth, and throat muscles to awaken and activate the neurology that makes those muscles continue to work correctly after the therapy. These retrained and strengthened muscles open airways and close the "open circuit" (awaken unstimulated nerves), calming the system and giving the body the oxygen it needs. This training and strengthening of muscles should also be performed before tongue tie release surgery on adults and older children and after the procedure.

Mouth breathing is a significant issue. Tongue-tie and mouth breathing lead to weak breathing, swallowing, and speech muscles. Tongue Lab® and Vivos® address these muscle and nerve weaknesses. She also instructs on Buteyko breathing techniques. Excellent information on Buteyko breathing is available in Patrick McKeown's book "The Oxygen Advantage."[366]

Here is a quote from Shirley on the subject of children and airway issues.

---

366 McKeown, Patrick. *The Oxygen Advantage*. Little, Brown Book Group, September 15, 2015. ISBN: 0349406707, 978034.

> Oral (or mouth) breathing is pathological breathing. It usually comes with a low tongue posture with/or without a tongue tie. In orofacial myofunctional therapy, we assess and find ways to examine position. When the tongue is up, the airway is no longer compromised by the volume mass of the posterior tongue. The brain will request constant contact between the tongue and palate by providing toning, strengthening, neurological, and proprioception exercises. The tongue is the support of the head.[367]

Shirley further explains there are two main goals in orofacial myofunctional therapy. One is to teach the tongue to rest in the palatal vault of the upper arch. This is key to holding the tongue out of the airway and closing the open neurological circuit between the tongue and palate. The second is to give better tone to the tongue muscles.

Not only are children unique, but those with sleep apnea present unique challenges, which can be considerably complex. Nearly all sleep apnea is accompanied by mouth breathing. Unlike adults, children affected by sleep apnea may exhibit distinct symptoms that can lead to potential misinterpretation. Rather than displaying drowsiness, they might show hyperactivity and may not show typical snoring signs. The implications of sleep apnea on children encompass various facets, including speech irregularities, aggressive behavior, reduced academic performance, bed wetting, weight gain, postural growth changes, depression, and anxiety disorders, frequent ear infections, crowded teeth, and the development of attention deficit disorders.[368]

This uniqueness of presenting symptoms is complicated because we are dealing with a growing person rather than a mature, non-growing adult. On the one hand, mouth breathing can deform the face and body. On the other hand, the fact that they are growing offers a tremendous opportunity to correct improper growth and behaviors because they are still presenting us with a growth redirection opportunity. Often, they can respond more easily and quickly than adults can with proper therapy.

---

367 Shirley Gutkowski, RDH, BSDH, *Primal Air LLC*, primalaire.com.

368 Chervin, R. D., Hedger, K., Dillon, J. E., et al. (2000). "Pediatric sleep questionnaire (PSQ): validity and reliability of scales for sleep-disordered breathing, snoring, sleepiness, and behavioral problems". *Sleep Medicine*, 1(1), 21-32.

In the *International Journal of Pediatric Otolaryngology*, a study on nasal breathing in children with adenoids and tonsils removed showed a significant improvement in forward head posture and body posture. After surgery, there was a notable reduction in forward head position, protrusion, elevation of the shoulders, and forward tilt of the shoulder blade compared to before the operation.[369]

These are the conclusions I summarized from their article: Adenotonsillectomy can improve head and shoulder girdle posture (the ring of bones supporting the arms) among children who habitually breathe through their mouths. These clinical observations carry significant implications, potentially enhancing the overall quality of life for children affected by mouth breathing.[370]

This further supports the concept that early intervention of breathing issues in children is a good practice and can redirect children's growth in the right direction or, better put, in the direction their genetic potential wants to take them. Don't assume that adenoid and tonsil removal is the first choice of care for children or even if it is needed. Studies looking at the sustained outcomes of these surgeries are disappointing. The best results come from collaborative care with airway-trained allergists, otolaryngologists, dentists, orthodontists, orofacial myofunctional therapists, sleep specialists, hygienists, chiropractors, the child's school teacher, and more.

Let's also consider that a child misbehaving may not just be exhibiting stubborn-willed defiance but rather an airway issue. If they have airway issues and are exhibiting behavior problems, they could also have neurological malfunction from cranial nerve compression and trappings that a chiropractor should examine. They could also be suffocating in their sleep! Be kind and try to rule out other causes of antisocial behavior.

A considerable percentage of children diagnosed with attention deficit hyperactivity disorder (ADHD) could potentially be impacted by sleep apnea. Estimates indicate that 50 percent of children diagnosed with ADHD may be demonstrating symptoms that align more with sleep apnea than with ADHD itself. [371]

---

[369] Neiva, Patricia Dayrell *et al.* (2018). "The effect of adenotonsillectomy on the position of head, cervical and thoracic spine, and scapular girdle of mouth breathing children." *International Journal of Pediatric Otorhinolaryngology*, 101-106.

[370] Ibid

[371] Marcus, C. L., & Brooks, L. J. (2013). "Diagnosis and management of childhood obstructive

A Boy Named Ridge (by Permission)

This story from a mother about her family's experience with her son illustrates some of the challenges faced by children with compromised airways. It is a story of the love, the trials, and the triumph of the whole family for a child in desperate need, undiagnosed with sleep suffocation.

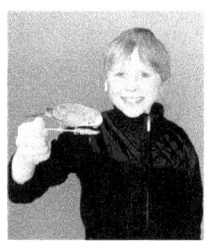

Figure 90: Ridge (with Permission)

It was September 2020, and things went wrong. Our family was suddenly filled with violence, uncertainty, and fear. It wasn't always like that. Jared and I had been happily married for over ten years, and we had four kiddos, ages two, five, six, and nine. Our family was full of snuggles, adorable voices, games, long days of bike rides, playing at the park, and reading more books than you can imagine. Over the years, we learned that eating healthy and developing healthy sleep habits were important to our family. We lived in Colorado for most of our lives and had a massive family support system. We moved to Florida in 2019 when Jared got a great job at Kennedy Space Center. We were a young family and ready for some beach adventures.

About a year after moving to Florida, we decided to go on a road trip to Colorado to spend a few weeks with our family. It was September 2020, and Jared could work remotely due to COVID-19. We were trying to maintain some sense of health even though we were on the road. We made the five-day trip while eating the healthy food we packed. The kids only watched two movies! I was proud of how well the trip went, but we were all tired from being on the road and sleeping away from home.

This is when everything changed. A few days after getting to Colorado, our six-and-a-half-year-old son, Ridge, had fallen asleep in the car on the way back from church. We were just a few minutes away from the house, and I wanted everyone to nap together, mainly because I was tired and wanted to lie down,

---

sleep apnea syndrome." *Pediatrics*, 131(3), e714-e725.

too! We woke him up, and it felt like a switch had flipped. He got really upset and was violent for hours.

We didn't know what to do, and none of our parenting techniques worked. I left the house with the other kids, and Jared stayed with Ridge. We were stunned at what had happened. Ridge had had normal tantrums or upsets before, but this was unlike anything we had ever experienced.

We didn't know it then, but this episode marked the beginning of a very difficult year for our family. His episodes would continue, although the triggers and time between episodes were unpredictable. Some episodes led to injuries, hospital visits with sedation, and visits from child protection services. All the episodes led to absolute heartbreak and insecurity. We consulted with over a dozen specialists throughout the next year to figure out why this was happening.

I wish we had known right then that he was tired, chronically exhausted from a lack of good quality sleep at night. His body was never able to detox, unwind, or heal, because his sleep was so disrupted. We didn't know that the added stress of our recent cross-country road trip would make his body unable to cope.

One night, he got furious, and it seemed he couldn't even hear us talking to him. He was throwing things, then weirdly moving his head and repeating himself. It was scary to see. We took him to the Emergency Department, and when we got to the hospital, they sedated him. He was frightened and angry, and nothing we did helped. We kept praying that he would calm down. This was terrifying, and I was physically and emotionally drained.

The episodes seemed unpredictable. We started meeting with providers immediately to figure out what was happening, but finding answers was a slow process. Sometimes, he would go days or weeks without a big problem, and during those breaks, we could maintain some sense of normalcy.

Ridge and his younger brother Charlie are seventeen months apart, and both have speech delays. While on our trip to Colorado, they had several appointments with an orofacial myologist. Orofacial Myology is like physical therapy for the muscles in your mouth. Orofacial Myologists help with many things, and they lead you in exercises to strengthen your muscles to help your mouth, tongue, and lips function correctly. We were hoping she could help the boys with their speech. She also recognized that the kids and I all had tongue ties, which could be problematic, and we had them surgically released. We learned from her that underdevelopment in the mouth can also lead to a compromised airway, which makes breathing at night difficult.

I told her about Ridge's recent aggressive behaviors and asked if it could at all be connected to the issues with his mouth. She said 'YES' and told me to watch a video on YouTube called "Finding Connor Deegan." It's a short video about a mom and her son and their journey of finding that his violent behaviors were tied to a compromised airway and a lack of quality sleep at night.

"Finding Connor Deegan," says that they found Connor's airway issues through a sleep study. After the two-months stay in Colorado, we went back to Florida and scheduled a sleep study for Ridge at the beginning of December. The sleep study found no significant concerns with Ridge's sleep.

We wanted to expand his mouth and airway through treatment with dental appliances. Still, the insignificant results from the sleep study led us to believe that there was another physical issue causing his aggression. Years later, we found out that the sleep study had been misinterpreted. The sleep study actually had shown that Ridge needed treatment, and I cried when I found out.

We saw a neurologist several times and did an MRI to check for a brain tumor. We were working with our new family care provider in Florida and regularly seeing a mental health therapist. Ridge also had regular chiropractic and craniosacral therapy appointments. We saw a psychiatrist, and she prescribed Lamotrigine, which can be used to treat mood disorders in kids.

My gut was telling me there was a physical issue going on and that this medication wasn't going to fix it, especially when I did some research and found that one of the side effects of the drug was aggression.

During an episode, Ridge sometimes got fixated on trying to hurt us or the other kids. Sometimes, we would have the kids go to a neighbor's house to separate them from Ridge, but a few times, we would have the other kids lock themselves in the bathroom so that Ridge couldn't get to them during an episode. My older daughter would even bring blankets, books, and snacks into the bathroom, and she would read to the younger kids while I was trying to help Ridge.

Once, Ridge got a hammer from the garage and was hammering at the locked door to the bathroom to get to them. Before I could stop him, he had hammered through the hollow core door and could reach in and unlock it from the inside. Nobody was hurt, and we got the kids out of the house until Ridge was calm again.

A few months into the episodes, I noticed that if I lay down with him during the day, he would instantly fall asleep and take a long nap. Ridge always had a quiet time but had recently started reading or playing quietly instead of sleeping. I made it a priority to lie down with him every day so he would sleep.

All the therapies we were doing, along with the daily naps, seemed to help him feel well for three months, and he was his usual, kind, and resilient self. We thought whatever was going on might have been resolved. Then we went on a short trip, and the episodes started again.

In the summer, he kicked out a second-story window and cut his leg. I was driving home when Jared called me in a panic, and the fire department was already on the way. I was terrified that Ridge was seriously hurt. When I got home, he was coherent and calm. The paramedics told us he was okay and we could transport him to the hospital. He ended up having seventeen stitches. While we were there, the hospital social worker interviewed us. I told her our story and how many specialists we were seeing, but I asked if she had any knowledge of resources that might help us. But she just cleared us, saying we were doing everything necessary.

One of the providers recommended that we look for mold in the home. We found a hidden leak in our bathroom that had grown mold. We did mold remediation in the house and worked on a mold detox for Ridge under the guidance of our healthcare provider. We were hopeful we would see behavioral changes but didn't notice a difference.

We met with another orofacial myologist in Florida, and she told us that Ridge could have a seriously compromised airway. She helped us connect with a dentist an hour away who used a dental appliance called Vivos Guide® to expand mouths and small airways in kids. I asked if I could talk to any of her patients, and she connected me with a mom who had four kids also using Vivos®. The mom shared how her son, a few years older than Ridge, faced similar challenges. He experienced huge improvements after starting treatment with the appliance. His issues stopped, including his aggressive behaviors and bed wetting, and he even underwent a noticeable growth spurt. Hearing about this was the final push we needed to commit to the treatment for Ridge.

Ridge started with his first Vivos® Guide appliance at the end of September 2021. It looked like a blue mouthguard. Wearing it at night and chewing on it during the day would grow his muscles and expand his mouth and airway. I was HOPEFUL. Hopeful this would work. I was hopeful that after everything we had been through and all the providers we had seen, this would finally be able to help. My sweet boy, I wanted him to be well.

It seems unbelievable, but Ridge started feeling better after wearing the mouth appliance for only a few days. About a week later, when we were traveling, he had one other major episode, and anything after that was mild. He also stopped peeing on the bed and consistently seemed more like himself.

We had found the answer! The solution was astounding, yet simple. Ridge's palate was too narrow, so his mouth was too small. His tongue had nowhere to go. His tongue bulged against his airway, making breathing difficult, especially at night. He never got good quality sleep. He was constantly sleep-deprived. Being sleep-deprived for years on end negatively impacted Ridge's body, daily behavior, and mental health. The positive effects, once he started sleeping properly, were significant.

I've learned that Ridge had many red flags pointing to his airway being compromised. I wasn't aware that these signs were abnormal, but now I recognize them as serious.

Ridge sucked on his finger until we broke the habit at age six.
He had bottles and didn't breastfeed enough.
He had a speech delay.
He wet the bed at night (sometimes during nap time).
He breathed through his mouth.
He snored, even though it was mild.
He had a lot of colds early on in life and had a stuffy nose often.
He had an open bite when his mouth was closed.

Parents don't know how important it is to have their kids' airways evaluated. I didn't. And most practitioners don't know either. Years before, we did have one practitioner early on who tried to alert us to an airway issue when our son Charlie was two years old. She was young and seemed inexperienced compared to our previous speech therapist. Charlie sucked on his thumb, and the speech therapist told us that he could be propping open his airway, and she urged us to see an ENT.

This was the first time we had ever heard about airway issues, and we had scheduled an appointment. The ENT said Charlie had a mild tongue tie but was not concerned. He said he wouldn't evaluate Charlie's tonsils or adenoids unless he was put under general anesthesia and that he didn't think evaluating them was necessary. I was very uncomfortable with the idea of general anesthesia, so we checked the box that we had seen a specialist and moved on.

It's incredible that we went through such a life-altering year with Ridge a few years later. If we had gone to a different ENT and believed the concerns of the young speech therapist, we might have been alerted to and believed the dangers of an underdeveloped mouth and a small airway sooner.

I hope our story will help other people schedule an evaluation with an airway-centric dentist. I hope speech therapists, ENTs, doctors, teachers, grandparents, and anyone who reads this will help the kids by educating their parents about airway issues.

I was never diagnosed with any airway issues, yet I should have been. I had a significant overbite and crooked teeth from sucking on my thumb as a kid. I had braces as a teenager but never had my small mouth expanded. I am currently going through expansion with the adult Vivos® appliance; I am about two months into my treatment. I have already noticed that I have a lot more space between my teeth, and I'm noticing good changes in my sleep quality and smile. I'm excited to see how much better I feel as I continue with treatment.

I'm beyond grateful for all of the help we had from family, friends, and neighbors during the tough times. I'm thankful for the mom who made the "Finding Connor Deegan" video and the mom I spoke with whose family was receiving treatment from the dentist in Orlando. It was courageous women sharing their stories that ultimately made us move forward with getting Ridge's airway evaluated and starting treatment. I hope that in sharing our story, every parent will be encouraged to find an airway-centric dentist and have their child's airway evaluated.

Things started going right in our family when we treated Ridge's airway. It's now 2024, and our family is much more stable and peaceful. Ridge is incredibly responsible, doing great in school, gets along well with his siblings, and adores his new baby sister. He is a fantastic person. He is loved, loving, strong, courageous, and I know he can have an amazing and successful life.

Ridge's story leads us to discuss two important therapies listed below.

Speech-Language Therapy:

Speech-language pathologists (SLP) have a wide range of specialties within the discipline. They work with individuals of all ages to address the functional mechanics of various facial and oral structures, including the face, lips, tongue, jaws, pharynx, and larynx. Their focus encompasses vocalization, speech articulation, biting, chewing, swallowing, facial expressions, oral sensation processing, and breathing.

Speech pathologists take a holistic approach that considers the importance of facial structure, core stability, diaphragm usage, and overall body posture in supporting oropharyngeal function. With their expertise, they collaborate on cases involving disordered breathing (such as sleep-disordered breathing, obstructive sleep apnea, and upper airway resistance syndrome), craniofacial pain (including temporomandibular joint disorder and trigeminal neuralgia, a stabbing pain in the face), dental misalignment, digestive issues, and nervous system regulation.

Speech-language therapy services are typically covered by medical insurance. One such group, BreatheWorks, offers virtual sessions across fifteen states and multiple locations to enhance access to care for individuals in need.[372]

Orofacial Myofunctional Therapy:

We are introducing this important subject with an introduction to what orofacial myofunctional therapy is and then a story of Kayla, who was treated by Shirley Gutkowski and her colleague Diane Romary. Shirley explains the profession and the need to work as a team with other healthcare professionals.

Orofacial myofunctional therapy, sometimes called oral myology, sometimes called oral myofunctional therapy, and never called myofascial therapy, is an integral part of any treatment plans for any sleep or breathing disorder. We'll be calling it OMT throughout the book. It is defined as a type of therapy that involves evaluating and treating the oral and facial musculature, including the tongue, lips, cheeks, and jaw muscles.

---

372 Jarvis, Corinne, MS, SLP. "BreatheWorks/SpeechWorks." Accessed May 9, 2024, from https://orofacialmyologist.org/corinne-jarvis/.

Children and Sleep Suffocation | 267

Before and after tongue tie extension.

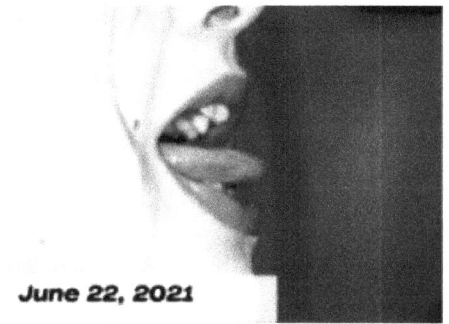

Figure 91: Pre-treatment tongue tie dysfunction

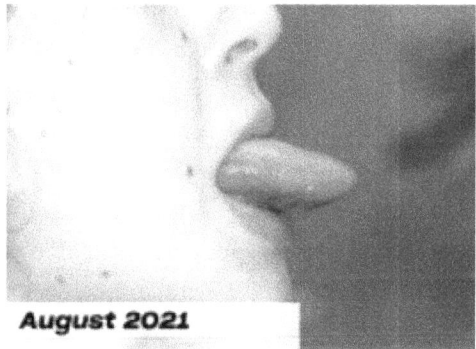

Figure 92: Myofunctional therapy and surgery.

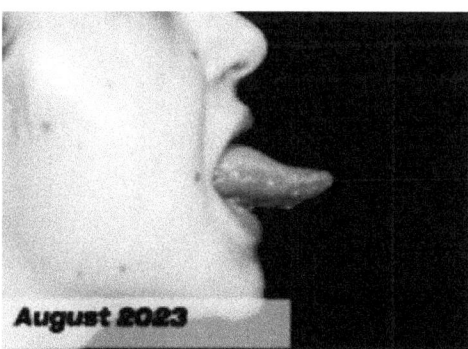

Figure 93: Myofunctional therapy with surgery, stable after two years.

As described earlier, without harmonizing the muscles in the mouth, the face won't grow to its genetic potential. One of the reasons we rarely see dental decay in ancient skulls is that there were no myofascial disorders. Myo is short for muscle, and fascial is about the face. If the muscles of the face don't work, chewing doesn't work. Chewing is critical for the facial and airway muscles. For instance, if the facial muscles don't work, the mouth doesn't clear of food that has been chewed.

Current thought about dental decay is that the diet changed 10,000 years ago to be more agrarian, more plant-based, and less meat-based. It's true that happened, but the problem occurred because of the lack of nutrient density. This lifestyle also began robbing humans of the space between their teeth. The lack of space trapped food and fed the oral microbiome, eventually favoring pathogens that caused dental decay. When there is space between the teeth, we can rest assured that the space for the airway is more significant.

The tongue's function for chewing, swallowing, and structuring the face is critical. People like dentists, ENTs, and hygienists now consider the tongue a respiratory organ, not just a speech and chewing muscle grouping. If the tongue and face muscle system doesn't work, it's hard for the rest of the body to function appropriately. At rest, the tongue needs to rest entirely on the palate, yes, against gravity. In that position, it's hard to block the airway.

Breathing starts from the nose, and when the air goes in, it swirls around the turbinates. We need some turbulence of this type in the nose. This slows down the air velocity and helps to warm the air. The cells surrounding the turbinates make mucus to capture the more giant molecules inhaled. The cells producing nitric oxide, if not covered by solidified mucus, kick out the gas that kills bacteria and viruses inhaled from the air. This nitric oxide also helps the lungs function better.

The air passes by the Eustachian tubes, and the adenoids veer down the back of the throat, past the tonsils and back of the tongue, past the vocal cords, and into the trachea. This right angle, which turns from the nose to the throat of the airway, is quite unique to primate humans.

Air that does not pass through the nose and instead passes through the mouth is unfiltered, unwarmed, and unconditioned air that passes the tonsils. Tonsils are not supposed to deal with large particles; they are intended to filter nanoparticulate (small particles) that pass through the nasal gauntlet and are sanitized by nitric oxide.

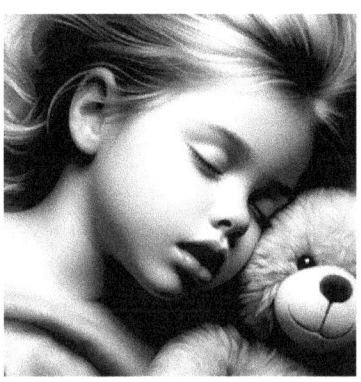 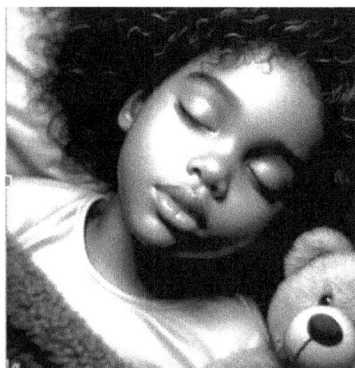

Figures 94 and 95: Dall E 3® Bing® and Copilot® AI images.

These children may look cute, but this is abnormal open-mouth breathing for the child on the left. We dentists also see crooked teeth, TMJ pain, ADHD-like behavior, migraines, speech development problems, high blood pressure, and more undergrowth development. The lips of the child on the right are closed.

The tonsils will grow to accommodate their new job of mouth breathing, further impeding the volume of the airway. Disuse of the nose and sinuses, such as by mouth breathing, was shown to stunt the growth of the sinuses.[373]

This begs the question: What will a forty-year-old man do with twelve-year-old-sized sinuses? There's little reason to delay getting to the bottom of tongue mobility issues as early as possible, say days old instead of years old, which is one of the best prevention strategies. This refers to a minor surgical intervention called tongue-tie release.[374]

The best way to treat these conditions is with a complete team approach as the child gets further from their first birthday. Before age one, most dentists and ENTs can release a tongue simply. It will likely need to be revised at a later age. Simply addressing a tongue tie by stretching the tongue or modifying the infant hold for breastfeeding is inadequate and detrimental to the growth and development of the craniofacial respiratory complex.

---

373 Agacayak, K. S., *et al.* "Alterations in Maxillary Sinus Volume Among Oral and Nasal Breathers." *Medical Science Monitor: International Medical Journal of Experimental and Clinical Research*, 21, 18–26. Accessed at https://doi.org/10.12659/MSM.89137

374 Tikku, T., *et al.* "Dimensional Changes in Maxillary Sinus of Mouth Breathers." *Journal of Oral Biology and Craniofacial Research*, 3(1), 9–14, Accessed at https://doi.org/10.1016/j.jobcr.2012.11.005)

The job of the OMT or speech and language pathologist is to find out what is interfering with nasal breathing and help develop the soft tissue contacts: lips together and tongue to palate. Achieving this in a young child is optimal.

Parents can start paying closer attention to the sounds the child makes when sleeping, the position of the child during sleep, and how they chew and swallow. All breathing should be silent, sleep positions should be still, and swallowing should be silent. If the mother is shamed into bottle feeding with comments about old nipples or the child being allergic to her milk, increasing awareness of these three things is super important. Keep the baby's nose clear, use a xylitol nasal spray and waft a bit of essential oil, or use a Neti Stick if the baby's nose is buggy. Nose hygiene is as important as oral hygiene, more so in infants. Cleaning the nose at each diaper change is a good habit to get into.

Close the baby's lips all day by lightly pinching them together. Teaching the child to motorboat their lips and to click their tongue is also essential. Babies can also make fish faces. Older children, aged four or later, can be reminded to sit straight and close their mouths when they eat. Always eat together at the table so you, the parent, can model good eating behavior. Move the schedule around and drop activities that interfere with family mealtime. Make sure the bites are small and the chewing is prolonged; make a game of it.

Snoring is not inert: it is incredibly damaging to the growing child, not just in facial development but also in the brain. As mentioned in chapter three, children who snore or make any sound during sleep have a much more challenging time in school and exhibit behavior problems throughout their lives.[375] Treating this before the first birthday also requires a team that includes a chiropractor. The trauma of birth can be exhibited in many areas; often, infants with tongue ties present with something called torticollis. The head is tilting or turning to one side. Too often, no one asks about the tongue's mobility and those who find the tongue immobilized by a tether of abnormal tissue.[376]

---

375 Galland, B., *et al.* "Sleep Disordered Breathing and Academic Performance: A Meta-analysis." *Pediatrics*, 136(4), e934–e946, https://doi.org/10.1542/peds.2015-1677

376 Eranhikkal, A., *et al.* "Neglected Torticollis: A Rare Pediatric Case Report." *International Journal of Clinical Pediatric Dentistry*, 13(1), 94-97. doi: 10.5005/jp-journals-10005-1730. PMID:

After age one, the child is challenged to manage for a tongue tie release. The result of an optimal release is only possible if the child is put under general anesthesia, and no one wants that. Secondarily, we wait until the child is four or older. By then, much damage has occurred in the oral cavity and brain development because of a lack of optimal oxygen.[377]

Kayla's story

The case of Kayla is an excellent example of how things fall apart and how ignoring the complaints of the mother created an expensive treatment plan that lasted nearly three years. Kayla's mother, Kelly, complained of nursing problems with Kayla since birth. She thought her child had a tongue tie, but no one confirmed it. Tongue tie releases lost favor in the 1970s. It was deemed a cosmetic or optional surgery because the child could gain weight and thrive based on infant formulas developed over the previous generations.

Infant weight gain is an extremely low-bar standard to gauge health. Today, we know that sleep apnea in children causes facial growth problems.[378]

Kayla and her family moved to three different states over her first decade of life, and although she had gone to many dentists, none had identified her tongue tie. In the mind of most physicians and dentists, once a child can talk and eat solid foods, the necessity for release is unnecessary, and the child is fine. They believe the procedure is optional, and at the same time, many dentists comment to parents that they may want to start saving money for braces. Like many in Kayla's situation, she did develop severe malocclusion (crowded teeth). Her upper right canine was trapped in the palate, and the rest of her teeth were jumbled. Her tongue was so restricted that she could not stick it out past her lip; she could not raise the tip of the tongue to the roof of her mouth without closing nearly completely. Her sleep was destroyed.

32581488; PMCID: PMC7299884.

[377] Isaiah, Amal, *et al.* "Association Between Habitual Snoring and Cognitive Performance Among a Large Sample of Preadolescent Children." *JAMA Otolaryngology–Head & Neck Surgery*, 147(5) (2021): 426-433. Doi: 10.1001/jamaoto.2020.5712) and Isaiah, Amal, *et al.* "Associations Between Frontal Lobe Structure, Parent-Reported Obstructive Sleep Disordered Breathing, and Childhood Behavior in the ABCD Dataset." *Nature Communications*, 12(1) (April 13, 2021). doi: 10.1038/s41467-021-22534-0)

[378] Huang, Y. S., & Guilleminault, C. "Pediatric Obstructive Sleep Apnea and the Critical Role of Oral-Facial Growth: Evidences." *Frontiers in Neurology*, 3, 184. https://doi.org/10.3389/fneur.2012.00184

Kayla remembers this: "I had a lot of dental work done last year. I had an oral surgeon exposed the trapped tooth so the orthodontist could pull it down into place; it's still in process."

Eventually, at age thirteen, Kayla and her family found a dentist who also provided orthodontic treatment for his patients. The dentist finally confirmed the tongue tie and identified the restriction as the reason for her malocclusion. Too many orthodontists have no idea why they treat malocclusion; they often don't say what caused the crooked teeth. Worse, they'll offer a pat answer of genetics. In Kayla's case, the tip of the tongue was tied to the floor of the mouth. A tongue tie is also called ankyloglossia or tongue tether. Simply put, the frenum or frenulum, a band under the tongue connecting the tongue to the floor of the mouth, was too short and tight. When it is too short, the tongue has lost freedom of movement. If it's attached too far forward, the tongue also loses freedom of forward movement. When the restrictions are in the back of the tongue, which is nearly invisible, the movement in a swallow is restricted, forcing the tongue to push forward against the teeth hundreds of times a day.

At age thirteen (and at every age past four), a person needs to have orofacial myofunctional therapy to get the tongue in an acceptable position and strengthened for the frenuloplasty. Functional frenuloplasty is the most precise procedure for tongue tie "release." It combines orofacial myofunctional therapy with surgical release of the tongue tie. Often a MyoMunchee® device is used with these patients. We will discuss this more later.

Frenectomy is a laser or scalpel removal of the frenum to the bone and the use of sutures to close the wound. Most people are more familiar with the less invasive frenotomy release,[379] where the result is a "nice diamond" tissue spread. If the tie is anterior (towards the front), there is little chance of excessive bleeding if the frenulum stands apart from the tongue muscles. For infants, a "quick" frenuloplasty is all that's necessary. On an infant, the dentist or ENT will likely use a little numbing gel, a snip with scissors, or a laser, and you're on your way. Frenuloplasty involves modifying or adjusting the frenulum, which may or may not include complete removal, depending

---

379 Aaronson, N. L. (2022, September 22). Frenectomy explained: Reasons, recovery, and what to expect. *Healthgrades*. Retrieved from https://www.healthgrades.com/right-care/oral-health/frenectomy

on the case. Frenuloplasty is a more general term encompassing multiple meanings and will often be used by our authors.

Let's not prioritize the instruments used for this procedure and overlook the surgeon's hands. You'll want to find a provider confident in their technique, not married to lasers or scissors. Trust the person to know what works best in their hands.[380]

For a functional frenuloplasty, the tongue must hold a tongue suction posture on the roof of the mouth for upwards of one minute and repeat that positioning over and over for ten to fifteen minutes, requiring strength and endurance of the tongue muscles. In the case of a functional frenuloplasty, OMT is there to help the tongue endure the repeated lingual palatal suction hold as the surgeon removes the restrictions. This is where the functional part of functional frenuloplasty lies. With the tongue in the position of the roof of the mouth, the surgeon can see the restrictions and remove them. The surgeon can also ask the patient about their perceived improvements and see bodily changes throughout the procedure.

Kayla worked with many practitioners, including a myofunctional therapist, a physical therapist, an orthodontist, and a periodontal (gum) surgeon, who provided functional frenuloplasty. We hesitate to guess the final financial investment with all these professionals and shake our heads when we know that a tongue tie release in an infant was about $500 back in 2010.

Myofunctional therapists often start by asking the tongue to do simple clicks to get people ready for functional release. In Kayla's case, even clicks were nearly impossible. She was diligent, for sure. Because the tongue will be numb during the frenuloplasty procedure, OMTs also use neurostimulation techniques. That is to increase awareness of the palate with the tongue against it. OMTs know how to ensure this imperative is satisfied, and it is helpful for them to be present during the release procedure.

Kayla could not produce the lingual palatal suction at all for two months. She had to work extremely hard doing tongue exercises multiple times throughout the day. Eventually, collaborating with the team, she was ready

---

380 Zaghi, S., et al. (2019). "Lingual frenuloplasty with myofunctional therapy: Exploring safety and efficacy in 348 cases." *Laryngoscope Investigative Otolaryngology*, 4(5), 489–496. Retrieved from https://www.zaghimd.com/_files/ugd/fd6d92_3efcaaaccc7e4256abad95529b908588.pdf?index=true.

to have her frenum released and repositioned to accommodate the full functionality of the tongue. Kayla reported this:

> I was incredibly nervous about the surgery. I had never heard of tongue tie therapy or anything to do about tongue ties before coming to Primal Air. It just wasn't anything that anyone had ever acknowledged. I had never heard of a tongue-tie release and had no idea what to expect. On the day of the surgery, I had Dr. Geivelis and Dr. Kelly, a craniosacral therapist who had been working on me for months, in the appointment. I had my tongue and buccal ties released.

Readers may be surprised that some tongue ties are deep into the tongue. The restrictions may be in the middle or last third of the tongue, requiring the manipulation of the muscles that many general practice dentists have no comfort in trying to reach. It takes confidence, know-how, and a good myofunctional therapist to prepare the tongue.

To add something to this section of the book, according to an interview with Dr. Geoffrey Skinner,[381] these posterior ties, or more properly mid-tongue ties, can be assisted in lengthening with a certain type of warming laser (ND Yag laser)[382] to be more elastic and relaxed so that the OMT can stretch them.

Lasers in other types of sleep treatment are also coming into the playing field. They are not just for cutting tissues. Laser therapy can help in other non-cutting wavelengths. Some dental offices offer laser treatment of the oral airway to shrink the soft palate tissue, for instance, opening the airway. Fat accumulation in the tongue can be reduced with laser therapy, too.

After the release, myofunctional techniques are employed to slow the healing process, completely countering most wound management norms. The body expects to remake the short frenulum as close to the way it was before the surgery as possible. The OMT's job is to help the patient stretch the frenulum to create a longer, more functional frenulum and prevent it from shortening again.

---

381 Skinner, G., Hillsboro, Dental Excellence. (Retrieved from (https://hillsborodentalexcellence.com/?y_source=1_MTAwNDY0NjI4MS00ODMtbG9jYXRpb24ud2Vic2l0ZQ%3D%3D))

382 Fotona. (n.d.). Fotona NightLase® Therapy. Retrieved from https://www.fotona.com/en/treatments/2019/nightlase-therapy/

As the tongue learns its new role, performing the contact between it and the palate, the lips naturally find their contact, too. When the tongue is up, it's impossible to breathe orally. A person must utilize nasal breathing, fulfilling the second objective of orofacial myofunctional therapy, obligate nasal breathing. This approach aims to streamline the process and reduce costs by incorporating OMT alongside mandatory nasal breathing.

The frenulum under the tongue is the beginning point of the fascia train from the tongue to the toes. It is crucial that someone also works with that fascia directly before and after the frenuloplasty, which is where Kayla's physical therapist comes in. The term fascia refers to the organ sheath surrounding muscles and dividing muscles from each other from the tongue to the toes. This collagen sheath is one piece that looks kind of like a thin plastic wrap around the muscles. The fascia "unwinds" with the frenuloplasty from the tongue to the toes. It needs help so as not to become trapped.

About 30 percent of Shirley's patients comment on improved constipation.[383] As she says, "Imagine being over sixty years old, having been constipated your entire life. The investments in digestive aids, doctors' appointments, eating foods that don't agree with your desires only to find that a tongue tie release procedure that solved the problem could have been done at birth."

According to Dr. Baxter, owner of the Alabama Tongue-Tie Center, there is a surprising link between tongue-ties and gastrointestinal symptoms like constipation and reflux. The mouth is the beginning of the gastrointestinal tract, and oral restrictions can affect what happens later in digestion. In infants, there's compelling evidence suggesting that infant gastroesophageal reflux (GER) is often linked to swallowing air, a condition known as aerophagia. Dr. Bobby Ghaheri conducted research on infant reflux and tongue-tie, revealing that a proper tongue-tie release can notably alleviate infant reflux symptoms. When babies can achieve a better latch on the breast or bottle and create a stronger seal, this substantially improves reflux symptoms. It also helps with gassiness, fussiness, colic symptoms, constipation, and normal stools.[384]

---

383 Baxter, R. (2023, February 23). "Tongue-Ties and the Surprising Link to Constipation & Reflux." Retrieved from https://tonguetieal.com/tongue-and-lip-ties-and-the-surprising-link-to-constipation-reflux/

384 Ibid.

Again, Shirley relates a story of success: after a lecture at a dental hygiene school in Eau Claire, WI, the program director talked about her grandbaby who, at eight days of age, was placed on Nexium for vomiting.

The director encouraged her daughter to have the child's tongue evaluated, and the tongue-tie was confirmed and released that day. The baby no longer needed medication. When studied on infants, this medication helps with vomiting. Still, there is little discussion about the detrimental effects, nor are they comparing the medication or acknowledging a tongue-tie procedure exists.[385] It's unfortunately too common.

Many pediatricians don't hesitate to give medications but are unaware that tongue restrictions cause many problems. Many have yet to give up on circumcisions yet fail to recommend a little frenuloplasty to improve the quality of life of the mother and the child.

Please note that tongue-tie release is not a guaranteed cure for constipation. If you are experiencing new, severe, or persistent symptoms, it is best to contact a healthcare provider.

Kayla suffered from a debilitating TMJ (jaw joint) flare after the tongue was released and needed a specialist physical therapist to work with her eighty-five miles away. Had she been older, the costs, in actual dollars, would have been even higher. Her debilitating symptoms would have been increasing even without the frenuloplasty. She would have spent thousands of dollars on TMJ appliances, paid for medications and Botox injections, and lost days of work and school[386] with no relief.

Time and Money

Airway problems turn into pain problems, brain fog, and coping problems. Think of a night when you don't sleep well. Are you pleasant the next day? Is it hard to manage your information/reaction filters? Do you answer more sharply than you want to? Do you roll your eyes more? How do relationships fare when people snore or are tired from secondhand snoring? For someone

---

385 Winter, H., et al. (2015, July). "Esomeprazole for the Treatment of GERD in Infants Ages 1–11 Months." *Journal of Pediatric Gastroenterology and Nutrition*, 60, S9-S15.

386 Riley, P., et al. "Oral splints for patients with temporomandibular disorders or bruxism: a systematic review and economic evaluation." Health technology assessment (Winchester, England), vol. 24, no. 7, 2020, pp. 1-224. doi:10.3310/hta24070.

like Kayla, managing all that was pretty taxing. She didn't know that life could be different and effortless.

Some providers talk about those who treat tongue restrictions as focused on unnecessary health procedures and fees they can charge for those procedures. Worse, they accuse those knowledgeable about myofunctional disorders of taking advantage of babies and their mothers' fears for their babies' health. In reality, it's the constant visits to get prescriptions or medical services, more resources spent on Individualized Education Programs (IEP) at schools necessitated by tongue-induced sleep apnea leading to learning disabilities, and so much more. A restricted tongue is not normal; it is only common.

The amount of money and time Kayla's parents put into her mouth is extreme. The time and energy her mother put into this project is also enormous. The practice of myofunctional therapy is truly preventive. Think of your health. If your tongue is not in a good position right now and you're suffering from many of the issues we've covered in this book, how much have you invested in solving those issues without getting to the root cause?

Orthodontic arch development in adults is possible, albeit not as easy as in growing children. There is a considerable time and financial commitment to do that, followed by another orthodontic treatment with comprehensive brackets and bands or aligners to finish the alignment of the teeth. Additional therapies may also be necessary to ensure sleep apnea is treated correctly. Much time and enjoyment of life could have been achieved for Kayla had that problem been addressed when her mother first started to complain that nursing was painful or impossible.

Migraines, restless legs, divorce, arguing, quality of life, teen police calls, stroke, heart disease, diabetes, and much more await those who could be helped early in life with simple and inexpensive interventions.[387] We do not claim you can avoid all these conditions with early OMT interventions. There are never guarantees of success in medical practice. There are too many variables, but why not rule out myofunctional disorders? The therapy is not painful or time-consuming. The results are very long-lasting.

---

[387] Wickwire, Emerson M. "Value-based sleep and breathing: health economic aspects of obstructive sleep apnea." *Faculty Reviews*, vol. 10, 19 April 2021, pp. 40. doi: 10.12703/r/10-40.

Shirley continues: If the tongue is restricted, we are often asked about the optimal time for OMT and frenum revisions. Our oldest case was a seventy-seven-year-old woman. If treating someone that old can help with sleep apnea, it is worth it. Getting less slow-wave sleep as you age may increase your risk of dementia; even a 1 percent drop can make a life-improving difference.[388] Slow-wave sleep decreases sleep apnea. Tongue-tie contributes to and may cause sleep apnea. It does so by forcing mouth breathing in adults and children.[389] Mouth breathing is destructive. Now that you know, don't delay. Treatment at the age of seven is better than at twenty-seven years of age, but not as good as at seven days of age.

Shirley wrote, "Recently, a seven-year-old girl visited for her fourth OMT appointment. Her overall posture was poor, and her mouth hung open at the assessment appointment. She spent two appointments with our therapist specializing in posture, focusing on a properly aligned back, tongue position on the roof of the mouth, and lips together. We had her start with a minute of posture therapy, and then built her time up to five minutes over a two-week time span. Along with some oral therapy techniques, this made a huge difference in her breathing. By session four, her mother reported that the previous night had been the first time the parents had ever gone into her room as she slept that they could not hear her breathing. The mother was alarmed until she saw her daughter's chest rise and fall."

Orofacial myofunctional therapy restores the function of the tongue. It retrains the tongue to support the upper jaw and the floor of the sinuses. With a wide dental arch and a low roof of the mouth, the tongue's mass can rest out of the direct stream of the airway. Restoring the tongue to palatal contact, we start getting the nose to work normally. When the nose works, the lymph tissue of the tonsils isn't taxed with unfiltered air and there is less chance of swelling requiring tonsillectomy. Patients even remark about the decrease of boogers after switching to obligate nasal breathing.

Kayla says: "They [medical providers] make the tongue tie seem unimportant. I'm sure there are people all across the U.S. and the world with unrecognized tongue ties. They are having issues they don't know are related

---

388 Himali, Jayandra J., et al. "Association Between Slow-Wave Sleep Loss and Incident Dementia." *JAMA Neurology*, vol. 80, no. 12, 30 October 2023, pp. 1326-1333. doi:10.1001/jamaneurol.2023.3889.

389 Rouse, Jeffrey. "Tongue Tie and Sleep Apnea: The Craniofacial Connection." Speareducation.com, 6 December 2022.

to the tongue. They will never get to the bottom of the issue because they're not looking in the right place."

Shirley says the incidence of tongue tie is under investigation. She says that nearly all her patients presently have a tongue-tie, some very obvious and some not. If the physicians are missing obvious ties like Kayla's, then the four percent reported incidence is an underreported statistic. In Brazil, they are purposefully examining every newborn for tongue restriction and are reporting eight percent of newborns are restricted, and they are seeing ties in up to seventy percent among babies where the mother is symptomatic during nursing.[390]

---

[390] Batista, C. L. C., and Pereira, A. L. P.. "Ankyloglossia severity in infants: maternal pain, self-efficacy, and functional aspects of breastfeeding." *Rev Paul Pediatr 42* (2023): e2022203. doi: 10.1590/1984-0462/2024/42/2022203. PMCID: PMC10593404.

CHAPTER 12

Nasal Breathing

Nasal Breathing and Cleaning

A team of doctors, including Clarke et al. (2018), looked at 1,906 patients who were having problems with their noses. They wanted to see what was causing the airway obstruction in their nasal airways. To do this, the doctors used a tool called the Nasal Obstruction Symptom Evaluation (NOSE) instrument to measure how severe the symptoms were. Their research showed three main reasons people had trouble breathing through their noses:

- Nasal Valve Collapse (NVC): Found in 67 percent of patients.
- Septal Deviation: Observed in 76 percent of patients.
- Inferior Turbinate Hypertrophy: Present in 72 percent of patients.

Among individuals with severe or extreme "NOSE" scores, indicative of those most likely needing intervention, the prevalence of nasal valve collapse, the prevalence of nasal airway obstruction, septal deviation, and inferior turbinate hypertrophy was 73 percent, 80 percent, and 77 percent, respectively.[391]

---

[391] Clark, David W., et al., "Nasal airway obstruction: Prevalence and anatomic contributors." Icahn School of Medicine at Mount Sinai. https://scholars.mssm.edu/en/publications/nasal-airway-obstruction-prevalence-and-anatomic-contributors-2 (accessed April 24, 2024).

It is very important to note that 82 percent of patients with severe or extreme NOSE scores had previously undergone septoplasty, and inferior turbinate reduction still exhibited nasal valve collapse.

These findings underscore the significance of considering the lateral nasal wall (the inside wall of the outer nasal opening) when devising treatment strategies for nasal airway obstruction.[392]

"No matter how wide you make your mouth or use oral sleep appliances, they are of no use if you are mouth breathing," observes Geoff Skinner, DDS. This is such an important statement by Dr. Skinner.

The objective of oral myofunctional therapy, explained by Shirley Gutkowski, is to get the person to breathe through the nose. As we have mentioned, mouth breathing is always detrimental to your health both during the day and at night. You must learn to breathe through your nose unless something blocks your nasal airway. Even if you have a dental sleep appliance that has opened your airway so that you have fewer suffocation events, what Dr. Skinner emphasizes is crucial.

One of the eye-opening books you can read on nasal breathing is James Nestor's book *Breath: The New Science of a Lost Art*. In this section, we will address nasal constriction and how it is addressed by ENT physicians, nasal airway widening by dental professionals, nasal cleaning, and maintaining nasal patency.

Nasal breathing is not just about breathing; it is about all nasal functions. Nasal breathing includes diaphragmatic breathing, pharyngeal elevator muscles activity, turbinate stimulation, deeper lung-enhanced breathing, tongue training, enhanced nasal cycling via nasal erectile cells, humidifying air, warming breathed air, and nitric oxide air.

We breathe 13,000 liters of air per day filtered by the nose (A railroad boxcar has 5,000 to 7,000 liters). That is roughly two box cars of air per day on average through our noses. This air is not only filtered but humidified, which helps oxygen absorption in the lungs.

---

392 Clark, David W., et al. 2018. "Nasal Airway Obstruction: Prevalence and Anatomic Contributors." *Otolaryngology–Head and Neck Surgery*. Baylor Scott & White Health, Texas A&M Health Science Center College of Medicine, Mount Sinai Beth Israel, ENT & Allergy Associates, University of North Carolina at Chapel Hill. https://journals.sagepub.com/doi/pdf/10.1177/014556131809700615

Eoleaf Greener Health summarized this well, and I will paraphrase their online article below and retrieve some of their footnotes.[393] I have added some information to it as well.

> When you breathe through your nose, the inhaled air enters the nasal passages through the nostrils. The nasal passages guide the air to the throat airway. In the nasal area, each breath undergoes filtration, removal of larger particles, humidification, and warming before continuing down the trachea into the lungs.[394]

The nose acts as a filter, capturing and trapping particles using the small hairs inside it to prevent larger particles from reaching the lungs. It also warms the air to body temperature before reaching the lungs.

Our airways are lined with sticky mucus to filter particles, a trap for pollutants and allergens. Your nose can make up to a liter of mucus per day.[395] This mucus is optimal at a certain thickness, or better said, when it is not too thick or too thin. The nose's shape causes a change in air direction; it does more than just divert it at a ninety-degree angle[396] from the nostril to the nasal cavity, but it also causes turbulence in the folds you can see when you look into the nose (the concha). These conchae are folded to create more surface area for the filtering, moisturizing, and warming functions. This alteration in direction, along with slowed airflow, results in the deposition of particulate matter onto the sticky surface inside the nose. Cilia, tiny hairs, then sweep away the mucus into the stomach for inactivation, preventing contaminants from reaching the lungs.

---

393 Eoleaf. "Air Filtration in the Human Nose." Eoleaf.com. Accessed January 16, 2024. https://eoleaf.com/pages/air-filtration-in-the-human-nose."

394 National Cancer Institute. "NCI Dictionary of Cancer Terms." Last modified 2023. Accessed January 16, 2024.. https://www.cancer.gov/publications/dictionaries/cancer-terms/def/nasal-cavity.

395 Allergy & Asthma Network. "Your Nose: The Ultimate Air Cleaner." (2023). from https://allergyasthmanetwork.org/news/your-nose-the-ultimate-air-cleaner/

396 Otrivine. (2022). "How Do We Breathe?" Retrieved from https://www.otrivine.co.uk/nasal-health/how-do-we-breathe.html

The human nose can filter out particles larger than 0.5 μm,[397] including pollen, pet dander, human sneeze particles, asbestos, vehicle emissions, mold and spores, smoke, and dust.

Eighty percent of lung infections are sourced from the nasopharynx[398]. Children are growing up in Daycare and get eight to twelve respiratory infections per year, says Joseph Zelk. This information is supported by the ENT physician Mandan Kandula, MD in his online website video presentations speaking about nasal airway issues.[399]

Viruses take about six to forty-eight hours to enter the cells.[400] It may take as little as six hours for some viruses, such as SARS-CoV-2, to infect nasal cells. Other viruses, such as rhinovirus, may take longer to enter the cells, up to forty-eight hours after exposure.[401]

Virus infections in the nose can result in ear infections, sinus infections, mouth breathing, lowered nitric oxide production, undeveloped facial bones with airway and orthodontic issues, smaller nasal opening, TMJ disease, inflammation, caries (dental cavities), weight gain, poor school performance, social aggression, depression, gingivitis, (gum disease), poor diets, ADHD, sleep apnea, lack of sleep, bad breath, forward head posture, spinal deformation, loss of facial symmetry and beauty, and social rejection.

These children then grow up with a lifetime of airway issues that are much harder to control: heart disease, cancer, stroke, and all the other diseases that result from chronic hypoxia we have spoken about in this book.

---

397 Breathing Retraining Center. (2023). "What your amazing nose can filter!" Retrieved January 16, 2024, from https://breathingretrainingcenter.com/blog/article-what-your-amazing-nose-can-filter

398 Thomas M, Bomar PA. *Upper Respiratory Tract Infection.* [Updated 2023 June 26]. In: StatPearls [Internet]. Treasure Island (FL): StatPearls Publishing; 2023 Jan-. Available from: https://www.ncbi.nlm.nih.gov/books/NBK532961/

399 Kandula, Madan. "Founder & ENT." *Madan Kandula, MD: Official Website.* Accessed April 8, 2024. from https://www.madankandula.com/.

400 Goldman, Bruce. "Stanford Medicine Scientists Pinpoint COVID-19 Virus's Entry and Exit Ports Inside Our Noses." *Stanford Medicine News Center.* January 5, 2023. Accessed April 8, 2024 Accessed April 8, 2024. https://med.stanford.edu/news/all-news/2023/01/covid-virus-infection-nasal.html.

401 Herndon, Kristina. "How Your Immune System Reacts to the Common Cold." *Verywell Health.* Last modified July 24, 2023. Medically reviewed by Jurairat J. Molina, MD. Accessed April 8, 2024 Accessed April 8, 2024. https://www.verywellhealth.com/what-is-the-medical-immunity-3955691.

Opening Nasal Airways
NASAL SPRAYS

Here is a list of the most common types of nasal treatments.

1. Saline (salt) and saline with baking soda
2. Xylitol
3. Nasal spray medications include
    a. steroids (corticosteroids) (Beclomethasone®) (fluticasone),
    b. Antihistamines (Nasalcrom®), (Astepro)
4. Antihistamines (Dimetane®) (Zyrtec®) (Benadryl®)
5. Decongestants (oxymetazoline) (phenylephrine) (Afrin®)
6. Combination antihistamine/decongestant (Allegra D®)
7. Antibiotics

Many nasal treatments and sprays are directed to patients diagnosed with nasal issues caused by allergies. A study indicates that many nasal allergy-diagnosed patients are misdiagnosed and have chronic rhinosinusitis (CRS). This paraphrased statement comes from *Health Day Magazine* in an online article and is summarized here:

> Dr. Ahmad Sedaghat, the lead author of the study, emphasized the significant number of patients enduring prolonged suffering due to the misunderstanding between allergies and CRS. He recounted instances where patients underwent allergy shots for extended periods, spanning decades, without experiencing symptom relief. However, upon identifying CRS and initiating suitable treatment, many patients reported relief within a few months.[402]
>
> Sedaghat is director of rhinology and allergy and professor of otolaryngology head & neck surgery at the University of Cincinnati College of Medicine. His team published its findings recently in the journal *Otolaryngology-Head & Neck Surgery*.[403]

---

[402] Mundell, Ernie. "Is It Allergies or Sinusitis? Many Folks Are Misdiagnosed." *Health Day*, Feb 28, 2024, 6:06 am. Updated on: Feb 28, 2024, 6:06 am. Retrieved from https://www.healthday.com/health-news/allergies/is-it-allergies-or-sinusitis-many-folks-are-misdiagnosed

[403] Houssein, Firas A. BS, Phillips, Katie M. MD, Sedaghat, Ahmad R. MD, PhD. "When It's Not Allergic Rhinitis: Clinical Signs to Raise a Patient's Suspicion for Chronic Rhinosinusitis." *Otolaryngology-Head and Neck*, 31 January 2024. doi:10.1002/ohn.646.

I will also introduce a new non-prescription nasal spray based on hypochlorous acid. Each of these different sprays is useful for specific areas of need. If prescribed, you should take them or discuss any concerns with your medical doctor. I will not go into the mechanism of action of each type. I will mention some of them that are common over-the-counter sprays which both Joe and I believe are useful for everyday use.

According to an article in epainassit.com, about 2 percent of all people are carriers of MRSA in the nose.[404] They can spread the infection to others through skin-to-skin contact or touching contaminated surfaces or objects.[405] Many of these individuals have MRSA on the surfaces of their cell phones.

Xylitol Nasal Sprays

An over-the-counter nasal spray that Joe and I recommend is Xlear.® Since it came onto the market, several companies have also created xylitol nasal sprays, including Neilmed®. Xlear® has made many versions and combinations of xylitol sprays.[406]

Dentistry has been promoting the use of xylitol for many years. It is a five-carbon natural sugar that bacteria cannot digest. It is used in toothpaste, mouth rinses, candies, and gum. It helps prevent tooth decay and has many other health benefits. Now it is being used in nasal sprays. It has the potential to help keep nasal passages open, help control microbes in the nose, and lower the incidence of earaches in children, which is called otitis media.[407]

Xylitol sprays hydrate the tissues, facilitating the removal of allergens, dust, and microbes. Simultaneously, they enhance the nasal tissues' ability to prevent bacteria from adhering to the nasal mucosa. Unlike prescription sprays that may dry out mucus, xylitol sprays thin the mucus without causing dehydration, ensuring essential moisture retention.

---

[404] "How Contagious Is MRSA in the Nose?" ePainAssist. https://www.epainassist.com/infections/how-contagious-is-mrsa-in-the-nose (accessed April 24, 2024).

[405] Kerkar, Pramod. "How Contagious Is MRSA In The Nose?" Epainassist.com. Accessed April 8, 2024. https://www.epainassist.com/infections/how-contagious-is-mrsa-in-the-nose.

[406] Xlear, Inc. (n.d.). Xlear | Sinus Care, Dental Defense, & Natural Sweeteners. Retrieved April 8, 2024, from www.clear.com.

[407] Xylitol.org. (n.d.). "Benefits of Xylitol Nasal Spray." Retrieved April 8, 2024, from https://xylitol.org/articles-about-xylitol/benefits-xylitol-nasal-spray/

Xylitol also helps control viruses and has been shown in a few studies to suppress their numbers in vitro[408] (in vitro means a study done on viruses in a lab, not humans). In a *USA Today* article, Dr. David Hamer suggested, based on several studies, that xylitol appears to be potentially safe and could serve as a beneficial antiviral nasal spray or rinse. However, definitive conclusions require large-scale clinical trials in humans. A study published in the *Journal of Allergy and Infectious Diseases* revealed the effectiveness of dietary xylitol in mice infected with the human syncytial virus (the RSV illness).[409]

At present, xylitol nasal rinse manufacturers can make no claim to help treat or prevent any disease. We like these rinses and hope more clinical trials will support that hope.

HOCL Nasal Sprays

Over-the-counter hypochlorous acid nasal sprays are new and have the potential to help nasal airways by cleaning them more effectively while at the same time not drying them out. I must make a disclosure because I am a developer of this type of nasal rinse and own a company that makes and sells these products.

First, a bit of information on HOCL. The white blood cells in our body make HOCL to combat viruses, bacteria, and yeasts. It also helps regulate our immune responses and reduces inflammation. Even though it is related to bleach, it is not caustic like bleach. If you take regular chlorine bleach at home, which is highly alkaline at a pH of about twelve, and if you move that pH down to a range of four to six, the formula turns into hypochlorous acid (HOCL) instead of chlorine bleach (sodium hypochlorite, NaCLO). They act very differently, and although bleach is a good killer of germs, HOCL is about 60 to 100 times more effective in this killing ability. Yet, you can place HOCL on your skin or throat[410] at the most useful concentrations,

---

408 Cannon, M. L., et al. (n.d.). "In Vitro Analysis of the Anti-viral Potential of nasal spray constituents against SARS-CoV-2." *Biorxiv.org*. doi: https://doi.org/10.1101/2020.12.02.408575

409 Fauzia, M. (2021, September 30). "Fact check: Xylitol may be helpful against viruses, but experts warn against hydrogen peroxide." *USA Today*.

410 Beattie, M., Lewis, F. C., & Gee, G. W. (1917). "Hypochlorous solution electrically produced from hypertonic saline as a disinfectant for septic wounds and for the throat in diphtheria, scarlet fever, etc." *British Medical Journal*, 1(2930), 256-259.

and it rarely irritates the tissues of humans or pets, while household bleach is caustic and would cause great harm. They are different.

How does it work? White cells, like neutrophils and macrophages, engulf a microorganism, and then once it is inside the white cell, our natural defense chemical HOCL is secreted, and the germ is destroyed.[411] Unlike antibiotics, bacteria, yeast, and viruses do not develop resistance to HOCL.

MRSA, a highly perilous antibiotic-resistant healthcare-associated infection (HIA), stands as the primary cause of serious infections among burn victims. The elimination of MRSA has proven to be very challenging. Research indicates that Hypochlorous Acid (HOCL) effectively kills MRSA and lowers the occurrence of infections. This can be achieved through environmental disinfection and wound bathing, involving the direct application of HOCL solution to the skin to inhibit bacterial growth.[412] And, as we mentioned before, 2 percent of people carry MRSA in the nose.

Most HOCL is made via electrolysis of salt water. Made this way, it is full of impurities and chemicals you do not want. In addition, this form of HOCL is not very stable. Once you make it and use it, it quickly begins to lose potency, so you cannot determine the concentration of the HOCL you are getting. I don't recommend this form of HOCL to be used in the nose or for anything.

To make more stable forms of electrolysis-generated HOCL, some companies filter their product and then add acetic acid to prolong its life. However, that process is fraught with other issues. It creates stability issues with the HOCL. The thought behind using acetic acid is that it will lead to a more stable pH—at least in low concentrations. However, this runs into several issues, as I discovered when speaking to scientists about this chemistry.

The first issue with adding acetic acid is the release of chlorine gas, which can occur and is problematic if you manufacture large quantities. The second is that technically, it is no longer considered "pure HOCL" as the addition of acetic acid is considered an additive, leading to some regulatory issues

---

411 Klebanoff, S. J. (1975). "Antimicrobial mechanisms in neutrophilic polymorphonuclear leukocytes." *Seminars in Hematology*, 12(2), 117-142.

412 Anagnostopoulos, A. G., et al. (2018). "0.01% Hypochlorous Acid as an Alternative Skin Antiseptic: An In Vitro Comparison." *Dermatologic Surgery*, 44(12), 1489-1493. doi: 10.1097/DSS.0000000000001594

with container labels and claims. The third issue is whether the antimicrobial activities come from the acetic acid vs. HOCL vs. a different chemical species. They have not found Raman spectroscopy (a measure of molecule vibration and rotation) data to confirm the final chemical species.[413]

Electrolysis-made HOCL also remains very salty. They taste salty, too, and if you use them to sanitize home or office countertops, hospital equipment, or door handles,[414] they leave a white film of salt.

Newer proprietary ways of making this HOCL in a pure form with over one year of shelf life are now available. These companies are keeping their process for making this pure HOCL confidential as a competitive edge. For example, one of USA-Guard's HOCL products is made with ion exchange, and the other uses a different proprietary process.[415] The ion exchange system has a slight amount of sodium, even though not made via electrolysis, and has a light chlorine taste and smell and nearly no salt flavor. Each of them is used in different ways. The concentration of HOCL in these products must be appropriate for the intended use. These are better suited to nasal and body use than electrolyzed salt water HOCL.[416] The pH of these products is intentionally higher than that of most HOCL products, yet the stability is over one year.

Studies of the use of HOCL in the nose are showing effectiveness. M. S Yu et al. (2017), writing in the publication *Infection Control & Hospital Epidemiology* about chronic rhinosinusitis (CRS) is one example. After four weeks of treatment, the bacterial culture rates in the HOCL group were slightly lower than the placebo group, but this difference was not statistically significant ($p > 0.05$). Their findings indicated that nasal irrigation with low-concentration HOCL improved CRS symptoms more significantly than saline irrigation.[417]

---

413 Lim, MD, PhD, Kenneth. Personal interviews and emails, Indiana University School of Medicine, March 2024.

414 Fertelli et al. "Effectiveness of an electrochemically activated saline solution for disinfection of hospital equipment." *Infect Control Hosp Epidemiol*, vol. 34, no. 5, 2013, pp. 43-44.

415 USA-Guard. "USA-Guard.com." Accessed April 7, 2024.

416 Ibid.

417 Yu, M. S., et al. (2017). "Low-concentration hypochlorous acid nasal irrigation for chronic sinonasal symptoms: a prospective randomized placebo-controlled study." *European Archives of Oto-Rhino-Laryngology*, 274(3), 1527–1533. doi:10.1007/s00405-016-4387-5

The fact that the number of bacteria culture rates from the nose in this nasal HOCL study is not significantly lower than the control group is a good thing. We want reasonable control of the rhinosinusitis but not complete removal of the bacteria in the nose.

While studies show the excellent killing power of HOCL on MRSA on surfaces and skin, we have no studies concerning how HOCL controls MRSA in the nose.

There is one study on SARS CoV-2 on the skin of the face and face masks. Applying the HOCL to a mask would likely involve breathing in the HOCL vapors. Here is a summary from that paper, which mentions the respiratory system.

> It mentions that using HOCL facial sanitizer alongside hand sanitizing and mask sanitizing enhances protection and prevention against SARS-CoV-2. This offers several benefits, including decreased microbial contamination, minimized risk of biofilm (bacteria formed into a sticky film rather than free-floating bacteria) formation, and lowered chances of respiratory tract and skin infections. The review concluded that it is ideally suited for this purpose.[418]

There is also a Spanish study on electrolyzed saline nebulized and breathed into the nose and lungs that showed efficacy on COVID-19.[419] This was not a study on nasal cleaning or health and is included here to show that the use of HOCL in proper concentrations in nasal applications seems well tolerated. We are not advocating the use of HOCL spray for the treatment or prevention of COVID-19.

We have one anecdotal cone beam radiograph of HOCL shrinking the size of turbinates in the nose and opening the airway. It is shown here, (Figure 96). We need a large-scale controlled study to verify this. Right now, reports of dentists using it are encouraging.

---

418 Nowbuth, A. A., et al. (2021). "A Potential Benefit of Hypochlorous Acid - Facial Sanitisation: A Review." Preprints.org. doi:10.20944/preprints202107.0129.v1

419 Gutierrez-Gutierrez, L., et al. (2021). "Safety and efficacy of a COVID-19 treatment with nebulized and/or intravenous neutral electrolyzed saline combined with usual medical care vs. usual medical care alone: A randomized, open-label, controlled trial." *Spandidos Publications*. Published online on June 29, 2021. doi:10.3892/etm.2021.10347

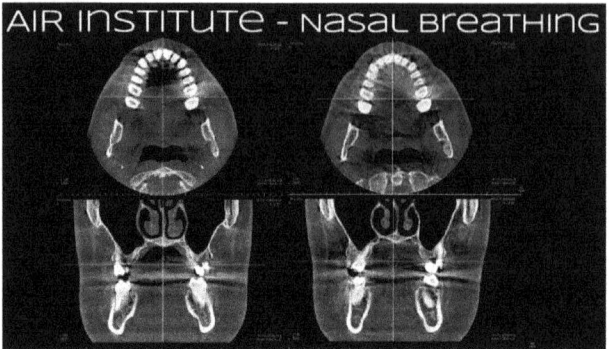

Figure 96: Image courtesy of Dr. Geoffrey Skinner

In this side-by-side photo, at the center of the figures, you see the turbinates in the nose have shrunk on the photo to the right, using the USA-Guard-like formula of HOCL spray.

At the present time HOCL nasal rinse manufacturers and resellers, including USA-Guard, can make no claim to help, treat, or prevent any disease. They are intended for general-purpose home and office cleaning, as well as skin and nasal cleaning only.

Saline Rinses

According to M. A. Pynnonen et al., saline rinses have at least five uses. They are commonly known as saline nasal irrigation or saline nasal sprays, involving the use of a saltwater solution to cleanse and moisturize the nasal passages. This practice has been recognized for its potential benefits in managing various nasal and sinus conditions.[420]

Saline rinses can help:

- **Clear Nasal Passages:** The saltwater solution aids in clearing mucus, allergens, and irritants from the nasal passages to relieve congestion.
- **Reduce Inflammation:** Saline rinses have anti-inflammatory effects, reducing swelling and promoting overall nasal health.

---

[420] Rabago, D., Pasic, T., Zgierska, A., et al. (2005). "The efficacy of hypertonic saline nasal irrigation for chronic sinonasal symptoms." *Otolaryngol Head Neck Surg*, 133(1), 3-8. doi:10.1016/j.otohns.2005.03.002

- **Improve Nasal Moisture:** By moisturizing the nasal tissues, saline rinses can alleviate dryness and discomfort.
- **Aid in Sinus Infection Recovery:** Saline rinses are often recommended as a complementary measure for sinus infections to promote drainage and reduce symptoms.
- **Enhance Postoperative Use:** Saline rinses are commonly used after nasal surgeries to aid in healing and prevent infections.[421]

As I understood an online lecture I listened to by the CEO, Nathan Jones, of Xlear®, the use of salt water over two weeks can cause people to get sick more often. It is because the flora (microbe family) is removed, and mucus too, and for two hours while these are being rebuilt, the pathogens are not filtered out. Salt goes into the tissue, then the water follows and thickens the mucus. This caution was supported in an article in the *Cochrane Database Syst Rev.* in which they said overuse of saline rinses could actually dry the tissues, and that is not helpful in preventing infections.[422]

Using contaminated water, even tap water, for nasal irrigation poses a slight risk of infection. Some individuals, hesitant about nasal irrigation, often cite news stories regarding "brain-eating" microbes. An amoeba known as Naegleria has the potential to cause a serious and life-threatening brain condition called primary amebic meningoencephalitis (PAM) if irrigated into the nose.[423] There is another similar parasite in tap water noted recently in the literature. Acanthamoeba can cause a condition known as granulomatous amebic encephalitis (parasites infecting the brain) (GAE).[424] Use boiled, filtered, or distilled water for saline rinses to help prevent this.

---

[421] Pynnonen, M. A., et al. (2007). "Nasal saline for chronic sinonasal symptoms: a randomized controlled trial." *Arch Otolaryngol Head Neck Surg*, 133(11), 1115-1120. doi:10.1001/archotol.133.11.1115

[422] Harvey, R., Hannan, S. A., Badia, L., & Scadding, G. (2007). "Nasal saline irrigations for the symptoms of chronic rhinosinusitis." *Cochrane Database of Systematic Reviews*, (3), CD006394. doi:10.1002/14651858.CD006394.pub2

[423] Cleveland Clinic. "Nasal Irrigation: Uses, Benefits & Side Effects." Accessed January 16, 2024. https://my.clevelandclinic.org/health/treatments/24286-nasal-irrigation.

[424] Centers for Disease Control and Prevention. "Free Living Amebic Infections." Last modified 2023. Accessed January 16, 2024. https://www.cdc.gov/dpdx/freeLivingAmebic/index.html.

Nasal Dilators:

A 14 percent increase in nasal valve opening (the opening of your nostrils) results in a 50 percent increase in nasal airflow. This statistic comes from Dr. Mark Abramson, DDS, who developed the Oasys® oral sleep device. This device received both an FDA clearance from the otolaryngology division of the FDA and an FDA clearance from the dental division of the FDA. The device has extension arms that push on the lips and cheeks from the mouth to open the nostrils and also has pads under the tongue to lift the tongue up and forward into the roof of the mouth where it belongs to open the airway behind the tongue.[425]

Many over-the-counter nasal dilators exist. They have been shown to increase the amount of air you can breathe through the nose. In a study conducted by Peter W. Hellings and Gilbert J. Nolst Trenité, the Airmax® endonasal dilator demonstrated a significant enhancement in mean peak nasal inspiratory flow (PNIF), registering a mean increase of 176.1 percent from baseline values.[426] Two other nasal dilators I and Dr. Zelk like are the Mute® and the NasalAid®. According to a study by Dr. Jerry Kram, founder of the California Center for Sleep Disorders and featured on the NasalAid® website, the NasalAid® nasal dilator can be adjusted to your nose and desired degree of dilation. Unlike other dilators, it can be used for up to a year. Dr. Kram also mentioned that he has found NasalAid® is more comfortable than other dilators since it only touches nasal soft tissue. This comfort is also something Dr. Zelk and I have noticed with NasalAid®. The reason is that it does not touch the middle septum in the nose. It does have an FDA classification.[427, 428]

These nasal dilators help with nasal valve collapse, too, and loss of properly developed nasal opening dilator muscles and cartilage. Some help can be gained from nasal adhesive strips.

---

425 Abramson, Mark, DDS. Online interview.

426 Hellings, Peter W., and Gilbert J. Nolst Trenité. "Improvement of nasal breathing and patient satisfaction by the endonasal dilator Airmax®." *Rhinology* 52 (2013): 31-34. doi:10.4193/Rhino13.061.

427 NasalAid. "Nasal Aid." Accessed April 7, 2024. nasalaid.com.

428 NasalAid. "Nasal Aid." Accessed April 7, 2024. nasalaid.com.

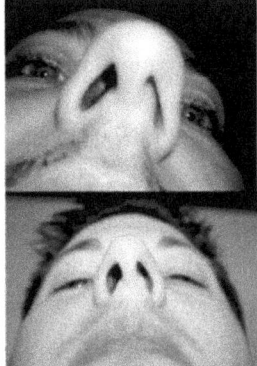

Figure 97: Relapse of Surgery/Allergy Treatment. Airway Compromised 50 percent. Photo courtesy of Joy Moeller, RDH

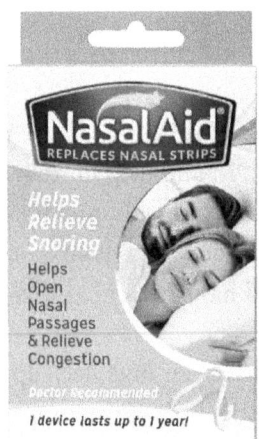

Figure 98: NasalAid®

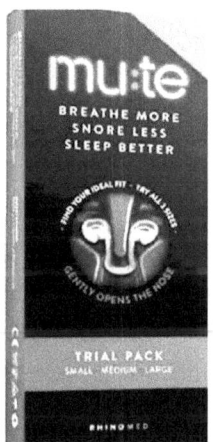

Figure 99: Mute®

Mute® also has FDA clearance and comes in three sizes. It can be used up to ten times.[429, 430]

We believe nasal dilators and sprays should be used routinely with any oral sleep appliance to increase oral appliance effectiveness.

---

429 Medical News Today. "Mute Snoring Review: What to Know." Medically reviewed by Kim Rose-Francis RDN, CDCES, LD. Updated on November 29, 2022.

430 Rhinomed. "Mute Receives Major Regulatory Approvals." Accessed March 22, 2024, from https://www.rhinomed.global/mute-receives-major-regulatory-approvals.

Dairy

When experiencing a respiratory infection such as a cold, the body increases mucus in the nose and throat as a defense mechanism to expel harmful germs. As noted by the Mayo Clinic, this heightened mucus production may result in symptoms like a runny or stuffy nose and a slimy, clogged, or irritated throat.

Despite common belief, consuming cow dairy products like milk, cheese, or ice cream during illness doesn't contribute to increased mucus. The perception of worsened phlegm may exist because some studies indicate it might thicken the mucus that is already there. It may also leave some milk products in the throat for a while. However, experts, including Michael Yong, MD, a board-certified otolaryngologist and neurorhinologist at Pacific Neuroscience Institute in Santa Monica, California, emphasize that research studies indicate no link between dairy consumption and congestion.[431]

Lip Seal

Effortless lip seal is necessary for nasal breathing, day or night. You may need to train yourself to breathe nasally, and help for that can come from chin straps, mouth tape, intraoral mouth shields, and lip pastes. Caution should be exercised when doing this if you have a nasal obstruction. You do not want to use these types of forced nasal breathing if you cannot easily breathe through the nose.

We also want to seal lips when using an oral sleep appliance if at all possible. Sometimes that requires elastics between the upper and lower oral trays, so your jaw does not fall open.

We want that, too, when you use a CPAP that is nasally delivered. If you do not do this, the air can escape through the mouth with a nasal CPAP, and an oral appliance is not doing half of its job, as Dr. Skinner has said.

I generally do not like the chin straps because they force the lower jaw back into the jaw joint sockets. This can create soreness and also may create a displaced jaw socket disc.

I do not recommend taping the lips of children. Adults must have good nasal patency to consider lip sealing. Some experts recommend no lip sealing

---

[431] Mayo Clinic. "Common Cold: Self-management." Accessed Feb 12, 2024 from https://www.mayoclinic.org/diseases-conditions/common-cold/diagnosis-treatment/drc-20351611

at all and recommend you practice lip closure during the day, and they believe this will translate to lips being together while sleeping. Working with an OMT or SLP can help you find unique ways to encourage labial occlusion or lip sealing.

Intraoral lip shields include devices that look a bit like a pacifier. The shield fits inside the lips, and the lips seal around it to stop air loss. iBreath® is the one we like. See image 100. There is a small tube with a hole that does not leak air, and if you suck on it, there is a negative air pressure created, which helps keep the tongue up and the lips sealed, so it does two important functions. At this time, the iBreath® is only sold as a snoring device. The Good Morning Snore Solution® is also a good lip seal device by MPowrx®. Myotalea® Lip Trainer™ by Myofunctional Research is also a good option.[432]

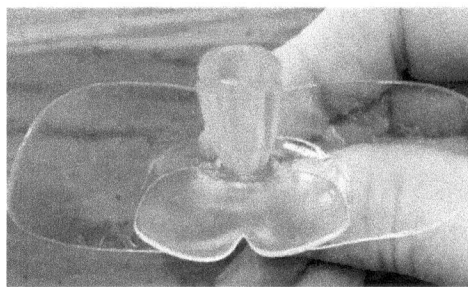
Figure 100: iBreath® by Somnics Health[433]

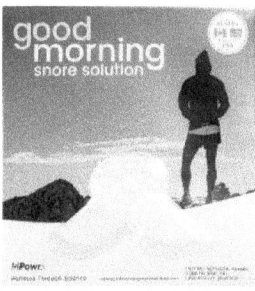
Figure 101: the Good Morning Snore Solution® MPowrx®

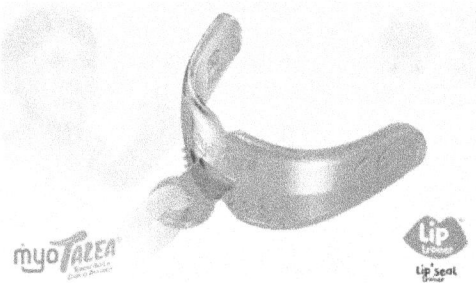
Figure 102: Myotalea® Lip Trainer™ from Myofunctional Research.

---

432 Myotalea Lip Trainer, Myoresearch, accessed 5-6-2024, from https://myoresearch.com/en-au/appliances/myotalea/lip_trainer

433 *Doctor Sleep Show*. Accessed Jan 13, 2024, from www.drsleepshow.com

One of the newer ways to help this is with a new Australian product called SleepQ+®. It is a gel that you put on the lips, and when they are closed, creates an excellent seal. It is easily loosened when you push your tongue through it. It then seals again once you put your lips back together.[433] These are also helpful for CPAP users who use nasal hoods or pillows to prevent air from escaping through the mouth.

Nasal Cycling

Many people do not know that the nose has a cycle of nostril use. In other words, one side of the nose will swell and close off while the other is open. They take turns opening and closing. There are erectile cells in the nose that help with the task; 70 percent to 80 percent of people have this. The cycle is every thirty minutes to four hours for most of them, and it is mostly controlled by blood flow increasing in one side or the other during the cycle.[434]

Buteyko and IHT

It seems counterintuitive but there is a therapy that improves oxygen delivery to the blood using intermittent hypoxia training (IHT). Related to the Buteyko nose pinching technique, in which increasing carbon dioxide in the bloodstream opens the nasal airway, IHT can improve the oxygen in tissues much like those living in high altitude, less oxygen-rich air regions of the world. They also use it to treat sleep apnea. It is a technique of breath-holding.

Intermittent Hypoxia Therapy is a novel approach for managing sleep apnea. It involves brief exposure to low oxygen levels in a controlled setting. The goal is to trigger the body's natural adaptations to low oxygen, improving its response to oxygen deprivation (hypoxia). This therapy aims to lessen the severity of apnea episodes, boost oxygen levels in the blood, and enhance overall sleep quality. By training the body to function better

---

433 SleepQ+. Accessed [Jan 13,2024], from https://sleepqplus.com/.

434 Aaronson, N. L., MD, MBA, CPE, FACS, FAAP. (2023, March 3). "What is the nasal cycle?" *Medical News Today*. Written by Santhakumar, S.

under low-oxygen conditions, IHT may help mitigate the adverse effects of sleep apnea.[435] However, as they always say, it is important to note that while IHT shows promise, more research is needed to fully understand its long-term effects and efficacy.[436]

---

[435] Lévy, P., et al. (2008). "Intermittent hypoxia and sleep-disordered breathing: current concepts and perspectives." *European Respiratory Journal*, 32, 1082-1095. DOI: 10.1183/09031936.00013308.

[436] Serebrovskaya, T. V., & Xi, L. (2015). "Intermittent hypoxia in childhood: the harmful consequences versus potential benefits of therapeutic uses." *Frontiers in Pediatrics,* 3, Article 44. doi:10.3389/fped.2015.00044.

CHAPTER 13

Child Growth & Facial Beauty
– Dr. Felix Liao

This chapter is credited to Dr. Felix Liao. Before his material is presented, there are several child growth strategies and appliances I want to introduce that help develop the genetic growth potential of our faces. Dr. Liao has his own unique approach. Here are a few of those approaches that you will see mentioned in the book.

The ToothPillow® is a company that sells the Vivos® Guide but has the added benefit of supervised care with that device (Figure 105). MyoMunchee® is from Australia, and the company is owned by a chiropractor.

The MyoMunchee® is a medical-grade silicone oral device that must be chewed on to work (Figures 103 and 104). It was initially designed as a teeth-cleaning device but was recognized later for its stimulation of jaw growth and widening. Some patients can wear it while sleeping if supervised by a dentist.

Myospots® were also developed in Australia and are made with seaweed to hold on the roof of the mouth to teach the tongue to be in that position. They dissolve and are all natural and edible.

The Myobrace® comes from Australia and is also a medical-grade silicone. It is not a device to be chewed on but instead worn for two hours per day to develop muscle tone. It is considered an orthodontic device.

HealthyStart® appliances are similar to Myobrace® and come in various sizes.

You will see throughout this book different ways to expand the mouth and tongue space with many kinds of techniques and appliances. Many use Vivos® and others use Invisalign® and Candid Pro® clear aligners. Some use traditional orthodontic brackets and bands. Dr. Liao will next show us how he approaches facial and airway development with his own appliances and methods with children and young adults.

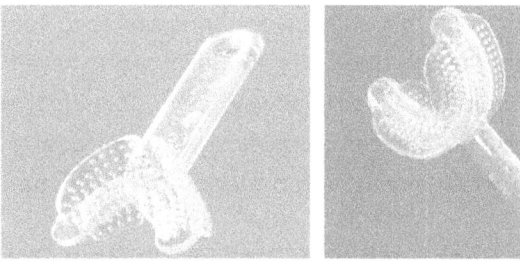

Figure 103: MyoMunchee®

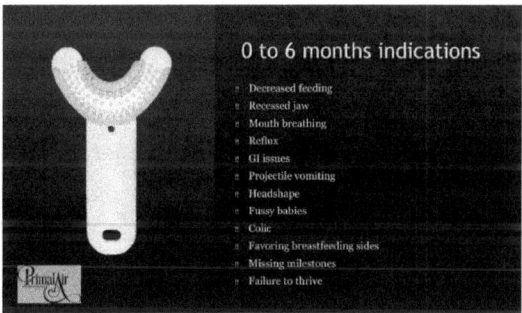

Figure 104: Courtesy of Shirley Gutkowski, RDH, BS

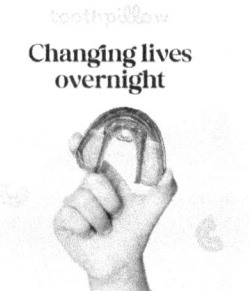

Figure 105: ToothPillow®

Dr. Liao is a general dentist focused on oral-systemic wellness in Falls Church, VA.

> Book authors note: Dr. Liao has spearheaded the guidance and training of many dentists in facial beauty and airway health. In this chapter, you will see many examples of his clinical expertise and valuable references. Please also read his books on this subject. Impaired Mouth Syndrome and Airway-centered Mouth doctors are Dr. Liao's terms similar to concepts we use throughout this book. We are delighted to have this important information about child airway health. Treating these conditions at a younger age can promote fuller dental facial growth, deeper sleep, wider airway, and better overall health naturally.

Your Child's Best Face and Top Health from Oral Facial Epigenetics

Dr. Felix Liao, DDS, MAGD, ABGD, D-ASBA

Epigenetics is the new science on how behavior and environment can influence how your genes work.[437] With three in four adults in the U.S. experiencing sleep disorder symptoms[438] and up to 84 percent prevalence of crowded teeth,[439] this chapter explores the connection between the two, focusing on children and young adults. It introduces a proactive playbook called Oral Facial Epigenetics, offering root-cause solutions for parents.

Crowded teeth and a bad bite have implications beyond just smiles, impacting whole-body health as illustrated in Figure 106. As discussed in the book 6-Foot Tiger 3-Foot Cage,[440] crowded teeth indicate deficient jaws, leading to a smaller airway, oxygen deprivation, sleep disruption, failure to thrive, premature aging, and increased healthcare costs.

---

[437] Centers for Disease Control and Prevention. "What Is Epigenetics?" Accessed May 10, 2024. https://www.cdc.gov/genomics/disease/epigenetics.htm.

[438] Liu Y, et al. "Sleep Disorder Symptoms Among Adults in 8 States and the District of Columbia, 2017." *Preventing Chronic Disease* 18 (2021): 210305. doi: http://dx.doi.org/10.5888/pcd18.210305.

[439] Cenzato N, Nobili A, Maspero C. "Prevalence of Dental Malocclusions in Different Geographical Areas: Scoping Review." Dent J (Basel). 2021 Oct 11;9(10):117. doi: 10.3390/dj9100117. PMID: 34677179; PMCID: PMC8534899.

[440] Liao, Felix. "6 Foot Tiger 3 Foot Cage: Take Charge of Your Health by Taking Charge of Your Mouth." Crescendo Publishing, 2017. https://www.amazon.com/Six-Foot-Tiger-Three-Foot-Cage-Charge/dp/1944177590. Accessed May 20, 2023.

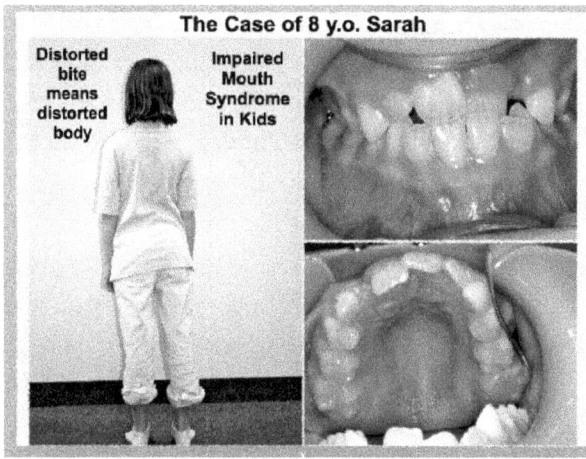

Figure 106: illustrates how crowded teeth in deficient jaws contribute to distorted posture.

There are nuances to consider between thriving wellness and failure to thrive. In the worst-case scenario, research has concluded that "Pediatric obstructive sleep apnea in non-obese children is a disorder of oral-facial growth."[441] This landmark finding pinpoints deficient jaws as the ultimate culprit.

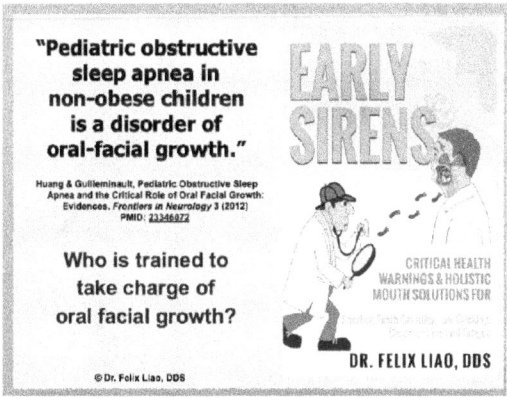

Figure 107

---

441 Huang YS, Guilleminault C. "Pediatric obstructive sleep apnea and the critical role of oral-facial growth: evidences." *Front Neurol*. 2013 Jan 22;3:184. doi: 10.3389/fneur.2012.00184. PMID: 23346072; PMCID: PMC3551039.

Who in healthcare is trained to oversee and guide oral-facial growth? The ideal answer is everyone, but the reality is that practically none are. This explains why the above-mentioned issues are so widespread. Dentists need additional training as Airway-centered Mouth Doctors® (AMDs) to connect the dots from mouth to face, tongue to airway, and sleep to school. With guidance and support from an AMD, you can avoid being vulnerable to health troubles such as dental crowding, teeth grinding, clicking jaw joints, ADHD, bed-wetting, frequent respiratory infections, anxiety, depression, social withdrawal, and more. These symptoms often have an Impaired Mouth lurking undiagnosed behind them.

Impaired Mouth Syndrome

An impaired mouth refers to structural deficiencies in size, form, or function. Impaired Mouth Syndrome encompasses many medical, dental, mental, and mood symptoms resulting from having a normal-sized tongue within undersized jaws, as detailed in the 6-Foot Tiger 3-Foot Cage. The case of HR depicted in Figures 108-110 illustrates this syndrome.[442]

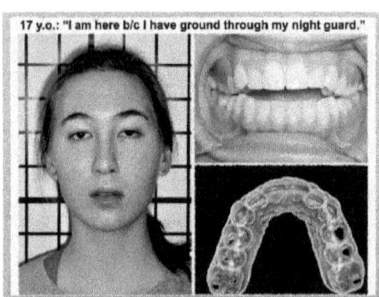 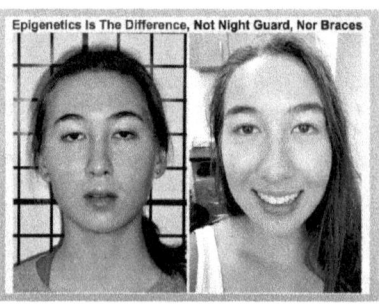

Figure 108: Left: HR three years after braces. Upper right: Big spaces between the front upper and lower teeth resulted from tongue thrust to stay out of the airway. Lower right: Holes in night guard.

Figure 109: Right HR three years after Oral Facial Epigenetics

---

442 Liao, F. "6 Foot Tiger 3 Foot Cage: Take Charge of Your Health by Taking Charge of Your Mouth." Crescendo Publishing 2017: https://www.amazon.com/Six-Foot-Tiger-Three-Foot-Cage-Charge/dp/1944177590.

At the age of seventeen, HR had already completed her growth spurt. Her facial structure and airway alterations can be credited to a fuller gene expression, potentially increasing from 60 percent to 90 percent.

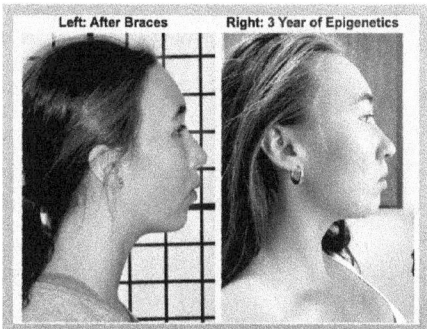

Figure 110: Right: HR three years after Oral Facial Epigenetics.

Originally presented as a case study to establish a connection between teeth grinding, airway issues, and sleep,[443] HR's case is a prime example of the efficacy of Oral Facial Epigenetics (OFE). Figure 111 illustrates the expansion of HR's airway through OFE. Upon identifying Impaired Mouth and treating deficient jaws, approximately 80 percent of associated symptoms naturally diminish, leading to improved functioning in academic, social, and professional domains for patients of all ages.

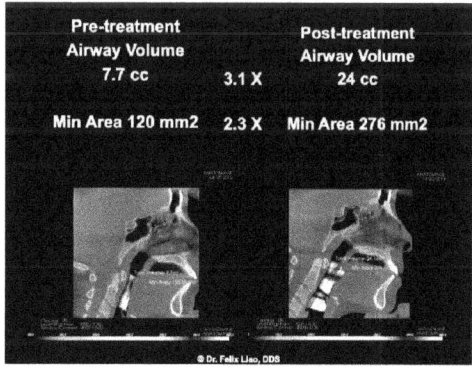

Figure 111: HR's airway minimal area increased by 230 percent with Oral Facial Epigenetics, resulting in cessation of teeth grinding, improvement in sleep depth, and enhancement of overall health. It also brought on her best face.

---

443 Liao F, Singh GD. "Resolution of Sleep Bruxism Using Biomimetic Oral Appliance Therapy: A Case Report." *J Sleep Disord Ther.* 2014;4:4.

Health relies on a series of physiological functions that depend on a specific body structure. Optimal sleep quality requires an unobstructed airway within what the author terms the "Best Face," characterized by sufficient jaw growth to accommodate straight alignment of all teeth.[444] Consequently, issues such as crowded teeth, narrow jaws, and compressed facial features indicate inadequate gene expression in the oral region, forming the face's foundation.

Achieving the Best Face isn't as simple as purchasing a product online or visiting an airway-centered dentist. Rather, it is earned through a diligent effort by parents committed to following the treatment plan prescribed by Airway-centered Mouth Doctors (AMDs). The cases discussed in this chapter demonstrate achieving the Best Face and optimal health requires additional parental involvement guided by qualified professionals.

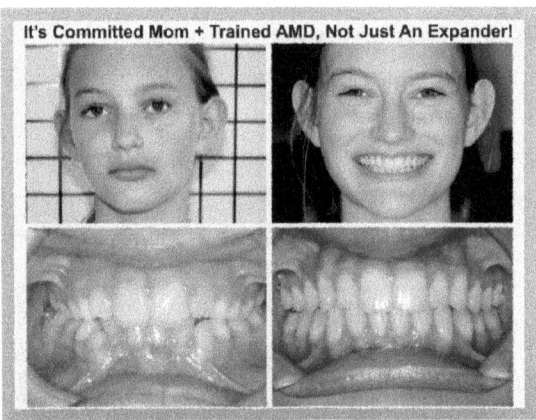

Figure 112: It takes a committed parent. This girl's mom drove three and a half hours each way to her AMD every two months for four years. This mom also ensured a bone-building diet for Best Face.

Oral Facial Epigenetics isn't suitable for everyone. It begins with having healthy, natural teeth in good condition, without infections or bleeding gums, and requires patient education. Success depends on strong compliance with dietary changes and doctor's recommendations.

---

444 Liao, Felix. "Your Child's Best Face: How to Nurture Top Health & Natural Glow. Holistic Mouth Solutions," 2022.

Epigenetics: A New Approach Beyond Medical and Dental Schools

According to the American Academy of Oral and Maxillofacial Surgeons, around 90 percent of people have at least one impacted wisdom tooth.[445] Wisdom teeth are the last to erupt, and they can become impacted when jaw growth is insufficient for them to come in properly.

From 2007 to 2016, approximately 80 percent of patients underwent the extraction of at least one tooth by age twenty-five, with about 50 percent undergoing the extraction of at least one wisdom tooth.[446] How can we improve jaw growth? Enter epigenetics.

The prefix "Epi-" in epigenetics is Greek for "over," "above," or "in addition to." First introduced by British embryologist Conrad Waddington in 1942, epigenetics doesn't alter a person's genetic code artificially. Here's a brief overview:

- According to the National Institute of Environmental Health Sciences, genes can be activated or deactivated by environmental factors such as diet, stress, aging, and pollutants.[447]

- Epigenetics is the complex developmental processes between the—genotype [the body encoded in your genes]—and phenotype [the body seen as gene expression].[448]

- If genes act as cells' guiding instructions, then epigenetic processes direct the cells to refer to particular "pages" of the manual at specific moments.[449]

---

445 American College of Oral and Maxillofacial Surgery. Wisdom Teeth FAQ. Retrieved from https://myoms.org/what-we-do/wisdom-teeth-management/wisdom-teeth-faq/

446 Schroeder, A. R., et al. "Estimated Cumulative Incidence of Wisdom Tooth Extractions in Privately Insured US Patients." *Frontiers in Dental Medicine*, 08 July 2022. Pediatric Dentistry Volume 3 - 2022. doi: 10.3389/fdmed.2022.937165.

447 Waddington, C. H. (1956). "The genetic assimilation of the bithorax phenotype". *Evolution*, 10(1), 1-13. https://doi.org/10.2307/2406091

448 Deichmann, Ute. "Epigenetics: The origins and evolution of a fashionable topic." *Developmental Biology* 416, no. 1 (2016): 249-254. doi:10.1016/j.ydbio.2016.06.005.

449 National Institute of Environmental Health Sciences. "Epigenetics." Accessed May 10, 2024, from https://www.cdc.gov/genomics/disease/epigenetics.htm.

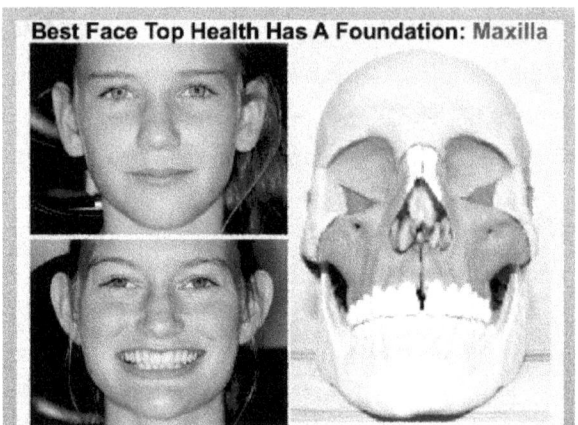

Figure 113: illustrates the concept of "Best Face," which is characterized by adequate jaw growth, depicted by the upper jaw in gray and the lower jaw in white, allowing all teeth to align naturally.

Oral Facial Epigenetics

If deficient jaws are identified as the underlying cause of crowded teeth, then Oral Facial Epigenetics (OFE) represents the author's solution by addressing three key factors outlined by the CDC:[450]

> A. Oral Behavior: This includes factors such as lip seal versus mouth breathing, normal versus abnormal swallows (typically around 2,000 times a day), chewing patterns, dietary choices, and the inclusion of bone-building nutrients.
>
> B. Oral Environment: This encompasses tongue size, jaw size, tooth positioning, lip strength, tongue posture, and the potential impact of past pacifier use on cheek and lip muscles.
>
> C. Surrounding Structures: Factors such as nasal breathing versus mouth breathing, facial symmetry, alignment of the head and neck, and even flat feet may also play a role in oral and facial development.[451]

---

[450] Centers for Disease Control and Prevention. "What Is Epigenetics?" Genomics and Health Impact Blog, CDC, https://www.cdc.gov/genomics/disease/epigenetics.htm. Accessed May 10, 2024.

[451] Liao, F. "Clinical Epigenetics: Solutions for Head-Scratcher." *Orthodontic Issues, Journal of*

Oral Facial Epigenetics activates entirely natural processes. Just as a body can change shape and fitness through exercise, a mouth can transform from crowded teeth and impaired airway through Oral Facial Epigenetics. No genes are artificially modified in this process.

Oral Facial Epigenetics contrasts with traditional braces in several ways:

- Braces primarily straighten teeth crowded into deficient jaws, while OFE focuses on jaw growth so all teeth can self-align naturally under larger, more natural-sized jaws.

- Braces mechanically align teeth along wires, following a standardized approach, whereas OFE aims to stimulate the natural growth potential of each individual's jaws and face.

- Braces involve artificial manipulation using wires, brackets, screws, and plastics, while OFE turns on the natural expression of genes inherited from both parents using epigenetic changes involving oral behavior and oral environment described above.

While braces can improve tooth alignment, OFE aims to enhance jaw growth, leading to a wider airway, deeper sleep, and achieving the "Best Face."

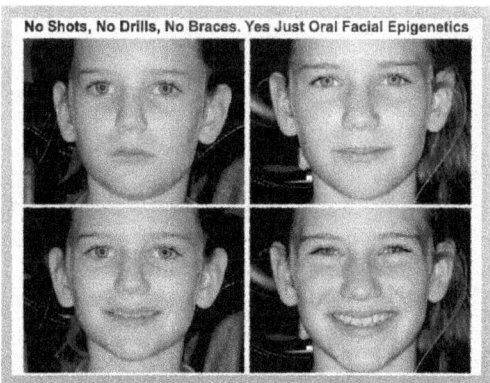

Figure 114: A painless patient-dentist relationship is part of Oral Facial Epigenetics.

Just as removing pressure from a garden hose allows water to flow freely for plant growth, genes can be influenced to promote the growth of jaws and facial structures that better support airway function, quality sleep, and optimal posture when provided with the right conditions.

Best of all, OFE treatment involves no injections, drilling, medications, surgical procedures, or screws. OFE can transform the patient-dentist dynamic from traumatic to joy, and from reactive to proactive care.

Oral Facial Epigenetics Rescue

SZ is the daughter of Dr. NMD, a naturopathic doctor from the Philippines and a dentist trained in the U.S. Dr. NMD observed her daughter experiencing difficulties with her homework, focus, and soprano singing shortly after starting braces with an orthodontist who coincidentally was Dr. NMD's best friend.

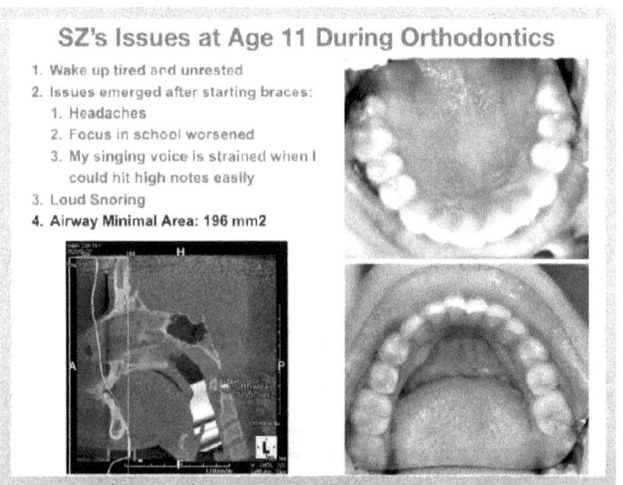

Figure 115

Dr. NMD had an "Aha!" moment after reading *Your Child's Best Face*. Her maternal instincts were validated when she underwent AMD training to become an Airway-centered Mouth Doctor. Despite her best friend's expert advice, Dr. NMD discontinued braces and initiated Oral Facial Epigenetics instead. Figure 116 illustrates the noticeable difference this decision made.

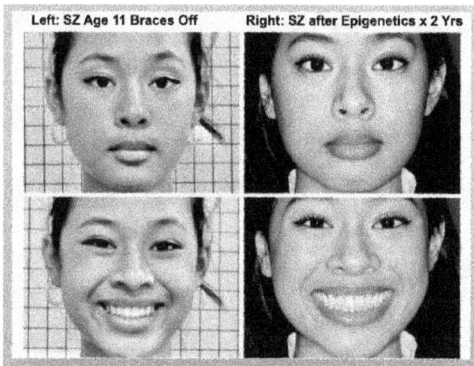

Figure 116: Fuller Gene Expression with Oral Facial Epigenetics instead of braces.

AMDs are trained in managing oral behavior and environment and collaborate with like-minded integrative healthcare professionals, such as physicians, chiropractors, physical therapists, myofunctional therapists, acupuncturists, etc. AMDs are also trained in the 3D Jaw Diagnostics® method to see which of the three dimensions of both jaws are malformed and deficient by how much, as shown in Figure 117. Solutions are then built into the epigenetic oral appliances used to target areas of deficiency for corrective growth. Not all expanders are created equal, even though they may look similar.

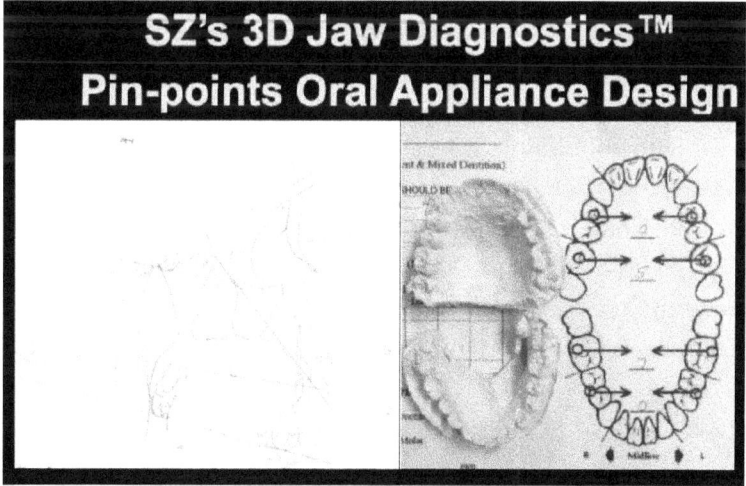

Figure 117: SZ's skeletal vertical (lower face height) is deficient; her maxilla is retruded (opposite of protruded) and too narrow for her mandible to fit like a foot into a shoe. The left drawing is called a cephalometric tracing.

Nurturing the Best Face begins with foundational jaw growth through epigenetics, followed by braces and/or integrative bodywork as necessary. In OFE, jaw growth is supported by a bone-building diet, as illustrated in Figure 118, which combines the best from both the plant and animal kingdoms to promote the growth of the Best Face.[452]

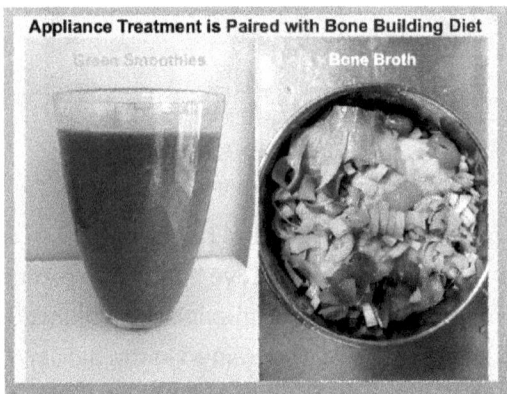

Figure 118: Bone-building diet is an essential part of Oral Facial Epigenetics.

Under the guidance of Dr. NMD, SZ diligently followed the recommended adjustments: adhering to a bone-building diet (oral behavior) and wearing her epigenetic oral appliance for fourteen to sixteen hours daily (oral environment). The outcomes are depicted in Figures 119-121. The Subjective Units of Distress Scale (SUDS), ranging from zero to ten, is a recognized measure for assessing anxiety and evaluating cognitive-behavioral treatments for anxiety disorders.[453] SZ experienced airway expansion through Oral Facial Epigenetics, which subsequently addressed 80 percent of her baseline complaints stemming from starting braces, as depicted in Figure 122 below.

---

452 Liao, F. (2017). *Licensed To Thrive: A Mouth Owner's GPS to Vibrant Health & Innate Immunity*. Crescendo Publishing, Chapter 23.

453 Wolpe, Joseph. 1969. *The Practice of Behavior Therapy*. New York: Pergamon Press. ISBN: 0080065635. PMID: 20509987.

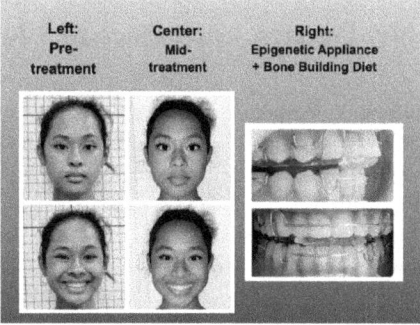

Figure 119: Eleven months of Oral Facial Epigenetics: bone-building diet and oral appliances.

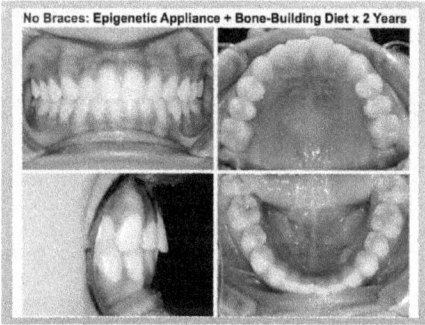

Figure 120: SZ's dental-facial growth is nearly finished in two years. Jaw growth results in a broader airway, deeper sleep, and vibrant energy, effortlessly facilitating high levels of achievement.

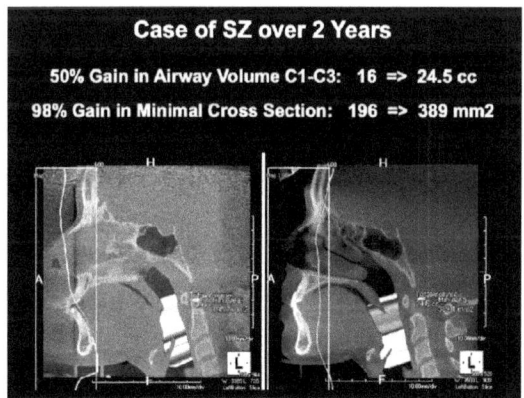

Figure 121: The left image is pre-treatment, while the right is 80 percent of the treatment after two years, resulting in a 98 percent gain in minimal area (where airway collapses in sleep apnea) and a 50 percent gain in airway volume.

No Pain | No Drugs | No Sweat | No Braces

SZ Symptoms	Before Treatment	Progress Week 4	Progress Week 10	Progress Week 20	Total Gain
Sleep Disruption	8	6	4	1	7
Snoring	8	6	2	2	6
Headaches	9	7	1	0	9
Inability to Focus	10	9	7	4	6
Vocal Stress	9	9	6	2	7
Fatigue	10	9	5	2	8
Total	54	46	21	11	**80%**

Figure 122: Subjective Units of Distress:
10 is "unbearably bad;" 0 is "Peace, total relief."

SZ went on to win the national speech and debate for homeschoolers and earned a full scholarship for four years of college at her chosen institution. However, is it all that simple and rosy for everyone? The outcome depends on each case, the parent's involvement, and the child's response. SZ's case, as depicted in Figures 115 and 116, was relatively mild due to her upbringing under a holistic dentist who became an AMD. More severe cases with a larger deficit will require greater patient compliance, parental effort, and clinical expertise.

Guarding Against Environmental Toxins

The mouth is the primary gateway for external elements to enter the body. Just as proper nutrition can activate gene expression, environmental toxins can inhibit it. During formative years, oral-facial growth can be influenced by various environmental toxins:

1. Environmental pollutants, even at low levels, have been linked to fetal growth retardation.[454]

2. Prenatal exposure to environmental chemicals has been associated with adverse health outcomes throughout life, including impacts on fertility, neurodevelopment, and cancer.[455]

3. Pharmaceuticals pass through water treatment processes, as noted by the U.S. Geological Survey.[456]

4. Hypothyroidism, characterized by an underactive thyroid gland, can affect the functioning of nearly every organ in the body.[457]

5. Xenobiotics, as detailed in "Big Chicken: The Incredible Story of How Antibiotics Created Modern Agriculture and Changed the Way the World Eats."[458]

6. Glyphosate contamination in food extends beyond oat products, as indicated in reports on breakfast with a dose of glyphosate.[459]

7. Umbilical cord blood analysis has revealed the presence of numerous chemicals, many of which are known to cause cancer in humans or animals and are toxic to the brain and nervous system.[460]

---

454 Carroll L. "Low Levels of Environmental Pollutants May Slow Fetal Growth." *Medscape*. December 31, 2017. URL: https://www.medscape.com/viewarticle/923218?src=wnl_edit_tpal&uac=175928DV&impID=2230161&faf=1. Accessed May 20, 2023.

455 Di Renzo GC et al. "International Federation of Gynecology and Obstetrics opinion on reproductive health impacts of exposure to toxic environmental chemicals." *International Journal of Gynaecology and Obstetrics*. 2015 Dec;131(3):219-25. doi: 10.1016/j.ijgo.2015.09.002. Epub 2015 Oct 1. PMID: 26433469; PMCID: PMC6663094.

456 "Pharmaceuticals in Water." US Geological Survey. Accessed May 20, 2023.

457 "Hypothyroidism." National Institute of Diabetes and Digestive and Kidney Diseases. Accessed May 20, 2023.

458 McKenna, M. "Big Chicken." *National Geographic*, August 18, 2017. ISBN: 978-1-4262-1766-1.

459 Temkin A, Naidenko O. "Glyphosate Contamination in Food Goes Far Beyond Oat Products." The Environmental Working Group. Feb. 28, 2019. Accessed May 20, 2023.

460 Environmental Working Group. "Body Burden: The Pollution in Newborns." July 14, 2005. https://www.ewg.org/research/bodyburden-pollution-newborns. Accessed May 12, 2024.

8. Studies have provided concrete evidence that newborns are exposed to BPA, a toxic plastic chemical, while still in the womb.[461]

This brief yet incomplete list sheds light on the prevalence of underdeveloped jaws, habitual mouth breathing, and obesity in modern America. Figure 104 illustrates air and water pollutants in a highly desirable suburb of Washington, DC.

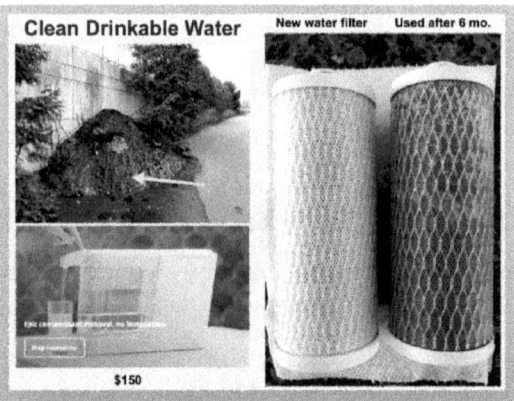

Figure 123: Top left: The arrow line points to a pile of snow that turned black from air pollutants one week later. Right: Water filter new vs. six month's use showing tap water contaminants.

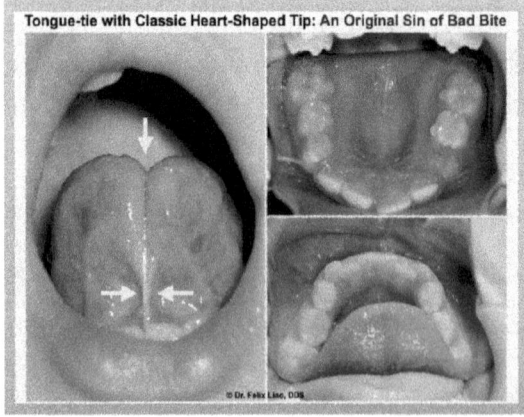

Figure 124: Tongue-tie inevitably leads to a bad bite and Impaired Mouth

---

461 Environmental Working Group. "Toxic Chemicals Found in Minority Cord Blood." https://www.ewg.org/news-insights/newsrelease/toxic-chemicals-found-minority-cord-blood. Accessed May 12, 2024.

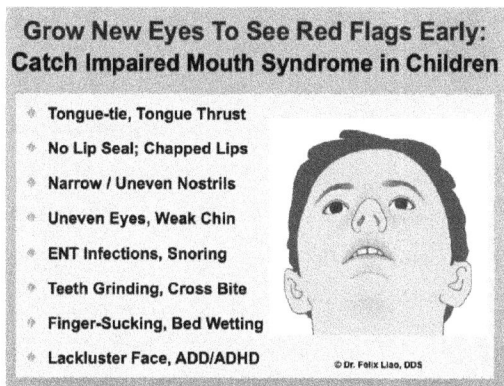

Figure 125

Red Flags re Your Child's Best Face

Mouth	Score	Body	Score
Lips chapped, peeling, or blue	0 1	Waking up tired or cannot get up	0 1
Mouth breathing (lips apart) habitually	0 1	Excessive daytime sleepiness	0 1
White shows between eye lid and pupil	0 1	Not sleeping through the night	0 1
Facial asymmetry: one eye higher, one mouth corner lower, ears uneven	0 1	Allergies, dark circle under eyes	0 1
Nostrils uneven, narrow, tiny	0 1	Stuffy/runny nose, ear tubes	0 1
Upper & lower dental midlines off	0 1	Uneven shoulders, scoliosis	0 1
Teeth grinding sounds or worn teeth	0 1	Bed wetting	0 1
Cavities-prone, red/bleeding gums	0 1	Under weight & height in growth	0 1
Swallow with gurgling sounds, bobbing head ("goose necking"), grimaced face	0 1	Obstructive sleep apnea diagnosed from sleep test	0 1
Tongue-tie, tongue thrust, tooth prints on the sides of the tongue	0 1	Slumped posture, head forward: ears ahead of shoulders	0 1
Frequent sighing or yawning	0 1	Learning or behavior problems	0 1
Thumb sucking, nail biting; narrow & high palate	0 1	Tired, listless, lethargic, cranky, depressed, anxious, moody	0 1
Weak chin, double chin	0 1	Overweight, low thyroid function	0 1
Malocclusion: crowded/crooked teeth, deep bite, open bite, cross bite, etc.	0 1	Snoring, snorting, choking in sleep	0 1
Total Score		Total Score	

Figure 126

Figures 125 and 126 are handouts that I provide to parents who are interested in fostering their children's Best Faces.

Ensuring optimal oral-facial growth requires ongoing vigilance from dedicated parents and continual learning from committed clinicians. Achieving Best Face and its associated benefits is an EARNED outcome, requiring diligent awareness of the harms of the standard American diet and environmental toxins. The great news: Best Face with top natural health is still achieving predictably.

The Case of Camilla

My son Franklin, a professional chef, asked me when my granddaughter was born, "How can I raise Camilla to her healthiest?" This question inspired me to write *Your Child's Best Face*.

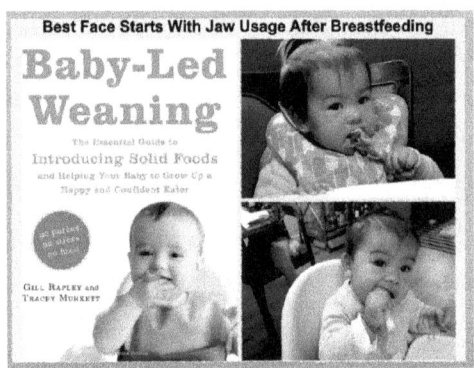

Figure 127: Crunchy whole foods at an appropriate age are my preferred way to stimulate jaw growth naturally in place of artificial devices.

Patients often juggle work and parental duties in today's busy world. The prevalence of fast and processed "convenient" foods has become the norm, contributing to skeletal malocclusion and nasal obstruction, which can lead to Impaired Mouth Syndrome.[462]

Considering the toxins in our environment and the abundance of fast and processed foods, mastering the skill of cooking whole, fresh

---

462 Liao, F. (2023). *Relaunch Your Vitality: Root Out Chronic Pain & Fatigue to Enjoy Life Again*. Holistic Mouth Solutions.

foods at home is arguably as important for personal wellness as regular toothbrushing.[463]

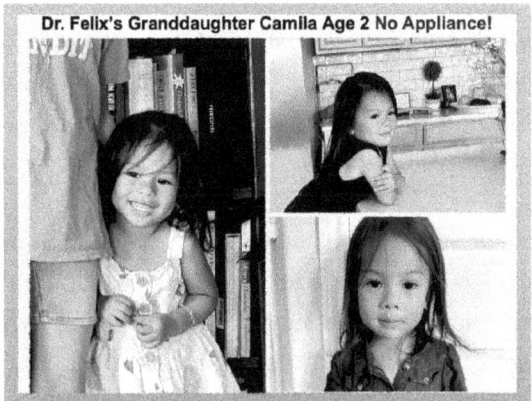

Figure 128

Camila has enjoyed the benefit of having 95 percent of her meals personally prepared by Chef Franklin at home, using organic ingredients and filtered water. Figures 128 and 129 show how Oral Facial Epigenetics works to bring on Camila's Best Face with top health. [These echo Chef Franklin's initial question earlier.]

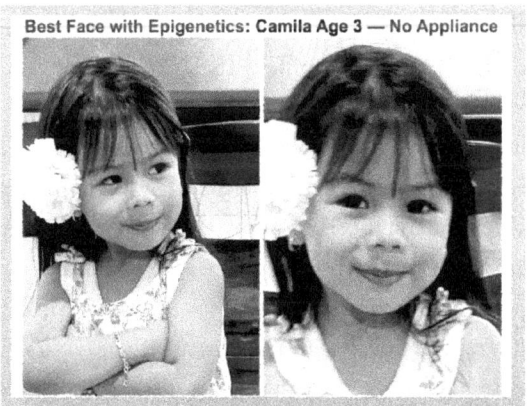

Figure 129

---

463 Liao, F. (2017). *Licensed To Thrive: A Mouth Owner's GPS to Vibrant Health & Innate Immunity* (pp. 19-31). Crescendo Publishing.

Conclusion

Oral Facial Epigenetics represents a groundbreaking, proactive, and painless solution for many prevalent medical, dental, and psychological symptoms stemming from an Impaired Mouth. The newfound understanding suggests that issues like crowded teeth, poor sleep, and ADD/ADHD may be viewed as consequences of incomplete gene expression, resulting in underdeveloped jaws, restricted airways, and disrupted sleep patterns.

In 2024, a new playbook has emerged to unlock the full potential and Best Face inherent in each child's genetic makeup. In this author's experience, Oral Facial Epigenetics can predictably improve or resolve up to 80 percent of symptoms rooted in Impaired Mouth with patient compliance.

CBCT Scans: (Dr. Downs' Note)

As you saw in Dr. Liao's cases, there is an X-ray image of the side of the head showing airway volume changes with treatment. In the next chapters, you will see many more. These are called CBCT or Cone Beam Computed Tomography images. You will see various views. Some are of the side of the head, others of the nasal structures, and some show just the airway volume isolated to look like a wrinkled pillar. These are similar to CT scans that might be more familiar to the general public. They administer much less radiation to the patient than CT scans do. Many dentists have adopted this imaging system because they are superior diagnostic images for implant placement and for the diagnosis of many types of oral and facial diseases.

While images cannot diagnose sleep apnea, they can provide dentists with valuable data regarding changes in airway volume over time. These images are not accurate representations of the airway when lying down or during sleep, as tissues tend to relax more in these positions. However, dentists can still observe the jaw joint health, dental arch width, yaw and cant. They can see nasal structures and, if needed, refer patients to an ENT physician for further examination of nasal obstructions. Additionally, some chiropractors use these images for spinal and TMJ evaluations.

CHAPTER 14

Case Studies by Kamran Fattah DMD, Airway and Vivos® Practitioner

Kamran Fattah, DMD, D-ASBA[464]

In 2003, I graduated from dental school with no training in sleep-disordered breathing; I enjoyed practicing dentistry and like many dentists, started my continuing education journey focused on doing everyday dentistry better. I quickly realized that fixing painful, cracked, and broken teeth and using night guards to protect teeth from wear was not solving the underlying cause of the damage to patients' teeth, joints, and muscles. At the time, the most prominent gurus of occlusion education did not discuss airway or sleep-disordered breathing as the potential source of these problems. Still, they were more concerned with reducing symptoms and restoring damaged teeth. It was not until I was introduced to education on treating sleep apnea. In this condition, breathing is stopped or reduced repeatedly while asleep, resulting in drops in one's blood oxygen concentration. I learned how much of an impact our airway has on our dental health. It is well known that sleep-disordered breathing increases our risk of heart attack, stroke, dementia, type 2 diabetes, metabolic syndrome, and cancer. However, sleep apnea and its variants also cause or contribute to multiple dental pathologies like

---

[464] Fattah, Kamran, DMD, Scottsdale Family Smiles, Scottsdale, AZ.

temporomandibular joint disease (TMJ problems), tinnitus (ringing in the ears), clenching, grinding, headaches and migraine, broken and cracked teeth, and muscle pain.

I started focusing my study and learning on sleep, its systemic effects, and how the midface, jaws, soft palate, and tongue affected treatment options and outcomes. I learned about sleep testing, the objective metrics of respiration during sleep, and the multiple and potentially life-threatening consequences of lack of oxygen during sleep. The main metric of apnea used for diagnosis is the Apnea Hypopnea Index or AHI. AHI is the number of times per hour someone has a reduction in respiration of 30% to 100% (complete obstruction), resulting in a drop of blood oxygen concentration that lasts at least 10 seconds. The higher your AHI, the more times per hour you have oxygen deficit events, the more severe your sleep apnea, and the greater the detrimental health consequences.

> Book author's note. The AASM defines hypopnea as a greater than or equal to 30% reduction in respiration airflow events and a 3 percent drop in oxygen saturation in blood or arousal from deeper stages of sleep (H3A). Medicare sets it at a 4 percent drop in saturation and does not count arousals in the definition (H4).[465]

I started treating sleep-disordered breathing in 2011 with dental devices that move the mandible forward called mandibular advancement devices (MADs), similar to the chin lift in CPR. My dental practice was across the street from a sleep physician who would refer his CPAP-intolerant patients to me for dental appliance therapy. CPAPs, or Continuous Positive Air Pressure machines, use air pressure to maintain the patency of the upper airway and keep people breathing while they sleep. They have always been considered the gold standard for treating severe sleep apnea, where at least 30 times per hour, a person's blood oxygen concentration drops by 3 percent for at least ten seconds. For mild to moderate sleep apnea, CPAPs and MADs are considered equally

---

465 Berry, Richard B., et al. "A Transition to the American Academy of Sleep Medicine–Recommended Hypopnea Definition in Adults: Initiatives of the Hypopnea Scoring Rule Task Force." *Journal of Clinical Sleep Medicine* 18, no. 5 (May 1, 2022). https://doi.org/10.5664/jcsm.9952.

effective with patient compliance and providing higher comfort with the mandibular advancement device.

In 2018, I attended a Breathing and Wellness Conference presented by Vivos® Therapeutics, which forever changed my perspective on breathing, sleep, airway anatomy, and dental therapies. There, I heard Dr. David Singh discuss biomimetic expansion therapy, Dr. Soroush Zaghi explain the impact of tethered oral tissues, especially tongue ties, on facial development, nasal breathing, and oral function, and Dr. Ben Miraglia discussed determinants of craniofacial development in modern man versus our ancestors and the epidemic of underdeveloped jaws and its impact on both children and adults.

These thought leaders opened my eyes to the possibility of helping people heal and not be tied to oral appliances or CPAPs for the rest of their lives. Altering anatomy to create lasting changes in breathing and sleep became my educational passion and the most rewarding aspect of my career ever since. Because of these passionate caregivers, I pursued and have since completed hundreds of hours of training and education on facial growth and development, airway physiology, surgical correction of tethered oral tissues, sleep-disordered breathing, temporomandibular joint disorders, and orthodontic and orthopedic expansion therapy.

Helping adults and children to breathe better while awake and asleep, to have adequate tongue space and mobility, reduce jaw pain, and normal facial growth has become my purpose as a dentist, where each patient I serve is an opportunity to improve, or even save a life.

The following cases are a sample of what I have found possible with modern non-surgical expansion techniques.

CASE 1: PATIENT J

Patient J came to our office as a new patient interested in routine dental care. She initially reported poor sleep and a history of anxiety and depression. She noted that she required trazodone to fall and stay asleep and had not had a good night's sleep without medication in as long as she could remember. J had frequent bouts of neck pain and had a persistent faint ringing in her ears. She reported incidents of restless leg and insomnia as well. Clinically, it was noted that J had right-side temporomandibular joint sounds, a high palatal vault, a narrow arch form, indents of her teeth on her tongue, and a mild tongue tie.

Anytime a patient shows clinical signs that may be related to sleep-disordered breathing or has a history of poor sleep, we recommend overnight pulse oximetry to see if oxygen saturation remains normal or if further testing should be pursued with the help of a sleep physician to diagnose a sleep-disordered breathing concern. The American Dental Association has recommended that all dentists screen for sleep-disordered breathing in their offices; unfortunately, it is not a common practice yet.

In J's case, the pulse oximeter reported that her blood oxygen had ten-second drops of 3 percent or greater twenty-two times per hour, and during the night, her blood oxygen went below 90 percent concentration twice. A physician-scored sleep test was recommended for J, where she was diagnosed with moderate sleep apnea; severe desaturations were noted, as were central sleep apneas, where the signal to breathe is not sent by the brain. Once the physician's diagnosis was reviewed with J, a 3D X-ray called a cone-beam computed tomography, or CBCT, of J's head and neck was acquired to see what areas of her anatomy were contributing to her obstructive sleep apnea and if they could be altered to improve her breathing and sleep. A comprehensive analysis of J's anatomy was completed, and J decided that rather than a CPAP or mandibular advancement device, she would like to address the underlying anatomy of obstructive sleep apnea through expansion therapy. Over the course of twelve months, J's obstructive sleep apnea scores were resolved, and her central sleep apnea scores went from 11.2 per hour to 0.2 per hour. Her minimum oxygen saturation went from 76 percent to 94 percent. By the end of treatment, J happily reported that all of her symptoms had resolved; her neck pain and ringing in the ear were both completely resolved, and she could sleep comfortably through the night without medications. She also reported that her once-chronic anxiety was gone. Obstructive sleep apnea increases the lifetime risk of heart attack, stroke, and cancer, and can reduce lifespan considerably. Eliminating these long-term health consequences improves the quality of life and adds years of healthy living for the patient.

Case Studies by Kamran Fattah DMD, Airway and Vivos® Practitioner | 323

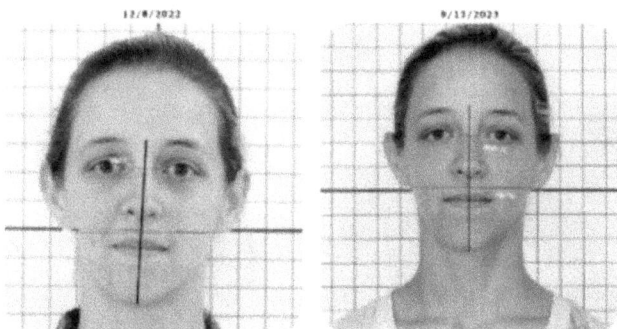

Figure 130: Through treatment facial symmetry and posture tend to improve. Notice the improved symmetry of the eyes, ears, and cheekbones.

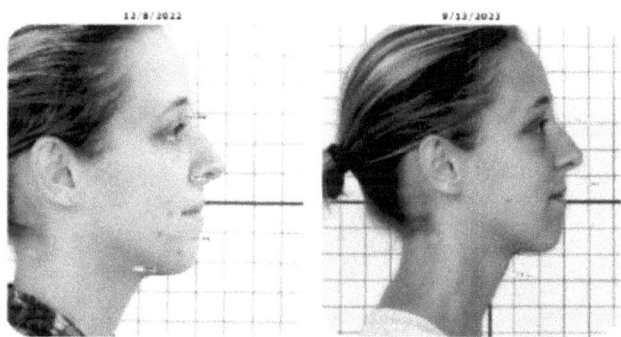

Figure 131: Forward development of the mid and lower face.

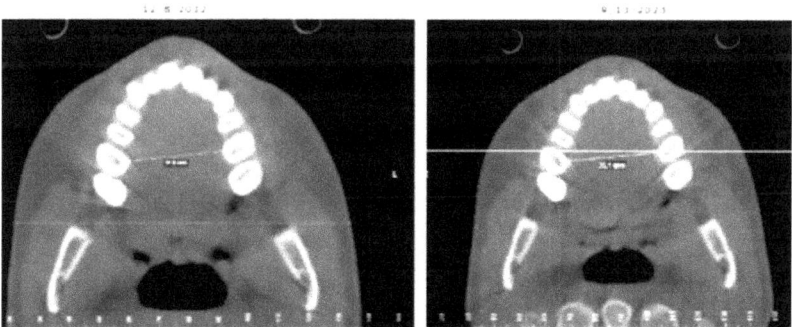

Figure 132: During treatment, the distance from the palate to the back wall of the pharynx increased by 25 percent. 12-8-2022 = 32.0 mm 9-13-2023 = 35.0 mm

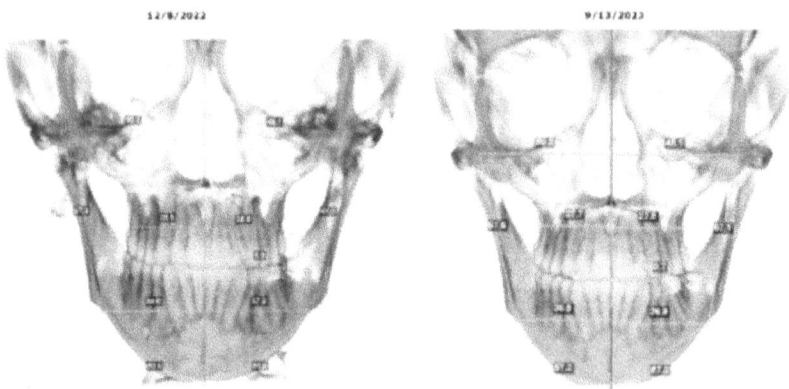

Figure 133: Facial metrics confirm that through treatment, symmetry and balance of the face were improved.

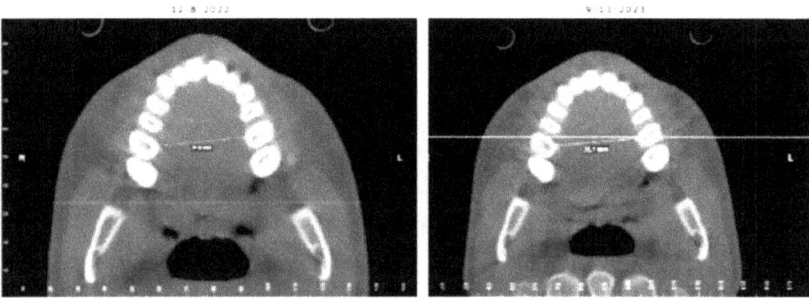

Figure 134: The expansion resulted in a 9.4 percent increase in trans palatal width, making more tongue space.

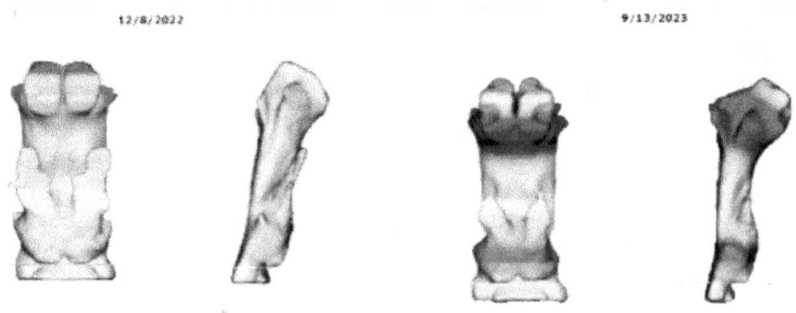

Figure 135

In J's case, airway volume was normal before and after treatment, but expansion resulted in a reduction of the expansibility of the airway which improved every metric of her sleep breathing by at least 48 percent. We perform myofunctional therapy in conjunction with our appliance care.

12-8-2022	AHI @3% = 25.3	RDI = 33.9
9-13-2023	AHI @3% = 3.9	RDI = 16.6
Change	AHI reduced -84.6%	RDI reduced -48.1%

CASE 2: PATIENT L

Our next case was referred to our clinic by a myofunctional therapist. They are professionals dedicated to the proper function and mobility of the tongue and masticatory system. They guide patients on improved breathing, tongue posture, head and neck posture, and swallow pattern. Our work would not be possible without their expertise, patience, and attention to detail. Myofunctional therapists are vital partners to the airway-centric dentist in supporting facial development, optimal sleep, and health.

Patient L had dealt with difficulty breathing her whole life. She reported as a child, she was chronically ill with a nose that was always stuffy, resulting in a lifetime of mouth breathing. She had frequent strep throat infections and had to have her tonsils removed as a child. As an adult, L revealed that she had been diagnosed with anxiety and depression, had frequent headaches when waking in the morning, and noted that both of her ears had continuous ringing in them (tinnitus). She felt like her sleep was not regenerative; she was fatigued throughout the day, even after a full night of sleep. L also experienced temporomandibular joint pain and sounds (TMJ dysfunction); she had her jaw locked in the past and felt her jaw muscles tire easily with persistent facial tension.

When asked what her primary treatment goals were, L said that she wanted better sleep, reduced jaw pain and tension, improved nasal breathing, her jaw to stop making sounds, and the ringing in her ears to improve or resolve.

L's treatment involved expansion therapy to increase tongue space, leveling of the upper jaw to improve facial balance, and advancement of the mandible to reduce pressures on the joint that can contribute to tinnitus, facial tension, and headache.

With ten months of treatment, L reported that she has no more TMJ pain or sounds. Her nasal breathing felt easier, allowing enough airflow so that she could comfortably mouth tape during sleep. She reported not waking fatigued or feeling tired during the day, and her jaw tension had resolved. Her tinnitus improved dramatically, which she frequently does not notice now. L's treatment is ongoing and will include further expansion and myofunctional therapy, as well as orthodontic treatment to bring the teeth and bite together after expansion therapy is complete.

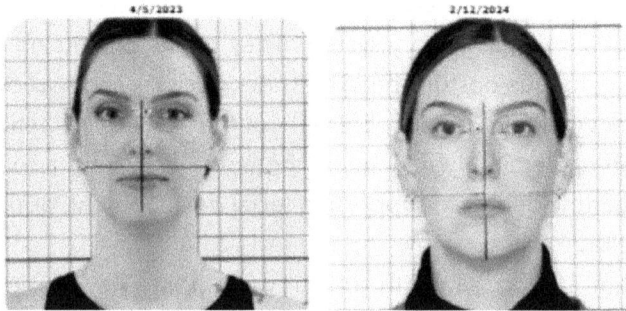

Figure 136: Improved facial symmetry—notice the leveling of the eyes, ears, corners of the lips, and bottom of the lower jaw, even the nose is straighter.

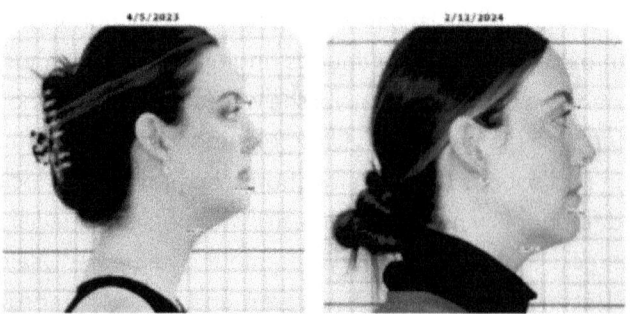

Figure 137: Lower jawline definition has improved, support of the lips has increased, and both jaws have developed forward.

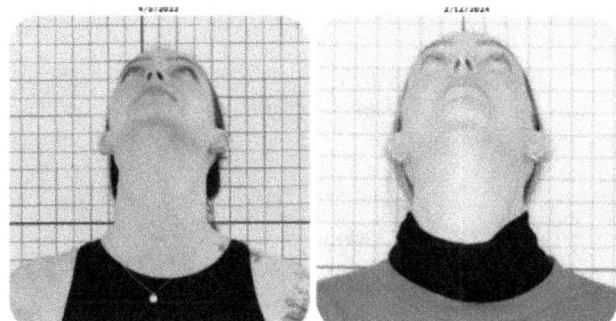

Figure 138: Cervical neck tension visible with the head tilt and sternocleidomastoid (this is a muscle) contraction in the before photos have improved along with the visible improvement to cheekbone, eye, ear, and nostril symmetry.

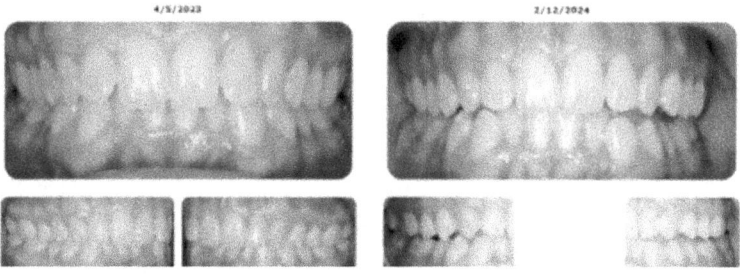

Figure 139: The lower jaw has changed position in relation to the upper jaw, reducing the deep bite present at the beginning of treatment. The lateral open bite, seen in the mid-treatment photos will be addressed with Invisalign® once all skeletal expansion has been completed.

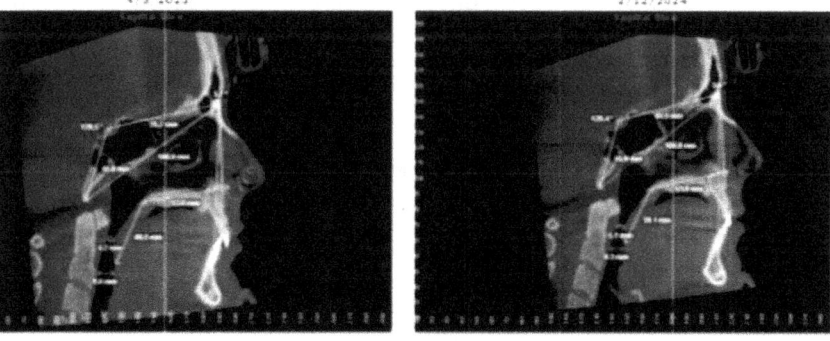

Figure 140: During treatment, the distance from the soft palate to the back wall of the pharynx increased by 25 percent. Notice reduction in overbite due to forward movement of the mandible.

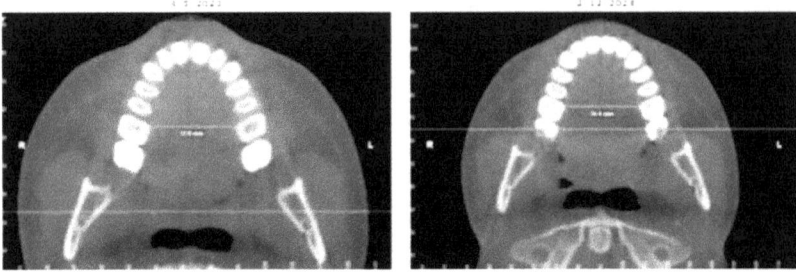

Figure 141: Tongue space measured by the distance between the upper first molars has increased by 7.8 percent.

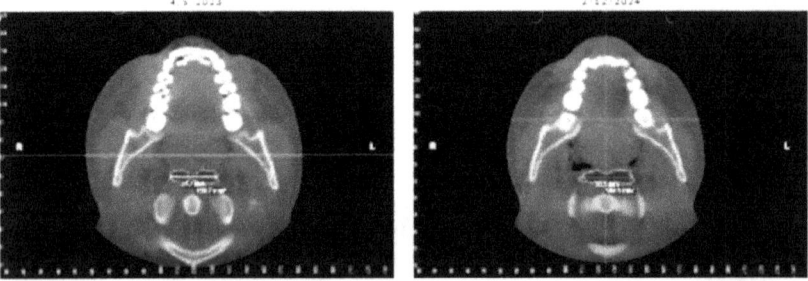

Figure 142: The cross-sectional area of the pharynx behind the soft palate has increased by 24.8 percent.

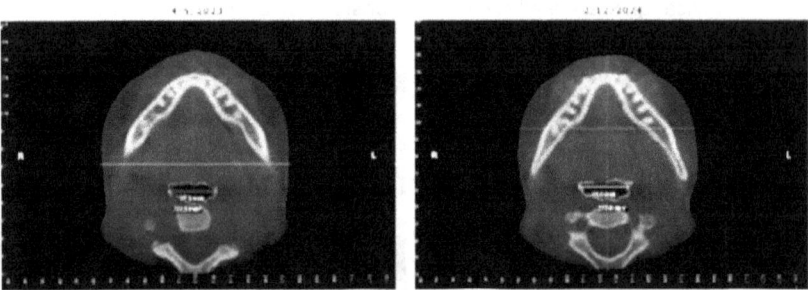

Figure 143: Another cross-sectional area of the pharynx behind the tongue has increased by 22 percent.

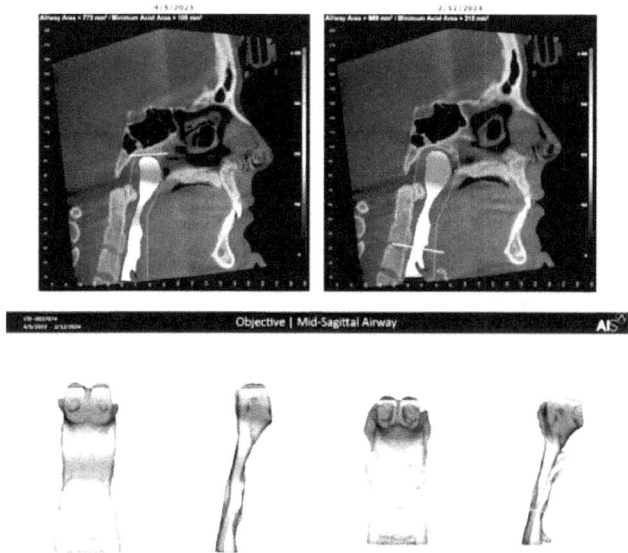

Figure 144: The total volume of the pharynx has increased by 30 percent during treatment.

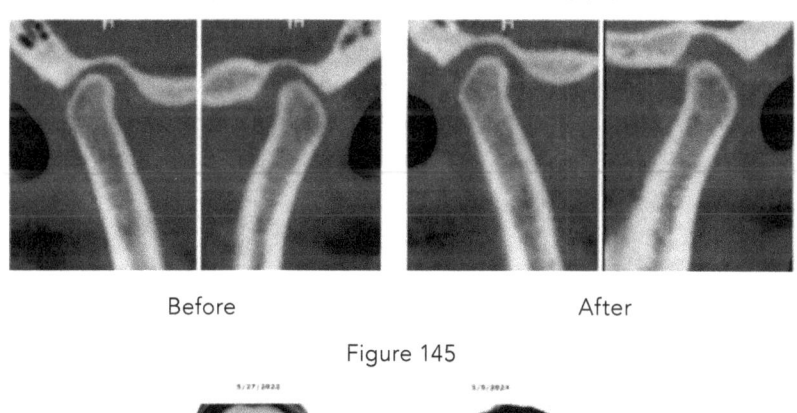

Before After

Figure 145

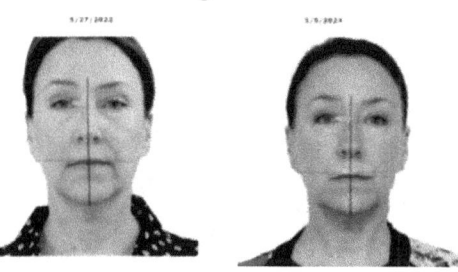

Figure 146: The image shows the leveling of the eyes relative to the ears and a decrease in the nasolabial folds (lines around the mouth).

This image 145 shows that prior to treatment, the lower jaw was pushed backward towards the ear, which is frequently associated with symptoms like jaw pain and tension, ringing in the ears, vertigo, and teeth grinding. It also reduces the size of the pharynx behind the tongue. In the after images, the joint is much more centered in the joint spaces relative to the base of the skull.

CASE 3: PATIENT K

Patient K came to us familiar with Vivos® Expansion Therapy and was looking for an alternative to a CPAP to treat the underlying causes of her obstructive sleep apnea. She had a history of congestion, brain fog, and clenching and grinding day and night. She was seeing a myofunctional therapist who recognized that K's anatomy was contributing to her sleep-disordered breathing and recommended evaluation for expansion therapy. K had a history of snoring and waking up fatigued throughout the day. For K, improving how she slept and felt during the day was a huge priority, along with reducing the systemic risks associated with sleep apnea, like, high blood pressure, diabetes, cancer, and dementia. K was committed to the process of expansion and airway improvement completely. By the end of her expansion phase of treatment, K reported normal sleep, almost complete resolution of snoring, no chronic fatigue, and no clenching or grinding. K's quality of life and longevity improved due to the resolution of her obstructive sleep apnea; she is a healthier and happier person with great sleep.

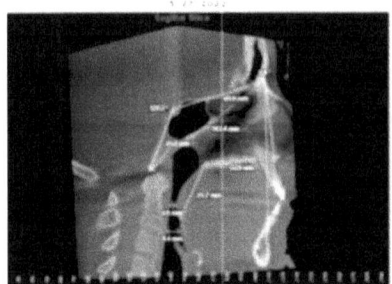 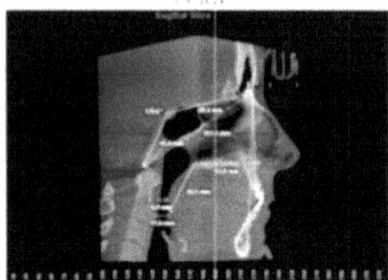

Figure 147: The minimal distance from the pharynx wall to the back of the soft palate increased by 55.6 percent, and to the tongue, it increased by 26.3 percent.

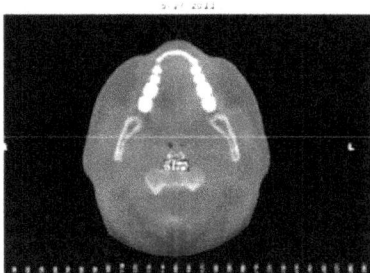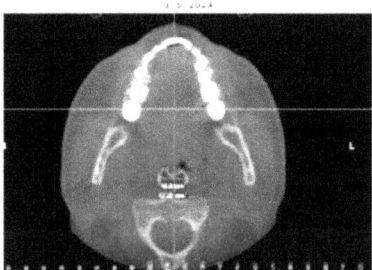

Figure 148: The area of the pharynx behind the palate increased by 129 percent.

K's sleep apnea decreased by 83.7 percent from an AHI of 10.4 to 1.7 through the course of treatment; her apnea metrics are now completely resolved.

CASE 4: PATIENT B

Our next patient is an eight-year-old male who came to us with a previous diagnosis of sleep apnea and a history of snoring. His tonsils had been surgically removed, but he still was waking with fatigue, restless sleep, and congestion that resulted in mouth breathing day and night. His mother's primary concern was airway-related; she wanted her son to have normal breathing, sleep, and growth.

Radiographic evaluation revealed narrow jaws, diminished airway volume, low tongue posture, diminished nasal passage volume, and a downward maxillary facial growth pattern frequently seen with patients that mouth-breathe. We can see in B's initial photos that his bite was very deep, hiding his lower front teeth completely, effectively trapping his lower jaw behind his underdeveloped upper jaw.

Imagine the chin lift of rescue CPR opening the airway of a trapped lower jaw that is in a backward position. A retruded jaw effectively shrinks the airway, making breathing more difficult, especially while sleeping. To free his jaw and breathe better, B was habitually posturing his jaw forward and to the side, which, over time can alter facial development and result in permanent facial asymmetry. This is a negative epigenetic influence on his genetic potential.

By intervening early, before B's facial growth had been completed (95 percent of maxillary growth is completed by age twelve in males), we were able to promote a more normal facial growth pattern and improve B's breathing and appearance. By the end of our phase-one treatment, B's growth pattern had been brought back to normal; his arches had been made wider, his nasal passage had become more patent, and his pharynx size had improved.

For B, we used a Rickonator® oral appliance that opens the bite, increases the vertical height of the lower third of the face, brings the lower jaw forward, and opens the airway. As B grows, his permanent teeth will have room to come in normally, his jaws will have space to grow, and he will have room for his tongue so he can breathe more easily. If orthodontic care is desired, it will be simple and for cosmetic purposes only, as his skeletal concerns have already been addressed.

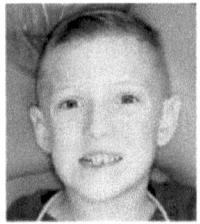 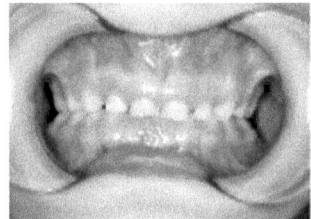 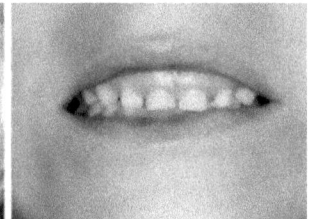

Figure 149   Figure 150

Pretreatment shows that B has a habitual forward and sideward posture to his mandible to free it from being trapped behind his upper jaw. Chronic mouth breathing has altered the growth trajectory of the upper jaw, resulting in a more gummy smile.

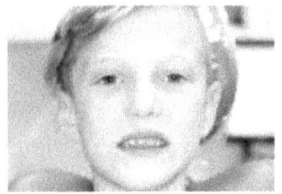 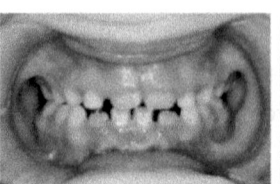 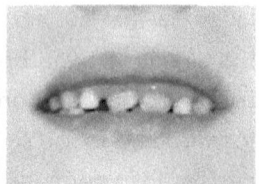

Figure 151

Post-treatment, B had a normal bite with his teeth overlapping the ideal amount. He is no longer posturing his jaw forward to breathe, and his facial symmetry and gummy smile have improved.

CHAPTER 15

Combination Vivos® & Clear Aligner Care by Kevin Goles, DDS, D-ASBA

As discussed in other sections of this book, our goal with our discussed treatment modalities is to maximize the ability to breathe. Ensuring your airway remains open during sleep is crucial for maximizing sleep quality. When your airway stays unobstructed, you can smoothly progress through the restorative stages of sleep, including REM and deep sleep, without fragmentation interruptions. This means your body doesn't need extra effort to keep the airway muscles toned, allowing for uninterrupted and rejuvenating sleep.

Current research indicates that getting low-quality sleep negatively affects nearly every aspect of one's brain and body.

That's the issue with the CPAP machine for most people—it doesn't always create better sleep; it just keeps your airway open. I often joke with my patients, "The way the CPAP fixes sleep apnea is that it doesn't let you sleep." Some individuals experience significant benefits from using a CPAP machine. However, for some people, my joke has a lot of truth to it. Up to 83 percent of people who are prescribed CPAP therapy do not use it as often as directed.

So what other treatment options do we have? I have been dedicating my career to sleep and airway since I graduated from dental school. My practice, the Breathing and Sleep Center in Colorado Springs,[466]

---

466 Goles, Kevin, DDS, Breathing and Sleep Center, Colorado Springs, CO.

focuses solely on sleep, airway, and breathing. During my residency, I focused my research on oral appliance therapy (OAT) for sleep apnea. However, despite these appliances being the typical mainstay for dental sleep medicine, the results provided by those appliances often weren't sufficient. So, that's when I started to explore other treatment options.

Transitioning from Traditional Dental Sleep Care to Airway Management and Facial Beauty with Vivos®

One of my most comprehensive forms of expanding the airway and maximizing sleep quality is through the Vivos® appliances. Since my contribution to this book, I have completed the most adult Vivos® cases within the Vivos® company since 2019, with a treatment number reaching into the thousands.

I quickly saw the magic these appliances could have on patient outcomes, with myself as my first patient (I cured my own obstructive sleep apnea). I have taken part in a few of their research articles, and these results have brought us to uncharted territory. These Vivos® appliances are the first dental appliances that have been FDA-cleared for obstructive sleep apnea. I knew these appliances had the ability to produce these results as we have been using this treatment as an alternative to CPAP for many of our patients who couldn't tolerate that therapy.

The big kicker in the publication of this approval is that, unlike CPAP therapy, this treatment might not have to be used for a person's lifetime. Instead, the expansion and airway remodeling created by these appliances create benefits that last for many people without further need for the devices once their treatment is completed. This is huge.

Compared to any surgery option, these appliances improve every aspect of the upper airway. Expanding the entire midface increases the airway size in the nasal region, behind the soft palate, and behind the tongue. It has drastically improved my patients' nasal breathing and sinus function.

To highlight the possibility of these appliances, I will show one case that demonstrates the expansion of the airway, jaw development, improved posture, improvement of nasal volume and sinus function, and increased space for the tongue in the roof of the mouth, not to mention the esthetic improvement as well.

336 | Beautiful Faces

Now, this case wasn't completed with just the Vivos® treatment. I use many adjunctive therapies, such as a soft-palate laser to shrink the tissue non-surgically and clear aligners to finish my Vivos® expansion cases.

CASE: PATIENT P WITH SEVERE OBSTRUCTIVE SLEEP

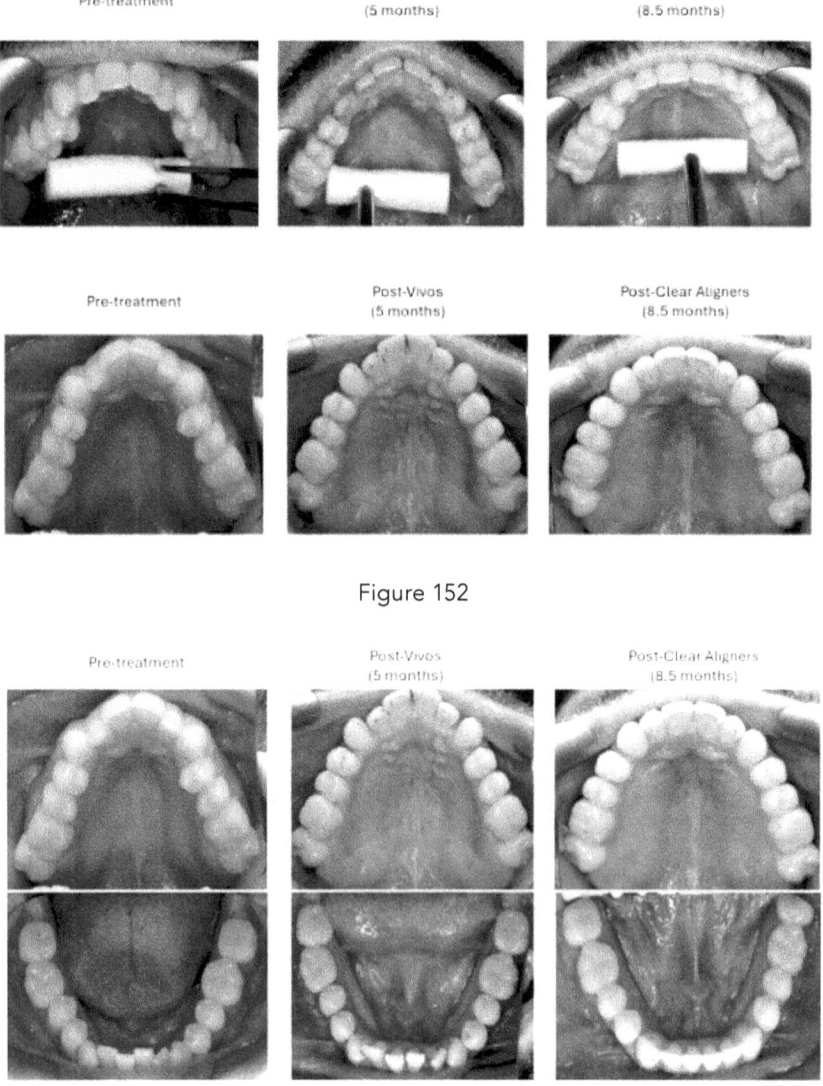

Figure 152

Figure 153

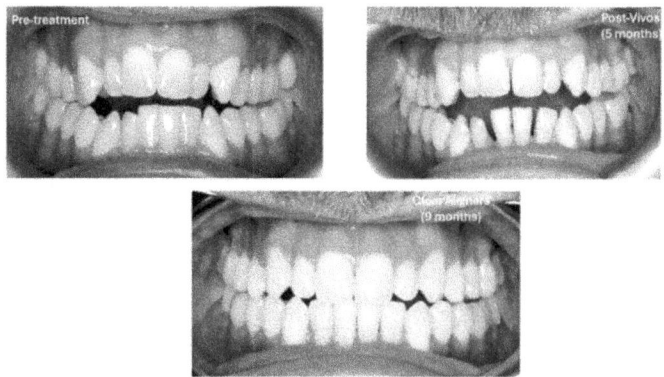

Figure 154

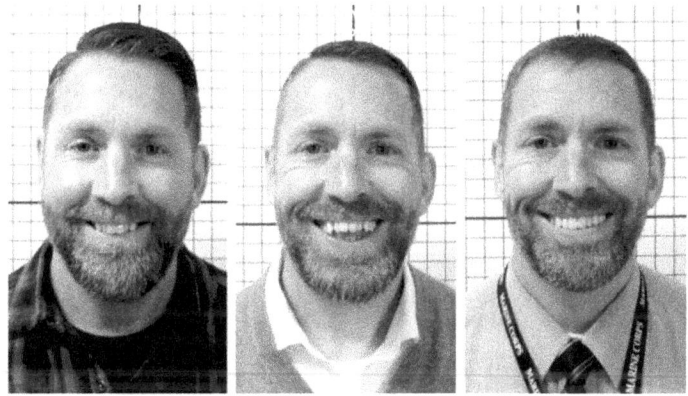

Figure 155

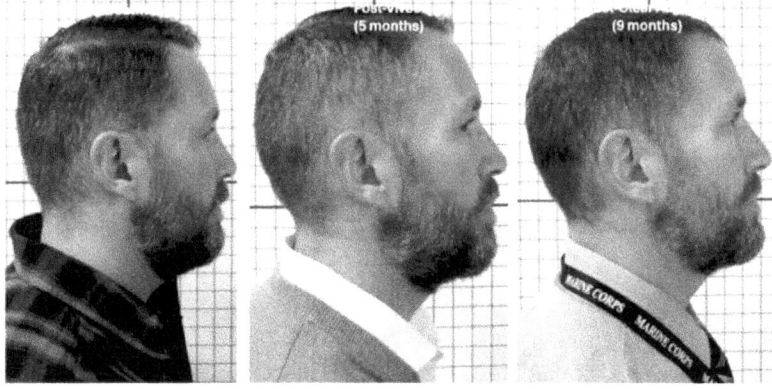

Figure 156

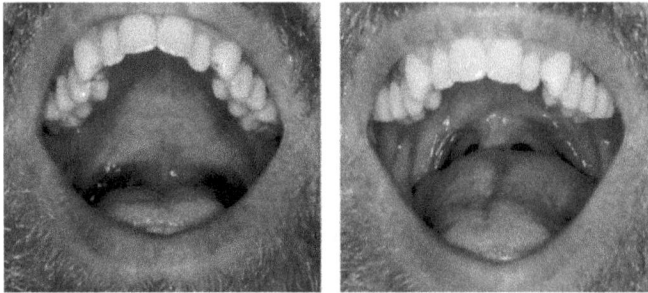

Figure 157: (Book author's comment. This is a before-and-after non-ablative laser treatment (NightLase®) to open airways.)

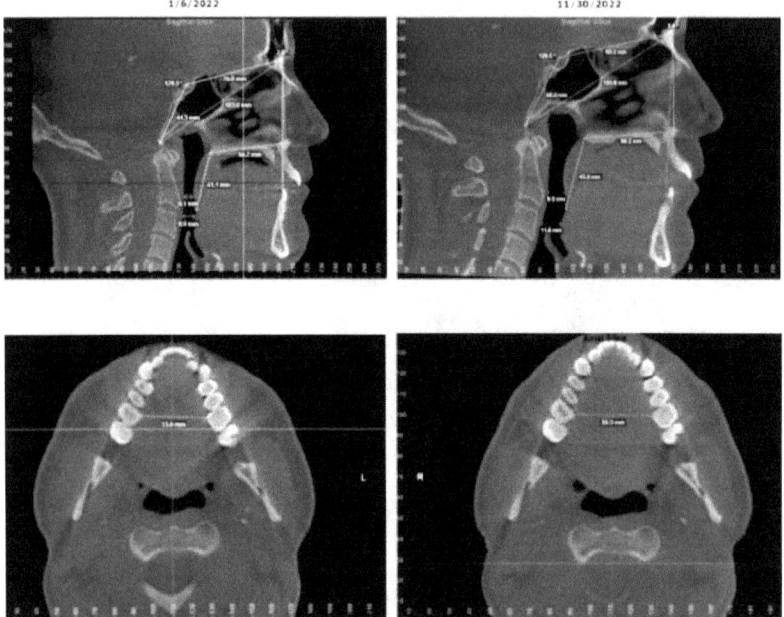

Figure158

	Transpalatal Width
1/6/2022	34 mm
11/30/2022	39.5 mm
% Change	16.2%

Figure 159

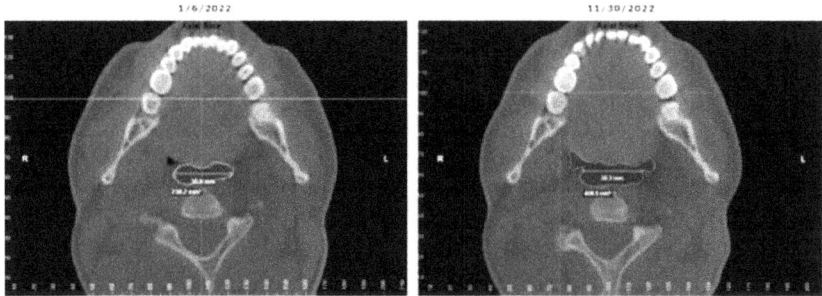

Figure 160

	Min RP Lateral Area
1/6/2022	238 mm²
11/30/2022	406 mm²
% Change	70.6%

Figure 161

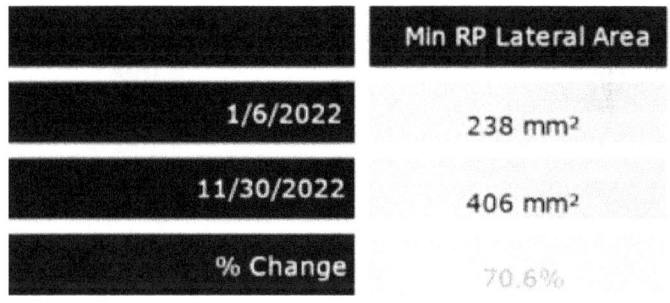

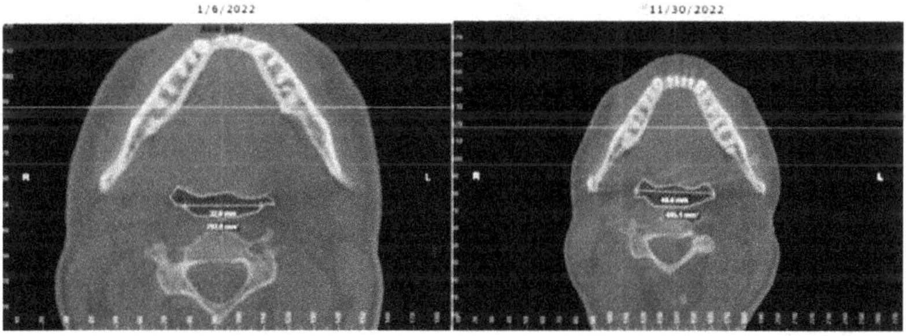

Figure 162

	Min RG MedioLateral Width	Min RG Lateral Area
1/6/2022	33 mm	292 mm²
11/30/2022	46.5 mm	485 mm²
% Change	40.9%	66.1%

Figure 163

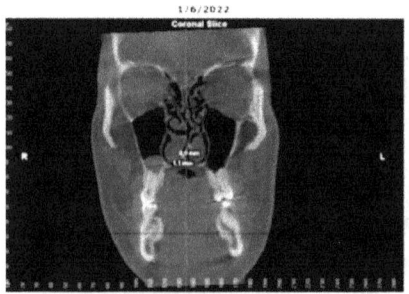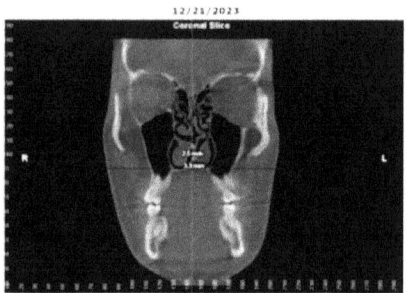

164

	Inferior Nasal Concha Right	Inferior Nasal Concha Left
1/6/2022	1.1 mm	0.9 mm
12/21/2023	2.5 mm	3.3 mm
% Change	127.3%	266.7%

165

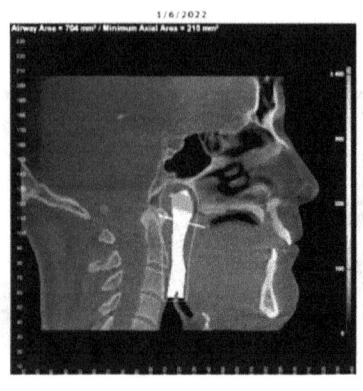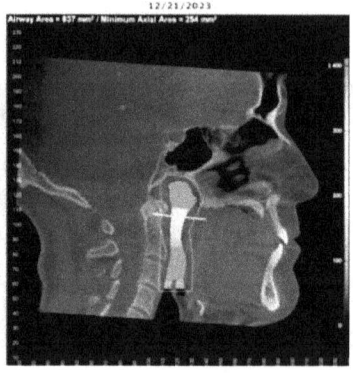

166

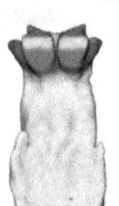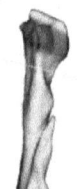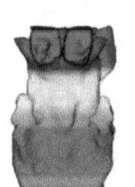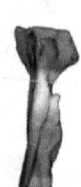

Figure 167

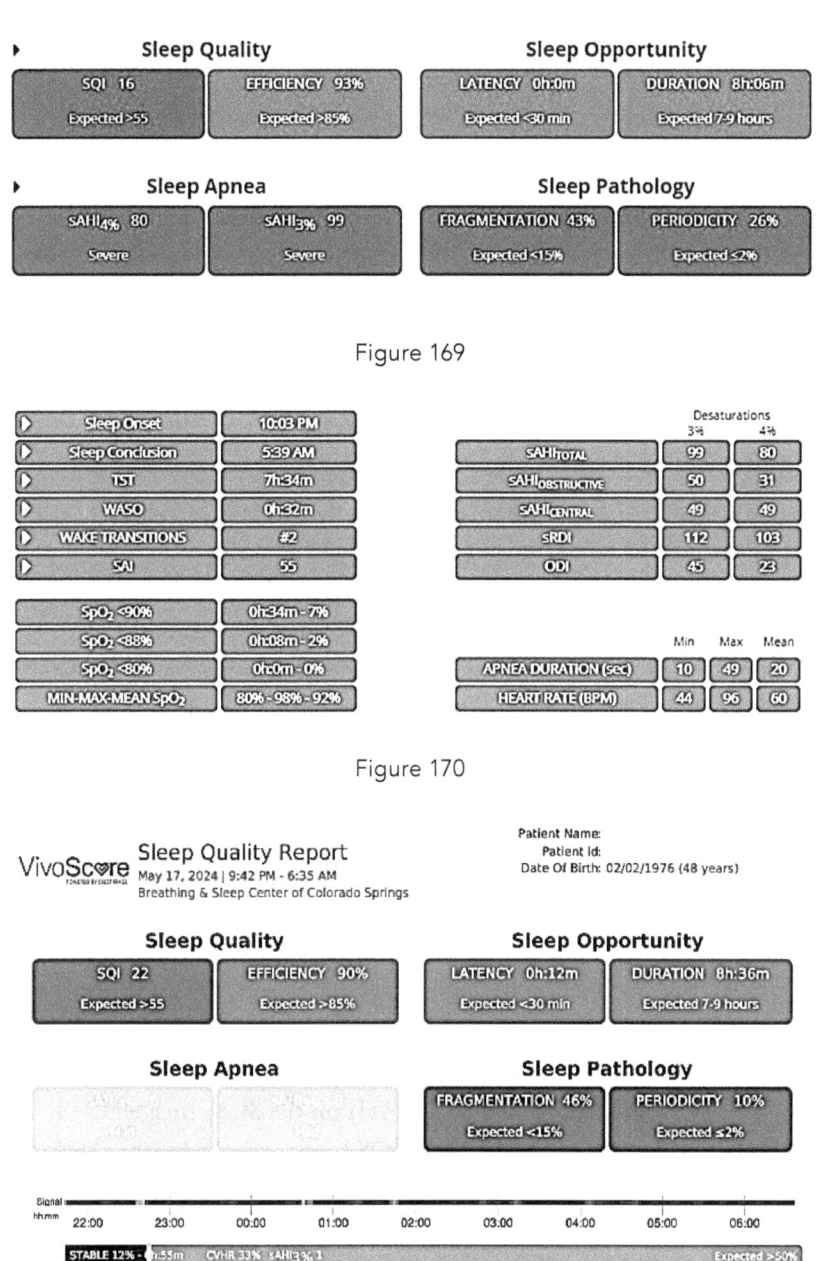

Figure 169

Figure 170

Figure 171

			Desaturations	
			3%	4%
Sleep Onset	9:55 PM	sAHI_{TOTAL}	8	6
Sleep Conclusion	6:31 AM	sAHI_{OBSTRUCTIVE}	8	6
TST	7h:57m	sAHI_{CENTRAL}	0	0
WASO	0h:42m	sRDI	11	11
WAKE TRANSITIONS	#12	ODI	2	1
SAI	47			

		Min	Max	Mean
SpO$_2$ <90%	0h:0m - 0%			
SpO$_2$ <88%	0h:0m - 0%			
SpO$_2$ <80%	0h:0m - 0%	APNEA DURATION (sec)	10	39	20
MIN-MAX-MEAN SpO$_2$	90% - 99% - 96%	HEART RATE (BPM)	53	107	68

Figure 172: For those who might get lost with all these numbers, just focus on one. The AHI went from ninety-nine suffocation events per hour to eight. (Comment by Dr. Downs.)

Here is the interpretation for this patient from Dr. Zelk:

> The most recent sleep testing was completed over three consecutive nights with the Sleep Image HSAT. The patient wore auto CPAP therapy for all three nights except for a split-night study on 5/17/24. From 9:55 p.m. to 12:50 a.m., the patient measured his updated untreated baseline AHI, and the rest of the test was performed using his standard auto CPAP therapy.
>
> There is no significant difference in treatment outcome between the three nights of testing based on AHI and low oxygen saturation. The average AHI of each night was 5/15 AHI 3% 7/hr, low oxygen 93 %, 5/16 AHI 3% 6/hr, low oxygen 93 % and 5/17 AHI 3% 8/hr, low oxygen 90 %.
>
> These findings demonstrate a dramatic improvement of OSA severity, from a very severe 99/hr. AHI on the Sleep Image HSAT 2021 baseline test to a mild level of OSA, approximately 7/hr. AHI.

Dr. Zelk's comments on this follow.

> This is a very significant improvement in the airway health of this patient, likely improving his breathing function twenty-four hours a day. Other treatments, like CPAP, only keep the airway open

while being used in sleep, which does not not necessarily improve daytime breathing function. This is a newer therapy option, and the treatment results can vary wildly from person to person. This area of study needs more research and investment by the sleep disorders community to better help identify appropriate candidates for this treatment plan.

This patient put in significant time and energy and was very compliant with the treatment plan. For significant improvements to be demonstrated in the adult population, superb compliance and patience are necessary for this treatment option to result in optimal results.

—Joseph Zelk, DNP, FNP, BC, CBSM, DBSM

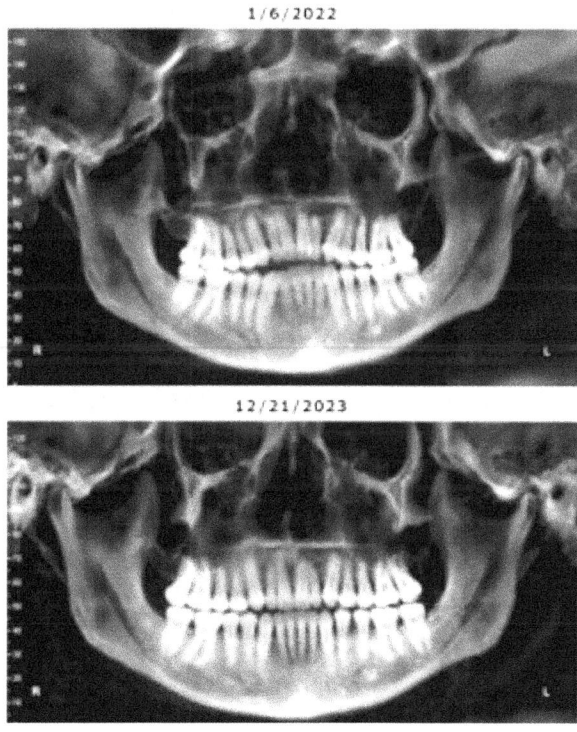

Figure 173: Not pushing teeth out of bone. No root resorption.

Child Patient Focus and ToothPillow®

With the completion and success of so many adult patients, our focus began to shift toward children. Instead of reactively treating this issue with adults who have struggled for decades, let's be preventative and create the foundation these kids need before dealing with these problems for the rest of their lives.

Unfortunately, however, many of these kids still have symptoms of airway and breathing issues. Bedwetting, ADHD, inflamed tonsils and adenoids, allergies, restless sleep, and teeth clenching are just a small example of symptoms children can deal with when their jaws are not properly developed, which leads to poor breathing and sleep.

These can all be drastically improved and often resolved with non-invasive treatment modalities. However, getting access to doctors who provide these treatments can be difficult. To address this access to care issue, the reseller company Toothpillow® was created to get the Vivos® Guide® appliance to those who need it. Essentially, these appliances are focused on children ages three to twelve. They encourage the proper functioning of the oral and facial muscles, which will be used for passive expansion and development of their jaws. They promote proper nasal breathing and support the jaw while a child sleeps.

All these aspects can drastically improve a child's breathing and sleep, resulting in significant improvement in the many symptoms they deal with. Moreover, we are addressing the issue at an early age and preventing so many other comorbidities that can occur as they age if they don't develop properly. In the patient photos below, only a Toothpillow®

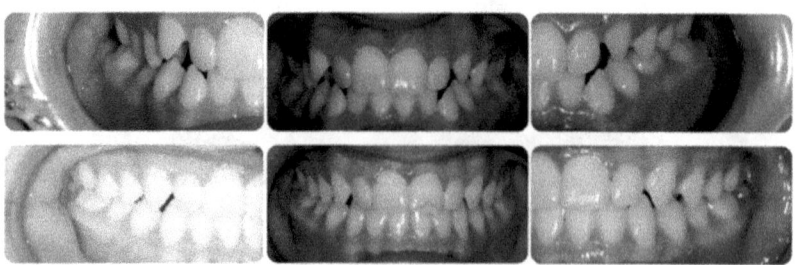

Figure 174: Toothpillow® guide was the only appliance used. The top image is pre-treatment, and the bottom is post-treatment.

is used, and it is a passive appliance, which means there are no active forces from the appliance pushing the teeth in any direction. It allows the teeth to move freely to their desired and genetically predestined locations. They are generally only needed for sleeping at night.

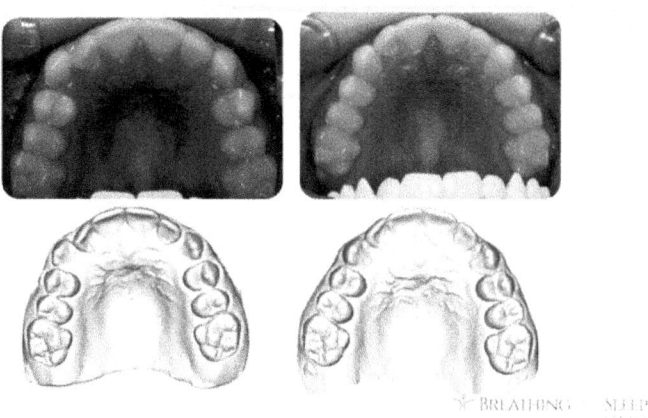

Figure 175: Pre-treatment Toothpillow® and post-treatment for the upper jaw.

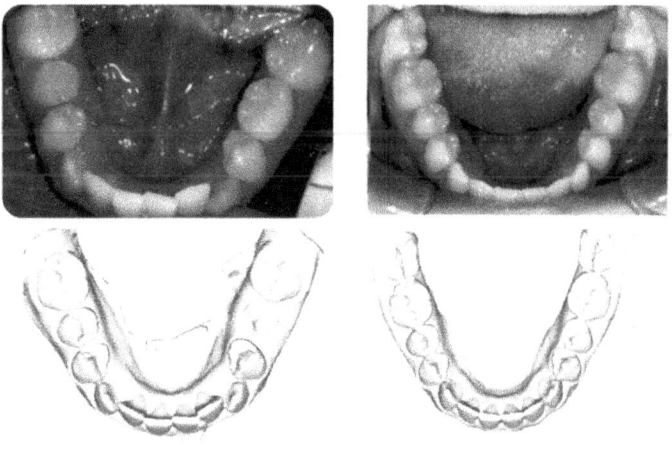

Figure 176: Pre- and post-treatment Toothpillow® for the lower jaw.

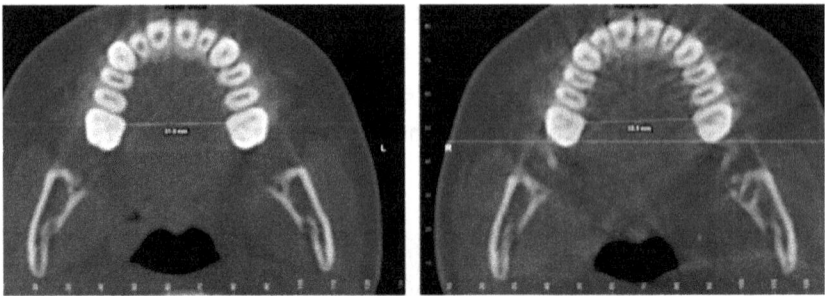

Figure 177: Toothpillow® results on the same patient.

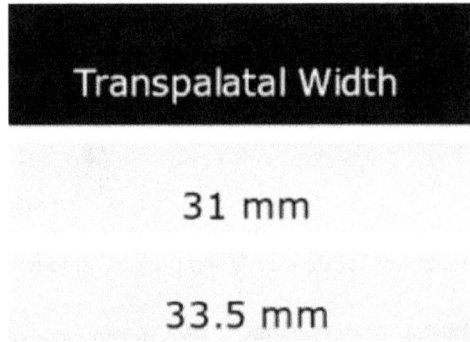

Figure 178: Toothpillow® results in a wider upper jaw.

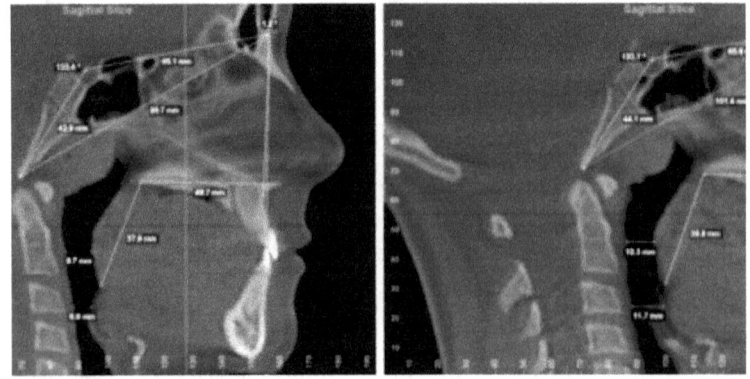

Figure 179: Toothpillow® increased retropalatal space from 9.7 to 10.3 mm. Night-time wear only.

Retroglossal distance, (posterior of tongue space) went from 6.8 to 11.7 mm.

The deep bite resolved and the head posture improved to a less forward position.

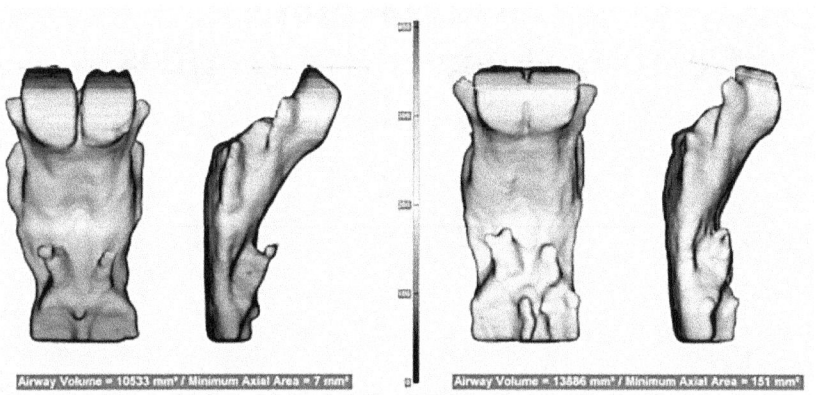

Figure 180: (Comment by Dr. Downs: These images are of a cone beam scan of the airway from the back of the tongue to the trachea. Airway volume increased from 10,533 cubic millimeters to 13,886 cubic millimeters. Minimum axial area increased from seven square millimeters to 151 square millimeters.) Toothpillow® results.

I hope this information and the results above help some people have a better life. Please note that these results do not necessarily happen for everyone. Always consult with your healthcare professional for specific recommendations for your situation.

Thanks, Kevin Goles, DDS

CHAPTER 16

The Air Institute: Geoffrey Skinner, DDS, D-ABDSM, D-ASBA

We are now ready to sum up much of the information that has been presented. Dr. Geoffrey Skinner[467] in partnership with Dr. Terry Coddington created an educational center and is working with Sleep Balance Academy to train and educate dentists to incorporate the newest information in treating patients with obstructive sleep apnea, abnormal growth of face and jaws, and optimal dental and orthodontic care. His name for this organization is the Air Institute—Portland Protocol. His medical director is Dr. Joseph Zelk. I have been privileged to work with him and contribute my areas of expertise. Dr. Mark Abramson is also a principal instructor at the institute. Other instructors and contributors have benefited from the educational programs, including Dr. Kimberly Santiago, Dr. John Bunkers, Dr. Lindsey Zeboski, and Dr. Terry Coddington.

Vivos® has given the approach of enlarging dental airways an FDA-cleared treatment modality on which to build. It is a landmark achievement that allows dentists to explore additional methods to enlarge airways. In this book, you will have noticed Dr. Skinner, Dr. Kamran Fattah, Dr. Kevin Goles, Dr. Felix Liao, Dr. Ilya Lipkin, and others are using different

---

467 Skinner, Geoffrey, DDS, Hillsboro Dental Excellence, Portland, OR.

jaw and nasal enlargement procedures, including clear aligners and mini implant-supported palatal widening, to get similar results. They document and research these therapies' effects on improving overall health and sleep disorders. NightLase®, NaseLase, and iNAP contribute to these new approaches with excellent data collection. New approaches to MARPE-like procedures, clear aligner therapy, and nasal cleaning are advancing rapidly and contributing effective results.

Dr. Skinner next shows his Portland Protocol approach to dental sleep treatment. He will show the sleep improvement data and increased facial beauty with his protocol.

The Portland Protocol: A Novel, Minimally Invasive Protocol for Treating Obstructive Sleep Apnea

Dr. Geoffrey Skinner, DDS, D-ABDSM, D-ASBA

Sleep-related breathing disorders, from snoring to obstructive sleep apnea (OSA), afflict 9-44 percent of Americans, and occasional snoring is nearly universal.[468, 469, 470] Although snoring does not increase a person's risk of dying as much as OSA, it does increase the risk of stroke by 300 percent.[471] Additionally, all significant sleep events inducing blood oxygen desaturation apply stress to the body in the form of cardiac arrhythmia and cardiac inflammatory events.[472] Obstructive sleep apnea also harms dental health. We must help our patients improve their airways and ability to remain fully oxygenated to help them live longer and healthier lives.

The Portland Protocol aims to minimize oxygen desaturation and snoring, improving total body health, well-being, and longevity. The

---

468 Senaratna, C. V., et al. (2017). "Prevalence of obstructive sleep apnea in the general population: A systematic review." *Sleep Medicine Reviews*, 34, 70-81.

469 Young, T., Palta, M., Dempsey, J., et al. (1993). "The occurrence of sleep-disordered breathing among middle-aged adults." *New England Journal of Medicine*, 328, 1230.

470 American Academy of Sleep Medicine. (2014). International Classification of Sleep Disorders, 3rd ed. Darien, IL: American Academy of Sleep Medicine.

471 Springs, D. A., et al. (1992). Snoring increases the risk of stroke and adversely affects prognosis. Q J Med, 83(303), 555-562.

472 Korantzopoulos, Panagiotis, et al. "Inflammation and atrial fibrillation: A comprehensive review." *J Arrhythm*. 2018 Aug; 34(4): 394–401.

Portland Protocol assesses the airway for potential sites of constriction or collapsibility. We systematically treat those areas once we get a diagnosis and prescription from our medical specialists.

First, we determine the primary causes of snoring or apneic episodes. We assess airway function with FDA-cleared sleep study measures. Once assessed and diagnosed, we develop and prescribe a multidisciplinary, minimally invasive approach to treat the areas involved in airway constriction and collapse.

Historically, patient compliance with oral sleep appliances is 93 percent,[473] and Continuous Positive Airway Pressure (CPAP) machines have a compliance rate of 50 percent percent.[474] Yet, despite their effectiveness in preventing cardiac events such as heart attacks and strokes, CPAPs have a low compliance rate of around 25 percent.[475] Most patients use their CPAP at the beginning of the night and take it off in the middle of the night. This is problematic because they take their CPAP off before they have most of their REM sleep and when their apneic episodes are typically more frequent and severe. Unfortunately, CPAP is considered successful if used four hours per night; therefore, official success rates are often listed at 50 percent.

Compliance with oral appliances and CPAP is directly related to airway improvements.[476] Yet, CPAPs and oral appliances only assist the airways of patients while they are being used. Compliance greatly improves when sleep apnea treatment is simple and requires minimal effort. Therefore, when requirements for compliance are minimized, as in the Portland Protocol, better airways and better long-term health outcomes should be more easily attained.

---

[473] Vanderveken, Olivier M., et al. "Objective measurement of compliance during oral appliance therapy for sleep-disordered breathing." *Thorax* 2013;68:91–96. doi:10.1136

[474] Wolkove, Norman, et al. "Long-term compliance with continuous positive airway pressure in patients with obstructive sleep apnea." Can Respir J. 2008 Oct; 15(7): 365–369.

[475] Meyers, David, et al. "Continuous Positive Airway Pressure Treatment for Obstructive Sleep Apnea." Agency for Healthcare Research and Quality, U.S. Department of Health and Human Services, April 2021. https://www.ahrq.gov/sites/default/files/wysiwyg/research/findings/ta/drafts-for-review/sleep-apnea-draftreport.pdf

[476] Vanderveken, Olivier M., et al. "Objective Measurement of Compliance During Oral Appliance Therapy for Sleep-Disordered Breathing." *Thorax*, vol. 68, 2013, pp. 91–96. doi:10.1136/thoraxjnl-2012-201949.

The Portland Protocol aims to provide an introduction and road map for practitioners who may or may not be currently treating sleep apnea to introduce an effective multidisciplinary approach to their practice. By including more providers in your treatment planning, you increase the size of your team and the number of clinicians looking for airway complications, leading to increased referrals to your practice. There is too much to know for any doctor or professional to be proficient in all facets of treatment. Airway management is a team sport!

Diagnosis, Documentation, Examination

The point of our examination of the patient for the Portland Protocol is to determine the constriction points of the airway and the points where the airway is likely to collapse. An initial dental examination and a comprehensive evaluation of the temporomandibular joint, the tongue and throat soft tissues, and the nasal complex are performed. After the initial screening and questionnaires, a sleep study may be conducted to determine if the patient is deemed at risk for OSA. The Epworth Questionnaire evaluates how tired or fatigued a patient feels. The Nasal Obstruction Symptom Evaluation (NOSE) questionnaire is often used to check the ability of a patient to breathe through their nose. The STOP-BANG Questionnaire is used to screen for the most prominent sleep apnea risk factors. Each of these questionnaires serves a purpose in determining the relative risk for sleep-disordered breathing.

Dental Exam:

The dental evaluation checks for the involvement of teeth in the airway problem. The examination also reveals if modifying tooth position could improve the airway and if they are healthy enough to move them to a better position. Teeth that are lingually tipped (tipped toward the tongue) apply pressure to the tongue, making it more likely for the tongue to collapse into the throat (i.e., look for scalloping in indents on the side of the tongue).

Having posterior interference means that the jaw can move more anteriorly and superiorly, but is held in a posterior position that is more likely to close off the throat. A worn dentition implies grinding. Airway problems are correlated with tooth grinding, especially in the anterior-posterior direction. This is likely why many patients with class II malocclusions (overjet with receded jaw), where the maxillary and mandibular anterior teeth do not touch, still demonstrate incisal (front teeth) wear.[477]

Periodontal Exam

The periodontal exam (gum tissue) identifies whether the patients have buccal recession due to malocclusion (bad bite) as another clue indicating the possible involvement of teeth in the airway problem. It also determines if the patient's periodontal health is suitable for the teeth to be moved into a position that is more beneficial to the patency (openess) of the airway.

Temporomandibular Joint Exam

Many patients with sleep apnea report jaw pain, so it is important to know if the patient has temporomandibular joint dysfunction or only pain from sore muscles. The temporomandibular joint exam reveals jaw tension or facial tenderness to palpation that could indicate teeth grinding during sleep while struggling for breath.

Soft-Tissue Exam

Patients with an enlarged tongue have a more constricted airway because the tongue takes up more space.[478] One method of changing the ratio of the tongue to oral cavity volume is myofunctional therapy. Toning the tongue with simple myofunctional exercises can lead to significant

---

[477] Wetselaar, Peter et al. "Associations between Tooth Wear and Dental Sleep Disorders: A Narrative Overview." *Journal of Oral Rehabilitation*, vol. 46, no. 8, 2019, pp. 765–775.

[478] Kim, et al. "Tongue Fat and its Relationship to Obstructive Sleep Apnea." *Sleep*, vol. 37, no. 10, 2014, pp. 1639–1648.

airway benefits. Myofunctional therapy decreases the apnea-hypopnea index (suffocation events per hour) by approximately 50 percent in adults and 62 percent in children.[479]

Tongue ties add resistance to the body of the tongue and make it more likely to fall back into the airway.[480] Deeper (longer) soft palates with higher Mallampati (this is a measure of how far your soft palate extends down your throat) scores are less supported and more collapsible.[481]

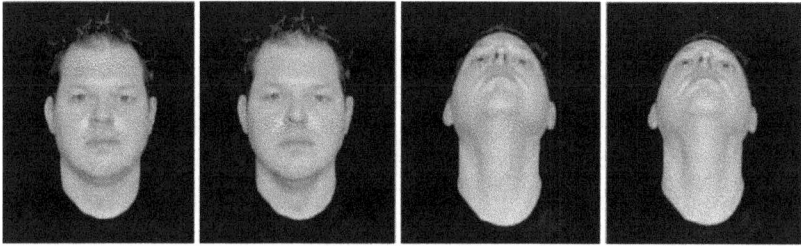

Figure 181

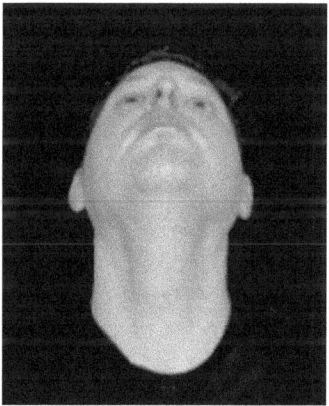

Figure 182: Nasal valve collapse of the left ala of the nose.

---

479 Camacho, Macario et al. "Myofunctional Therapy to Treat Obstructive Sleep Apnea: A Systematic Review and Meta-analysis." *Sleep*, vol. 38, no. 5, 2015, pp. 669-675. doi: 10.5665/sleep.4652.

480 Guilleminault, Christian. "A Frequent Phenotype for Pediatric Sleep Apnoea: Short Lingual Frenulum." *ERJ Open Research*, vol. 2, no. 3, 2016, pp. 00043-2016.

481 Liistro, G. et al. "High Mallampati Score and Nasal Obstruction Are Associated Risk Factors for Obstructive Sleep Apnea." *European Respiratory Journal*, vol. 21, 2003, pp. 248-252.

Nasal Exam and Nasal Breathing

The nasal exam is meant to look for areas of constriction of the nasal airway (Figure 182). We ask the patient to breathe in quickly and deeply to check for nasal valve collapse that reduces airflow through the nose. Visual examination of the inside of the nose also allows you to search for polyps, inflamed turbinate tissues, and deviation of the septum, which could increase the likelihood of mouth breathing. Mouth breathing leads to a 250 percent increase in upper airway resistance compared to nasal breathing.[482] Nasal breathing allows 10-20 percent more oxygenation of the blood than mouth breathing. This is due to a slowing of the air intake, increasing the oxygen exchange, and the intake of nitric oxide, a potent vasodilator that is released by the nasal turbinates.[483] We must do everything possible to help patients breathe through their nose because otherwise, they are more likely to have a higher risk of apneic events from breathing through their mouth. Daily nasal cleaning is a part of this important pillar of airway health.

Nasal decongestants can be an important tool in helping patients breathe through their noses by decreasing congestion and inflammation of turbinates. Nasal decongestant usage is associated with a decreased AHI, along with improvements in sleep efficiency and non-REM and REM sleep in apneic patients.[484] I use xylitol and USA-Guard's HOCL formulation rinses for routine nasal cleaning for my patients.

Nasal decongestants are only half of the equation because the use of nasal decongestants only temporarily shrinks the tissues. An overall nasal hygiene regime is indicated to help reduce the incidence of upper respiratory disease as well as prevent the tissue from puffing up again once the decongestant medication finishes its time of efficacy.

Many patients who have nasal valve collapse can also benefit from the same laser we use for NightLase in a procedure called NaseLase. The laser is used on the collapsable side of the nose, and a nasal cone is placed to support it while it heals. This increases collagen formation

---

482 Fitzpatrick, M. et al. "Effect of Nasal or Oral Breathing Route on Upper Airway Resistance During Sleep." *European Respiratory Journal*, vol. 22, no. 5, 2003, pp. 827-832.

483 McKeown, Patrick. *Oxygen Advantage*. William Morrow, November 2016. ISBN 0062349473.

484 McLean et al. "Effect of treating severe nasal obstruction on the severity of obstructive sleep apnoea." *Eur Respir J*. 2005 Mar;25(3):521-7.

and firmness so the tissue does not collapse when breathing in through the nose. NaseLase is typically done by a medical provider.

Many patients with airway problems demonstrate a narrow and raised palate. Raised palates are associated with deviated septums.[485] Depending on the patency of the nose, a referral for a septoplasty may be indicated to improve nasal patency and airflow.

Buteyko breathing exercises and mouth taping may be indicated to help patients learn to breathe through their noses, particularly if they have a previous history of mouth breathing.[486]

Nasal dilators can stretch the nasal valve open and prevent its collapse during breathing. Nasal dilator usage is associated with an 18 percent average increase in nasal airflow, a significant reduction in snoring, and a 47 percent reduction in AHI.[487]

Airway-Centric Orthodontics

Clear aligners can increase space in the mouth, particularly for the tongue. When the teeth are tipped towards the tongue, they apply pressure to the tongue, increasing the likelihood of pharyngeal collapse.[488] By up righting and tipping the crowns of teeth to the buccal (cheek), we are expanding the dental arch. Expanding the dental arch makes more space for the tongue and prevents pharyngeal collapse caused by the tongue, improving the airway and the patient's smile at the same time.

To maximize expansion, sometimes it is necessary to intrude the molars of the top jaw. The reason we intrude the posterior molars is important to note: it is to offset the "wedge effect." (Figure 183). As we tip the crowns of the teeth outwards, we simultaneously increase the height of the teeth. This, unfortunately, can increase the relative height of the back teeth and prevent the front teeth from touching in a process known as the "wedge effect" or "clockwise rotation" of the

---

[485] Sapmaz, Emrah et al. "Impact of Hard Palate Angulation Caused by Septal Deviation on Maxillary Sinus Volume." *Turk Arch Otorhinolaryngol*. 2018 Jun; 56(2): 75–80.

[486] Sano, Masahiro. "Increased oxygen load in the prefrontal cortex from mouth breathing: a vector-based near-infrared spectroscopy study." *Neuroreport*. 2013 Dec 4; 24(17): 935–940.

[487] Höijer. *Arch Otolaryngol Head Neck Surg*. 1992 Mar;118(3):281-4.

[488] Sunny, Sunil. "Three-Dimensional Control on Lingually Rolled in Molars using a 3D Lingual Arch." *J Clin Diagn Res*. 2017 Aug; 11(8).

mandible. By intruding the molars, we avoid the wedge effect and bring the anterior aspect of the mandible into a more appropriate position at the finishing of the case. This is called autorotation.

The intrusion of the posterior teeth is simple and predictable with clear aligners.[489] Temporary anchorage devices, mini-plates, and elastics can be used if significant posterior intrusions are indicated.

Posterior intrusion can relieve the teeth' strong posterior contacts, allowing the jaw to auto-rotate counterclockwise to a more advanced and superior position. Forward movement of the mandible in a counterclockwise way improves patency of the airway because the tongue is moved forward with the mandible and out of the throat.[490]

Our strategy for orthodontic cases involves a preference for leaving maxillary space to restore instead of making the mouth smaller with interproximal (the space between your teeth) reduction (IPR). Our strategy maximizes the available space for the tongue.

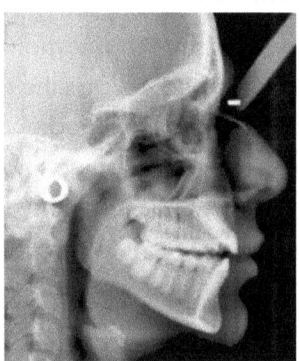

Figure 183: The wedge effect

CASE: RAYMOND

Raymond is a fifty-year-old male whose chief complaint is, "I wake up with headaches a few times a week and have been having jaw pain." The patient had class I occlusion bilaterally with V-shaped arches and

---

489 Glassick, Andrew et al. "Aligner Corner: Evaluating the Efficacy of Lower Incisor Intrusion with Clear Aligners." *J. Clin. Ortho.*, April 2017. Retrieved from [https://www.jco-online.com/archive/2017/04/233-aligner-corner-evaluating-the-efficacy-of-lower-incisor-intrusion-with-clear-aligners/]

490 Mehra, P. "Pharyngeal airway space changes after counterclockwise rotation of the maxillo-mandibular complex." *Am J Orthod Dentofacial Orthop.* 2001; 120: 154.

an anterior open bite (Figure 184). Based on the exam, we made a plan for orthodontic expansion and intrusion using Invisalign® (Figure 185). The results of orthodontic treatment are shown in Figure 186. Tables 1-3 list sleep study data at baseline, after Invisalign®, and after a third treatment step, NightLase®, a non-ablative laser uvulopalatoplasty described below.

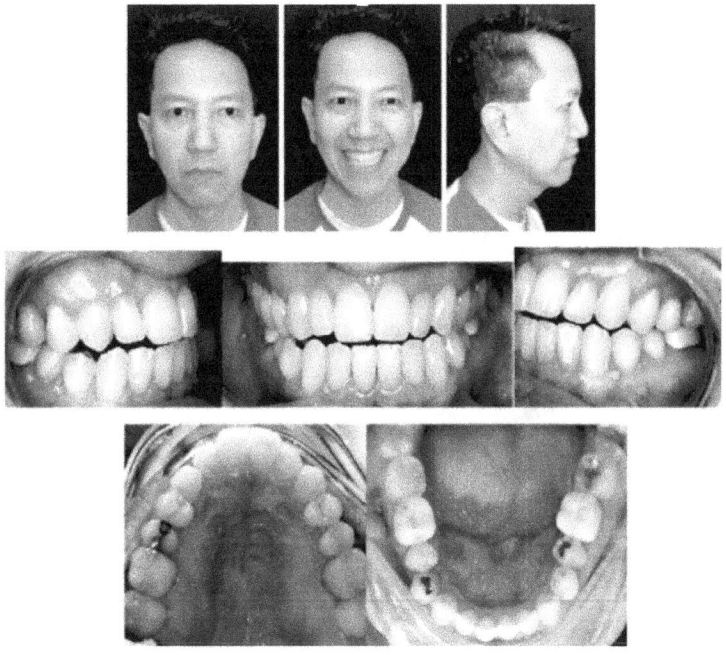

Figure 184: The patient's presentation at baseline was of bilateral class I occlusion, V-shaped arches, and an anterior open bite.

As seen in Figure 188, after clear aligner therapy, the patient had greatly improved AHI, snoring, and arousal indices (RDI, REI), as well as lower maximum heart rate during REM sleep (Table 1). However, stopping breathing for ten seconds or more six and a half times per hour indicated that the patient was still suffering from mild sleep apnea. In addition, the patient was experiencing clinically significant oxygen desaturation events after clear aligner therapy (Tables 2-3). We performed a simple, non-ablative, laser-assisted uvulopalatoplasty procedure called NightLase® to correct these issues.

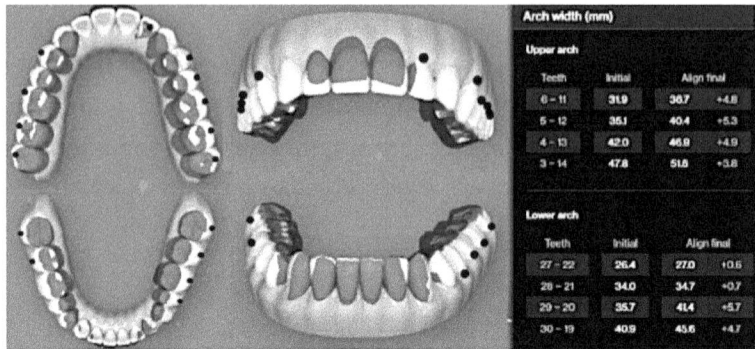

Figure 185: Invisalign® treatment plan to expand and intrude the posterior teeth and tip all the other teeth out. The trays were worn for thirteen months.

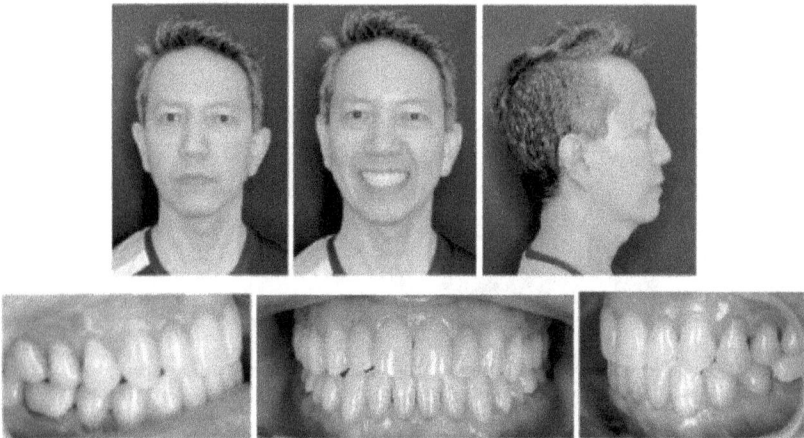

Figure 186

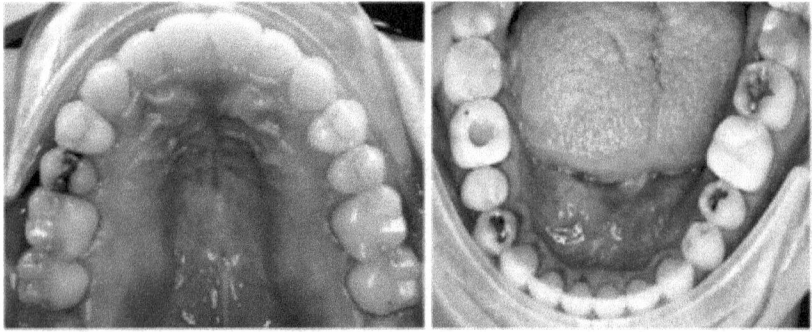

Figure 187: Patient after clear aligners. More space is available for the tongue following Invisalign® treatment.

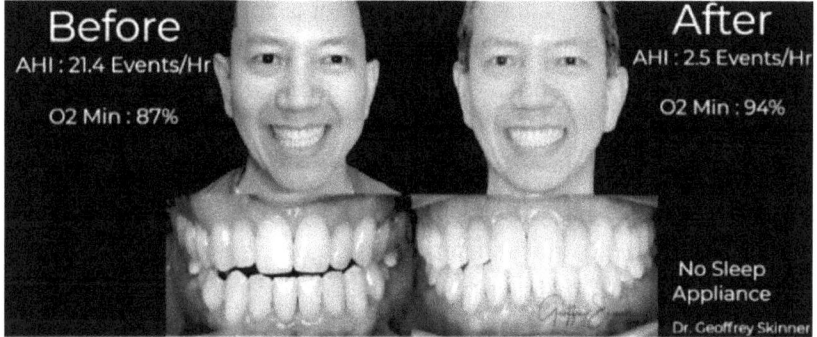

Figure 188: This is part of Figures 156 and 157. Note also improvement in facial beauty.

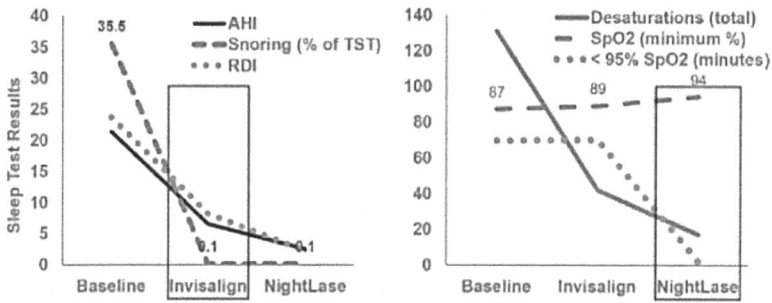

Figure 189: Sleep test results at baseline, after Invisalign®, and after NightLase®. Left: Snoring and apneic episodes decreased after Invisalign®. Right: Respiratory measures and oxygen saturation were clinically impaired even after clear aligners, which were in a healthy range after NightLase®. AHI, apnea-hypopnea index (number per hour); RDI, respiratory disturbance index (number per hour); TST, total sleep time; SpO2, (oxygen saturation).

Laser Airway Management with NightLase®

The most well-established and researched laser airway and snoring procedure over the past decade is NightLase®. NightLase® is a non-ablative laser tightening and elevation of the uvula, soft palate, and surrounding tissues. It does not remove or cut any tissues. Each NightLase® case consists of three to five sessions of laser treatment, each session lasting approximately thirty minutes in length. The sessions are conducted three to four weeks apart to allow maximum neocollagenesis (the formation of new collagen). Because NightLase® is non-ablative, anesthetic is unnecessary. The NightLase® procedure uses both wavelengths of the Fotona LightWalker laser: Nd:YAG and Er:YAG (these are two types of laser). The effect of these lasers is to tighten collagen,[491] thereby making the soft palate more open and less collapsible. The deeper tissues are pulled together via mechanical tension between the layers. These mechanisms result in a 66 percent average decrease in AHI,[492] which is on par with what would be expected with an oral appliance but without the need for compliance or the potential risk of complications like jaw pain or unwanted changes to the bite.

NightLase® decreases snoring,[493] increases airway volume,[494] and decreases AHI.[495] The tightening of collagen in the soft palate moves it more anteriorly and allows for better airflow even through the nasopharynx (the space behind your tongue where food and air pass through), resulting in improved nasal breathing.[496] The tightening of collagen can also lift the soft palate and change the Mallampati score. Many patients have an immediate, visible rise in the soft palate (Figure 193). The average snoring improvement after one session is about 50 percent, and after the third session, 85 percent.[497] The effects of the NightLase® procedure last nine to twenty-four months.[498] Patients are encouraged to return annually or sooner if needed for a single session to maintain their airways.

---

[491] Unver, T. et al. "Histological effects of Er: YAG laser irradiation with snoring handpiece in the rat soft palate." *Photomed Laser Surg* 2016;34:321–325.

[492] Shiffman, H. S., Khorsandi, J., & Cauwels, N. M. "Minimally-invasive combined Nd: YAG and Er: YAG laser-assisted uvulopalatoplasty." *Photobiomod Photomed Laser Surg* 2021; 39: 1-8.

[493] Miracki, K., & Vizintin, Z. "Nonsurgical minimally invasive Er: YAG laser snoring treatment." *J Laser & Health Acad* 1: 36-41.

[494] Lee, C. Y. S., & Lee, C. C. Y. "Evaluation of a non-ablative Er: YAG laser procedure to increase the oropharyngeal airway volume: a pilot study." *Dent Oral Craniofac* Res 2015; 1:56–59.

[495] Shiffman, H. S., Khorsandi, J., & Cauwels, N. M. "Minimally-invasive combined Nd: YAG and Er: YAG laser-assisted uvulopalatoplasty." *Photobiomod Photomed Laser Surg* 2021; 39: 1-8.

[496] Shiffman, H.S., & Lukac, M. "NightLase: minimally invasive laser-assisted uvulopalatoplasty." *J Laser Health Acad* 2018; 1:39–44.

[497] Monteiro, L., et al. "Treatment of snoring disorder with a non-ablative Er: YAG laser dual-mode protocol. An interventional study." *J Clin Exp Dent* 2020;12:561–567.

[498] Shiffman, H. S., et al. "Breakthrough non-surgical laser sleep applications in dentistry and medicine." *Journal of Dental Research and Reports*, 2020.

Figure 193 shows the clinical improvements after Invisalign® and two NightLase® sessions, as only two sessions were needed to get an average SpO2 over 96 percent and minimum SpO2 to 94 percent (Tables 2-3). The patient will be returning for maintenance sessions, and we will likely see further improvement at follow-up.

Invisalign® decreased snoring, AHI, and arousal measures but had minimal effect on respiratory indices (Figure 189). Subsequent treatment with NightLase® decreased AHI even more and improved respiratory function. The minutes the patient had <95 percent oxygen saturation was significantly reduced by NightLase®. This was associated with decreased maximum heart rate during REM sleep and improved sleep efficiency (Table 1).

The patient reported better nasal breathing and no pain or adverse effects from the treatment. He was using the USA-Guard HOCL nasal rinse formula, too. However, the patient came in for an exam after the first NightLase® session, complaining of "non-painful, non-fluid-filled areas on the back of his tongue." Examination suggested that he was seeing his normal circumvallate papillae (these are normal bumps on the tongue near the back), which were now visible after the inflammation of his tongue was reduced with the NightLase® procedure.

Although clear aligners brought him from moderate to mild apnea, clear aligners like Invisalign® alone were not adequate to bring respiratory measures into a healthy range. Further treatment of the soft tissues using NightLase® is an essential component of the Portland Protocol that we have seen eliminate the need for CPAP or oral appliances in many patients.

Expiratory Positive Airway Pressure (EPAP)

EPAPs apply positive pressure upon exhalation, keeping the airway open until the next inhalation.[499] EPAPs are helpful for patients who have collapsible nasal valves and a collapsible pharynx and are unwilling or unable to go through NightLase®. One EPAP device FDA-cleared to treat obstructive sleep apnea is called the Bongo Rx.

---

499 Rosenthal, L., et al. "A multicenter, prospective study of a novel nasal EPAP device in the treatment of obstructive sleep apnea: efficacy and 30-day adherence." *J Clin Sleep Med*, vol. 5, no. 6, 2009, pp. 532-537.

Table 1. Sleep test data at baseline, after Invisalign and after NightLase.

	Baseline	Invisalign	NightLase
Lights Off (Date, Time)	2/29/2020 22:43	9/15/2020 22:33	9/1/2021 21:13
Lights On (Date, Time)	3/1/2020 6:31	9/16/2020 5:52	9/2/2021 6:02
Total Recording Time (minutes)	860.7	915	931
Time in Bed (minutes)	467.7	437.8	528.4
Time in Bed (TIB; hours, minutes)	7, 48	7, 18	8, 48
TIB (% of total recording time)	54.3	47.8	47.8
Total Sleep Time (minutes)	437.4	407.4	517.4
TST (% of TIB)	93.5	93.1	97.9
Sleep Efficiency (% of TIB)	93.5	93.1	97.9
Apnea Hypopnea index (AHI, number per hour)	21.4	6.5	2.5
Respiratory Event Index (number per hour)	22.3	7.7	2.7
SpO_2[1] < 89% (cumulative minutes)	3	0	0
SpO_2 < 89% (longest span, minutes)	1	0	0
Snoring (minutes)	155.2	0.3	0.1
Maximum heart rate, REM (bpm)	100	93	86

[1]SpO_2, oxygen saturation

Figure 190

Table 2. Sleep study measures for all sleep stages and total time in bed at baseline, after Invisalign and after NightLase.

	All Sleep Stages			Total Time in Bed		
	Baseline	Invisalign	NightLase	Baseline	Invisalign	NightLase
Average SpO_2[1] (%)	95.5	95.1	96.4	95.5	95.1	96.2
Desaturations (number)	131	42	17	133	43	18
Minimum SpO_2 (%)	87	89	94	87	89	94
<95% (minutes)	69.5	70.0	2.1	71.8	77.4	10.4
<90% (minutes)	1.1	0.1	0	1.3	0.1	0
<85% (minutes)	0	0	0	0	0	0
No Signal/Artifact (minutes)	0.0	0.2	0.1	0	0.5	0.2

[1]SpO_2, oxygen saturation

Figure 191

Table 3. Sleep study measures during REM and non-REM sleep.

	REM			Non-REM		
	Baseline	Invisalign	NightLase	Baseline	Invisalign	NightLase
Average SpO$_2$¹ (%)	95.7	95.1	96.1	95.5	95.0	96.0
Desaturations (number)	44	23	9	87	19	8
Minimum SpO$_2$ (%)	89	89	94	87	90	94
<95% (minutes)	18.2	22.7	3.7	51.3	47.3	4.3
<90% (minutes)	0.1	0.1	0	1.0	0	0
<85% (minutes)	0	0	0	0	0	0
No Signal/Artifact (minutes)	0	0	0	0.0	0.2	0.1

Figure 192

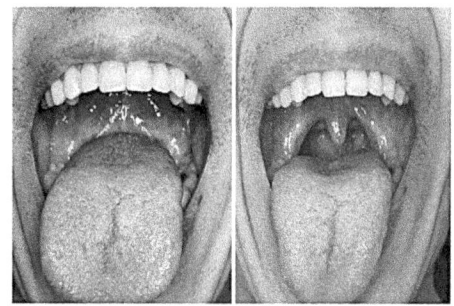

Figure 193: Before (left) and after (right) NightLase® non-ablative uvulopalatoplasty, lingual pyroptosis, and photo biomodulation using Er:YAG and Nd:YAG lasers. You can see the tongue center is depressed due to fat loss of laser pyroptosis. The soft palate has been raised as well.

Mandibular Advancement

Patients with residual obstructive desaturation (these are remaining suffocation event readings resulting in lower oxygen levels in the blood) events after orthodontics, NightLase®, or nasal breathing aids may require a mandibular advancement appliance to prevent the jaw from falling back during REM-associated atonia (a deficiency of usual or expected tone in the muscle) Advancing the mandible or increasing the vertical dimension may be helpful to treat the patient thoroughly.

A study by Anuita et al. found that 81% of patients get a maximal decrease in AHI from jaw protrusions less than or equal to 3 mm and that 39% of patients experienced a greater than or equal to 50% reduction in AHI with advancement of zero mm.[500] This study suggests that oral appliance therapy is less about advancing the mandible and more about preventing the jaw from falling back and collapsing the airway. We use oral sleep appliances only if needed rather than as a first choice in our protocol.

Expanding the arch before oral appliance therapy helps create space and may decrease the advancement needed to resolve airway constriction. Decreasing the amount of protrusion means that the patient is less likely to experience appliance-related complications like changes in the bite and/or temporomandibular joint dysfunction or pain.[501] We use Invisasleep® oral appliance therapy nighttime wear for some cases.

In summary, adding simple techniques like non-ablative laser uvulopalatoplasty that is highly tolerable by patients and has predictable results to the Portland Protocol can eliminate the need for CPAP or oral appliances in some cases of sleep apnea, thereby removing issues of patient compliance.

We have found that opening space for the tongue does much of the work in eliminating snoring and apneic episodes but may not fully resolve sleep apnea in some patients. As there are compliance issues with CPAP and oral appliances, and they only help with airway issues while they are being used, NightLase® should be considered a first-line treatment. NightLase® improves breathing twenty-four hours a day and requires no compliance.

A multidisciplinary approach considers orthodontic alignment, expansion, NightLase®, and, as a last resort, compliance-dependent CPAP and oral appliances. Patent nasal airway support, supplemented with nasal rinsing, is the best way to offer additional simple, customized sleep apnea treatment. It also improves facial beauty, which is a very important additional benefit.

---

500 Anuita, Eduardo, et al. "Minimizing the mandibular advancement in an oral appliance for the treatment of obstructive sleep apnea." *J Sleep Medicine*, vol. 34, 2017, pp. 226-231.

501 Sheats, Rose, et al. "Management of Side Effects of Oral Appliance Therapy for Sleep-Disordered Breathing." *J DSM*, vol. 4, no. 4, 2017.

CHAPTER 17

Conclusions

You've embarked on a journey through this book, exploring a contemporary health challenge that we consider the cornerstone of all other health issues. Despite its magnitude, it is often disregarded by almost all healthcare fields. Along the way, you've explored the correlation between facial beauty and underlying health, gaining insights into how they intertwine. You've been introduced to trailblazing individuals and organizations reshaping airway healthcare, pioneering innovative approaches with promising and remarkable outcomes. This journey offers hope and a platform for revitalized radiance, beauty, and vitality, shaping a future where health and energy for life take center stage.

You will notice that the therapies presented in this book largely rely on recapturing the growth potential that we have lost in our modern world. There is a great deal to do. We have just begun. You have seen that the dental profession has a huge role in this epidemic that they are uniquely positioned to carry out partnering with our medical colleagues.

You may have noticed that the approach we are advocating not only helps with sleep breathing issues, but has the potential to improve daytime breathing and overall health as a result. We are convinced that this new awareness and treatment philosophy will reduce the incidence of many diseases that most people don't know stem from our deformed modern faces and restricted airways.

You should have noticed that some of the cases presented showed patients with advanced care strategies we advocated in the book. Amazing results in both health and beauty were achieved. Others had variable and partial resolution of sleep, beauty, and health issues. No one protocol for treatment works for everyone. It's clear that intervening early in life for individuals experiencing airway issues and their effects on facial structure is key. By addressing these issues early, we can guide their growth trajectory to align with their genetic potential, promoting optimal aesthetic and healthy outcomes. It is much more difficult for adults.

For parents who have been puzzled and confused by their children's behaviors and illnesses, we encourage you to consider the potential negative impact that your child's disrupted sleep and narrow airway issues might be having on their optimal growth potential and appearance. In addition, consistently shorter sleep durations throughout childhood increase the risk of developing psychosis later in life. One potential mechanism for this association could be inflammation, as indicated by elevated levels of IL-6.[502] IL-6 is an inflammation marker.

To schoolteachers, guidance counselors, social workers, and mental health professionals, we hope you consider the role of possible undiagnosed deficient facial and airway development in addressing the challenges you're trying to solve.

Additionally, we encourage you to utilize the information in this book to guide your children's health and facial development, ensuring they grow unhindered by unrealized genetic potential. This can be compromised by various factors such as modern diets, untreated tongue ties, habitual mouth breathing due to chronic nasal congestion, poor posture, inflamed adenoid and tonsillar tissue, limited breastfeeding opportunities, weakened swallowing strength from improper bottle nipple use, frequent nasal congestion from viral infections, inflammation from pollution, unhealthy sleep habits, excessive screen time leading to late bedtimes and sleep deprivation, early school start times, misguided medical and dental interventions, delayed orthodontic/orthotropic treatment until preteen years, and overlooked spiritual and emotional support.

---

502 Morales-Muñoz, I., Marwaha, S., Upthegrove, R., et al. (2024, May 08). "Role of Inflammation in Short Sleep Duration Across Childhood and Psychosis in Young Adulthood." *JAMA Psychiatry*. https://doi.org/10.1001/jamapsychiatry.2024.0796

You've been given a wealth of footnotes, references, and citations to delve into. We encourage you to make use of these resources and explore the numerous insights they offer. As knowledge evolves and our information becomes outdated, new authors will continue to forge ahead in the quest to find the most effective ways to assist our fellow human beings.

We recognize that those non-healthcare individuals who have taken the time to understand this information may now know more about airway health and sleep health than their dentist or family doctor. Our hope is that instead of avoiding or obscuring a patient's questions and concerns, healthcare professionals, including ourselves, will be inspired to research and educate themselves about these fundamental aspects of health. Doing so allows us to catch up with the latest findings and guide our patients toward improved aesthetics, health, and healthcare. We believe this will also reduce the burgeoning cost of healthcare and save lives in this country and worldwide.

To the sleep medicine professionals, we hope you will see this book as a resource for raising awareness about sleep health. We aim to be your collaborators in addressing a problem that is too vast for you to tackle alone. Educating allied healthcare providers and primary care providers to assist responsibly is a shared goal. As consumer wearable health devices become more sophisticated, there is a concern that people may falsely believe they have no health concerns when they do, or they may mistakenly believe they have a health issue they don't have. We also acknowledge that too many allied health professionals and primary care providers need to gain the knowledge they should have in airway health. Let's work together to overcome this deficiency.

At the same time, I hope the profession of sleep medicine will recognize the contributions other allied health professionals can make, especially that of dentistry. Dentistry is advancing treatment options that no other profession does as well. It's incredible that dentists successfully treated obstructive sleep apnea in up to 26 percent of patients using the most commonly available measuring tools just a few years ago, while dramatically improving facial beauty.

We believe the reliance on the limited treatment models in the medical profession in the United States has not been adequately addressed. Rather than clinging to the traditional scope of practice boundaries and insurance coverage restrictions, let's seek eyes that see beyond each profession's discipline and adopt the binoculars of far-reaching vision. We applaud those medical sleep professionals who have already embraced these new treatment approaches and are working with allied health professionals to address this need.

For dentists focused on dental sleep medicine, or even those who have limited their practices to dental sleep medicine and have primarily relied on oral sleep dental appliances, it's crucial to recognize the evolving landscape of the field. Knowledge in the field and the practice of dentistry is rapidly changing, and even those with a diplomate credential in dental sleep medicine may fall behind if we don't stay updated. As times change, we must set our egos aside and remain open to continuous learning and adaptation.

While we owe a debt of gratitude to those who have paved the way in dental sleep medicine, it's essential to acknowledge that the information presented in this book will quickly become outdated. Dr. Zelk and I have had to change information in the book as new insights have emerged, even in the nine months it took to write it. We acknowledge that there may be areas where our knowledge is lacking, and we recognize that other educators may be teaching and writing about topics with equal or superior expertise to what we are presenting. We welcome the contributions of those advancing the field with their knowledge and insights. This realization should motivate us to stay abreast of the latest developments in the field. Our patients deserve the best.

Finally, we want to thank those who contributed to our shared information. These people are blazing the way toward a better future of health and beauty for everyone.

Dr. Kamran Fattah, Dr. Kevin Goles, Dr. Felix Liao, Dr. Geoffrey Skinner, Shirley Gutkowski, RDH, Joy Moeller, RDH, Corinne Jarvis, MS, SLP, Dr. Karen Hannah, Dr. Shane Smith, Dr. Rus Kort, Joanette Beibesheimer, Dr. Mark Abramson, Dr. Terry Coddington, Dr. Lindsey Zeboski, Dr. Kimberly Santiago, and the AIR Institute.

I also want to acknowledge Pearl Maisiri, my invaluable executive assistant, who knows how to organize and arrange a book better than I do and who has a better understanding of the English language. Though she resides in and has been raised in Zimbabwe, my sole influence on her editing and writing abilities has been advising her to use "while" instead of "whilst" for American readers. Without her assistance and assistance from Grammarly®,[503] Dall E 3® Bing® and Copilot®, Open AI®, and Chat GPT 3.5®,[504] I would never have gotten this project done.

I am immensely grateful to Taajah Phenezy (Goddess), whose inspiration prompted me to write this book. She even offered to be a ghostwriter for us, a gesture that initially did not register importance in my mind. However, her encouragement ignited a passion within me that I didn't realize existed. Her dedication to patient advocacy is a constant source of inspiration, as her primary focus is always on the welfare of patients.

I cannot thank enough those CEOs and heads of companies who contributed information vital to the book. Kirk Huntsman's information on Vivos® and Vivos® Guide was crucial, and his company has changed dentistry and the world for the better.

Neil Friedman, COO of Bodimetrics®, provided vital information on state-of-the-art innovative ring diagnostics, including his information on Circul+® and Circul IQ®.

While we didn't conduct interviews with the head of Invisalign® or Candid Pro® clear aligner orthodontic care providers, we recognize their growing role in creating airway space and beautiful faces for patients. Our case presenters acknowledged their essential contributions to the outcomes they are achieving.

Lastly, we are immensely grateful to the patients who shared their stories and images in this book. Without their images, stories, and statistics, the impact of what we wrote about would have been diminished precipitously. You cannot really get a message about improved faces without photos. You cannot convince healthcare professionals without statistics. These brave individuals shared all that and more. Their altruism is pure. They really want to help others to better health and lives. God bless them all.

At the beginning of this book, we wrote,

---

503 Grammarly. "Chicago Citation Generator Hub | Grammarly." Grammarly, December 17, 2021. Accessed May 25, 2024. https://www.grammarly.com/plagiarism-checker.

504 ChatGPT 3.5. *OpenAI*. Accessed March 2024. ChatGPT 3.5.

Imagine a world where every breath you take, whether awake or asleep, contributes to your vitality and the sculpting of your facial features. As you embark on the pages that follow, prepare to unlock the secrets that connect the rhythm of your breath to the radiance of your face. This journey is more than a quest for beauty; it is an exploration of the profound harmony between developmental and conventional airway wellness, sleep, and facial elegance.

We hope you have found some help in unlocking the secrets that connect the rhythm and health of each breath to the beauty and radiance of your face.

About the Authors

DR. RICHARD DOWNS

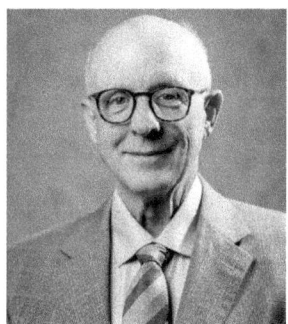

Dr. Richard Downs is an accomplished dental professional with a career spanning decades in general dentistry, research, and innovation. He graduated from the University of Iowa, earning a B.S. in 1971 and a D.D.S. in 1975; Dr. Downs began his career serving as a Navy dental officer at the Great Lakes Naval Base. Over his professional journey, he has made significant contributions to dental and sleep medicine. He is retired from active dental practice.

Key Professional Achievements:

- **Credentials:**
  - Diplomate of the Global Mini Dental Implant Association and the American Sleep and Breathing Academy.
  - Fellowships from institutions including the Academy of General Dentistry, Misch International Implant Institute, and International Congress of Oral Implantologists.

- **Professional Memberships:**
  - American Dental Association, Iowa Dental Association, and the Fortune Practice Management—Platinum Circle division.
  - Former affiliations include the American Academy of Cosmetic Dentistry and the International Association of Breath Odor Research.
  - Dr. Downs was the editor of the Iowa Academy of General Dentistry newsletter for four years and is past President of the Iowa Academy of General Dentistry.
  - Faculty of Air Institute, Portland, Oregon.

- **Research Contributions, Published Works, and Lectures**
  - Published works and lectures on topics such as cytokine immune response, wound healing, nitric oxide and microbiome balance in the oral cavity, and oxidative molecule therapeutics in dentistry.

Entrepreneurial and Charitable Efforts:

Dr. Downs co-founded **ProBreath MD, LLC**, which developed **OraCare**, a cutting-edge chlorine dioxide mouth rinse for enhanced oral health. His entrepreneurial ventures also include:

- Sleep dentistry platforms such as **Sleep Balance Academy and USA-Guard HOCL Nasal Rinse**.
- Efforts to diagnose and treat obstructive sleep apnea through innovative partnerships.

Charitable Initiatives:

Dr. Downs is dedicated to humanity, exemplified by his founding of the **Haiti International Dental Institute**, which focuses on dental implant training and providing much-needed care in Haiti. This initiative aligns with **Hosean Ministries International**, promoting education, healthcare, and economic development in the region.

Dr. Downs continues to inspire and lead through his dedication to advancing dental science, health-interprofessional collaboration, improving public health, and championing humanitarian causes.

JOSEPH ZELK

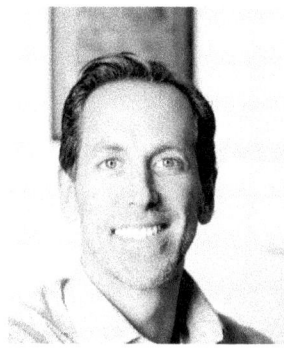

Dr. Joseph Zelk is a highly accomplished expert in sleep medicine with an extensive career focused on treating and educating about sleep disorders, particularly snoring and obstructive sleep apnea (OSA). He is double board certified in Behavioral Sleep Medicine and holds a Doctor of Nursing Practice (DNP). Over the past two decades, he has innovated oral appliance technologies, including the patented Hybrid Positive Airway Pressure (HPAP) therapies.

Dr. Zelk's efforts emphasize removing barriers to care by integrating home sleep testing, diagnostics, and personalized treatment options. His contributions extend to training medical and dental professionals in mandibular advancement therapy and oral appliance management. As Medical Director of the Sleep Balance Academy and the Sleep Medicine Group, he has dedicated his career to advancing sleep medicine.

He is also deeply committed to early airway development education, underscoring its importance in fostering healthy, happy, and well-rounded children. His work advocates for prioritizing Phase 1 treatments, ensuring optimal growth and development during critical formative years.

Key Highlights of Dr. Zelk's Career:

- **Education & Credentials:** Earned his DNP from Oregon Health and Sciences University and holds board certifications in Behavioral Sleep Medicine.
- **Experience:** Over 20 years in oral appliance therapy, specialized training in Sleep Disorders and Dental Sleep Medicine.
- **Professional Roles:**
  - Medical Director at Sleep Balance Academy and Sleep Medicine Group.
  - Adjunct faculty at OHSU for seven years.
  - Faculty of the Air Institute, Porland, Oregon.

- **Research & Innovations:** Co-inventor of oral appliances, extensive work in hybrid therapies, and advancements in CPAP alternatives.
- **Licenses:** Licensed in Oregon, Washington, Colorado, and Arizona.

Dr. Zelk continues to contribute significantly to sleep medicine through research, education, and patient-focused innovations, helping shape a healthier future for all ages.

www.ingramcontent.com/pod-product-compliance
Lightning Source LLC
Chambersburg PA
CBHW060450030426
42337CB00015B/1535